# An Introduction to Psychopharmacology for Counselors and Psychotherapists

Mark Stanford, Ph.D.

An Introduction to Psychopharmacology for Counselors and Psychotherapists

Lightway Centre Publishers
P.O. Box 7902
Santa Cruz, CA 95061

Copyright © 2024. Lightway Centre. All rights reserved

No part of this publication may be reproduced, stored in a retrieval system, or transmitted, in any form or by any means, electronic, mechanical, photocopying, recording, or otherwise, without the prior written permission of the publisher.

*Dedicated To Professor Raphael Mechoulam*

## About this book

There are a number of very good books about psychopharmacology but most of them are not very relevant to the work of counselors, psychotherapists and recovery workers. The books are generally either too technical, seemingly preparing the reader for medical school or the Pharmacy Boards, or they're entirely too simplistic and not covering the material in a very useful or meaningful way. For over thirty years, Dr. Stanford has worked alongside counselors, psychologists, nurses, social workers and therapists in outpatient and hospital care settings. He has seen firsthand, that armed with a working knowledge of psychopharmacology, these staff are better able to embrace an integrated whole person approach to patient care.

Thus, the purpose of this book is to provide a more reasonable, in-depth, moderately technical review of the psychopharmacology of addiction, substance use-related, and co-occurring disorders. Becoming more co-occurring competent, which is the understanding about the nature and treatment for clients with co-occurring conditions (both addiction and mental health issues), is now more the norm for behavioral health programs and clinical staff. The material presented in this book contains current information about the basic and essential aspects of psychopharmacology from a clinician's perspective. From basic concepts in pharmacology to pharmacodynamic and pharmacokinetic actions, to understanding a drug's "mechanism of action" (how it works) to applying these concepts to psychoactive drugs, both legal (medicines) and illegal street drugs are the focus of the book's contents.

Since 1987, Dr. Stanford has researched and taught psychopharmacology at the college and university levels. From community colleges, including San Mateo and Cabrillo Colleges, to graduate schools, including San Jose State School of Social Work, Stanford University School of Medicine, UC Berkely Extension, as well as training residents in an addiction medicine rotation. The skills gained from this material can greatly enhance the clinician's skills as a helping professional.

## Table of Contents

Chapter 1: Introduction ..................................................................................... 1

Chapter 2: Pharmacology Basic Concepts ........................................................ 7

Chapter 3: How the Body Deactivates Drugs .................................................. 27

Chapter 4: The Nervous System & How it Works .......................................... 47

Chapter 5: Functional Neuroanatomy .............................................................. 64

Chapter 6: The Chemistry of Behavior: Neurotransmitters ............................. 83

Chapter 7: The Neuroscience of Substance Use Disorders ........................... 105

Chapter 8: Alcohol and Sedative Drugs ........................................................ 125

Chapter 9: Stimulant Drugs ........................................................................... 154

Chapter 10: Opioid Drugs ............................................................................. 176

Chapter 11: Cannabis Pharmacology ............................................................ 201

Chapter 12: Hallucinogenic Drugs ................................................................ 225

Chapter 13: Inhalants .................................................................................... 242

Chapter 14: Methods of Drug Testing ........................................................... 249

Chapter 15: Schizophrenia: Symptoms, Causes and Treatments .................. 272

Chapter 16: Bipolar Disorder: Symptoms, Causes and Treatments .............. 288

Chapter 17: Depression: Symptoms, Causes and Treatments ....................... 302

Chapter 18: Anxiety: Symptoms, Causes and Treatments ............................ 322

Appendix: Principles of Drug Addiction Treatment ..................................... 341

# CHAPTER 1. INTRODUCTION

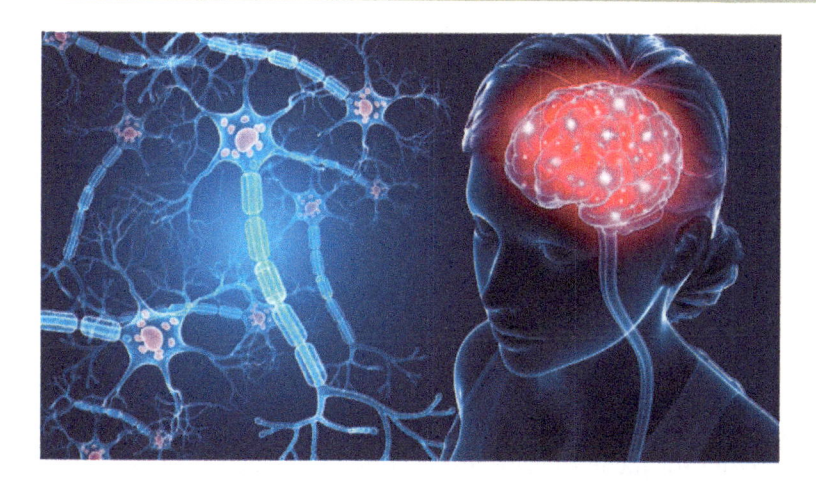

The overall objective of this book is to help healthcare providers, primarily counselors and psychotherapists, gain a working understanding of the neurobiological and pharmacological factors which contribute to addiction, substance use-related and mental health disorders. Over the last decade, an enormous amount of data began pouring in from the various findings of long-term neuroscience research and clinical practice experience. This material focused on discovering more of the biogenetic, neurobiological, biochemical and pharmacological determinants that are significant in substance use and mental health disorders.

From this information, virtually every discipline within the helping profession experienced a dramatic influence as a result of these discoveries. This ultimately led to the incorporation of the information, in varying degrees, into their given disciplines, and changed the traditional psychodynamic viewpoint considerably. Take for example, the evolution of the Diagnostics and Statistics Manual, Fifth edition (DSM-5TR), where yesterday it was largely psychodynamic, but today includes a significant amount of the neuroscientific and biological aspects of behavior.

Previous to this occurrence, therapists and counselors could exist within their own philosophical or ideological domains without having to understand different perspectives from other behavioral health areas including physiology. Now however, the profession as a whole has incorporated many of the new research findings across various disciplines including social work, psychology, psychotherapy, counseling and recovery work. Indeed most providers view behavior from a whole person care perspective as a result of the impact research had made. The neurobiological aspect brings a critical component into the health care mix, providing therapists with important tools that would not be available otherwise.

As the behavioral health care industry continues its mysterious journey of continued change, case management requires a multidisciplinary treatment team to provide for their patients. This requires a much greater degree of cross-communication between medical and non-medical providers. The healthcare industry also continues to expect social workers, psychologists, recovery workers, counselors and therapists to monitor acute behavioral signs of substance use, withdrawal management, and side effects of medications their clients are taking for mental health. Especially is this the case today with the emphasis properly being placed on co-occurring disorders. Providers are embracing a multidisciplinary approach to treatment, not simply because of changing healthcare, but in response to the dramatic impact neuroscience has made on understanding behavioral problems.

Therefore, while all health care professionals do not have a background in biochemistry, neurobiology and pharmacology, they should have a basic and practical knowledge of these perspectives as they pertain to behavioral health – a foundation in behavioral pharmacology. This book will help enhance the reader's understanding about these important areas to whole person care.

Toward this end, there are five objectives I am hopeful the reader will achieve:

1. To better understand the pharmacological and neurobiological factors that influence involvement in and patterns of substance use disorders;

2. To understand the biochemical and pharmacological aspects of substances of abuse, which in turn, determines vulnerability to substance use disorders;

3. To gain a working knowledge on the nature of addiction, substance use-related and co-occurring conditions;

4. To competently and confidently respond to questions frequently asked in a counseling/psychotherapy clinical treatment setting regarding substance use and mental health disorders;

5. To be able to articulate the neurobiological basis for behavioral problems and be able to articulate the pharmacological rationale for current medical and psychiatric treatment interventions for substance use and co-occurring disorders.

**Dynamics of Brain Chemistry and Behavior**

Behavior has no clear beginning or end. The analysis of behavior starts out innocently enough to describe the interactions of the organism with the environment. More specifically, it is the interaction of the organism's brain with the environment. The environment includes not only the outside world, but also the organism's internal environment. Of course, the brain is a part of that internal environment and the behavior itself becomes a part of the environment. Lest we become tempted to pursue the logical proof that the universe is made up of behavior, let us return to some more direct issues to illustrate that these considerations are not just idle philosophical musings--we must understand the implications of these interactions in order to appreciate the dynamics of brain chemistry and behavior. These interactions are presented as six principles for understanding behavioral pharmacology

Principle 1. *Changes in brain chemistry produce changes in behavior.*

This is perhaps the most straightforward principle and the one that has guided most of the research in behavioral pharmacology. Manipulation of the biochemical system that controls behavior will change behavior.

Principle 2. *Changes in behavior produce changes in brain chemistry.*

This principle is a bit more subtle and offers the opportunity to confuse cause and correlation. The fact that behavioral change is correlated with the chemical changes that produced it is simply a restatement of Principle 1. The important point here is that behavioral change can actually produce changes in brain chemistry. One type of change is an increase in the efficiency of the biochemical system that produces the behavior (analogous to increased muscle efficiency with exercise). This change may, in turn, produce changes in related chemical systems that were not directly involved in the first bit of behavior.

Principle 3. *Changes in the environment produce changes in behavior.*
This principle is the simple definition of behavior and requires little in the way of explanation. The major point that needs to be made is that the environment is quite extensive. It includes not only the relationships and contingencies of the external world, but also the internal milieu--blood pressure, gastrointestinal activity, level of energy stores, memory of past experiences, etc.

Principle 4. *Changes in behavior produce changes in the environment.*
In some sense, the only role of behavior is to change the environment. In the simplest case, the behavior is operant and results in opened doors, captured prey, warmed cockles and the like. But just as the environment was expanded, so must our notions of the effects of behavior be expanded to include, for example, changes in the internal environment either directly (as in the case of autonomic responses to a fear arousing situation) or indirectly (as in the case of nutritional changes).

Principle 5. *Changes in the environment produce changes in brain chemistry.*
We begin to complete the circuit through brain, behavior, and environment by noting that environmental changes can produce changes in brain chemistry. In some cases, the environment has tonic influences on brain chemistry as exemplified by responses to seasonal changes, temperature fluctuations, lighting changes and so forth. Other environmental changes are more closely interactive with behavior, and include responses to crowding, members of the opposite sex, complexity of the physical and behavioral environment, etc. These and many other types of environmental manipulations have been shown to alter the status of the neurochemical transmitter systems.

Principle 6. *Changes in brain chemistry produce changes in the environment.*
On the surface, this seems to be the least likely of the principles. Changes in brain chemistry obviously cannot directly perform operations like opening doors. It can, however, produce significant changes in the internal environment and set the stage for such operations to occur.

The listing of these six principles is a formal way of stating the major considerations that must accompany our study of psychopharmacology. Drugs indeed change behavior. But the effect of a drug can be altered by the organism's behavior, which in turn has been produced by current and past changes in the environment. Drugs do not possess some essence that magically induces a change in behavior. They act through the normal channels of our physiological response to the environment. As human organisms in a complex environment, we are fortunate that these interactions are complicated.

In the spirit of research, and to introduce this work, I offer the following questions as a general outline. Periodically, as you are reading through the chapters, you may wish to revisit some of these questions and see if your response to them might have changed.

**General**
- What are the biobehavioral processes of drug-seeking behavior?
- How is "addiction" currently defined? Refer to the American Society of Addiction Medicine (ASAM)
- Who are the susceptible host populations for substance use disorders and addiction?
- How are pharmacodynamic processes important in the abuse of specific drugs (half-life, absorption, distribution, metabolism, excretion, etc.)?
- What biochemical properties gives a drug an abuse potential?
- What are basic pharmacological "mechanism of action" of alcohol.
- What are the principle treatments for the spectrum of substance use disorders?

**Psychiatric Medications**
- Describe the advantages/disadvantages of the newer antipsychotics and antidepressants over the more traditional medications.
- Describe current theories on the neurobiological aspects of depressive disorders, bipolar illness and schizophrenia.
- What is behavioral toxicity and how can it be identified from a primary illness?
- Where does the future of medications for mental health need to go

There are several excellent books that provide a rich and detailed account of the historical perspective of substance use disorders and psychiatric illness, but that is not the purpose of this work. There are even more great books written on the many psychosocial theories and dynamics about substance use and mental health disorders, but these also are not the focus of this book. Rather, the principal focus is to provide an accurate yet understandable, current and practical account of the neurobiological aspects which add to the whole person perspective of behavior, with an emphasis on psychopharmacology of addiction, substance-related and co-occurring disorders.

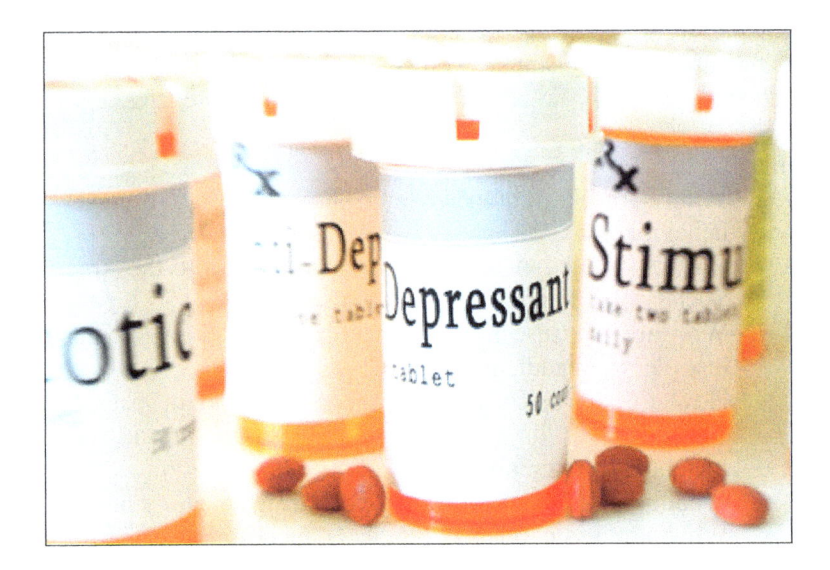

# CHAPTER 2. THE FOUNDATION: PHARMACOLOGY BASIC CONCEPTS

## Key Concepts

| | |
|---|---|
| Absorption | The process of how a drug is absorbed and enters into a system. |
| Administration | The process of how a drug enters the body. |
| Blood-brain-barrier | A membrane that impedes the distribution of certain molecules into the brain. |
| Down regulation | Decrease in neuron receptor site sensitivity due to excessive activity causing over stimulation. |
| ED50 | The median effective dose (ED) that is effective in 50% of the individuals studied. |
| Enteral | The route of administration by way of the intestine (gut). |
| Half-life | This pharmacokinetic principle describes the time it takes for the body to eliminate 50% of a drug's concentration. In other words, once the half-life is reached, the concentration of the drug in the body is half of its starting dose. The concept of half-life helps to determine excretion rates. Different drugs have different half-lives; however, the same rule applies to all of them: after one half-life has passed, 50% of the initial drug amount is eliminated from the body. |
| LD50 | The lethal dose range that causes death in 50 percent of the studied population. |
| Placebo effect | Drug effects that have nothing to do with its pharmacological aspects. |

| | |
|---|---|
| Pharmacodynamics: | Pharmacodynamics (PD) is the study of how drugs affect the human body given their mechanism of action. |
| Pharmacokinetics: | Pharmacokinetics (PK) is the study of what the body does to the drug and describes information about administration, absorption, distribution, metabolism, and excretion. |
| Potency | A drug's ability to produce an intended effect at the lowest dose possible (different than a drug's purity). |
| Tachyphylaxis | The rapid onset of tolerance to a drug's effects - perhaps as soon as after a first dose. |
| Therapeutic index | The range between minimum effective dose and the maximum dose without toxicity. |

# CHAPTER 2

# THE FOUNDATION: PHARMACOLOGY BASIC CONCEPTS

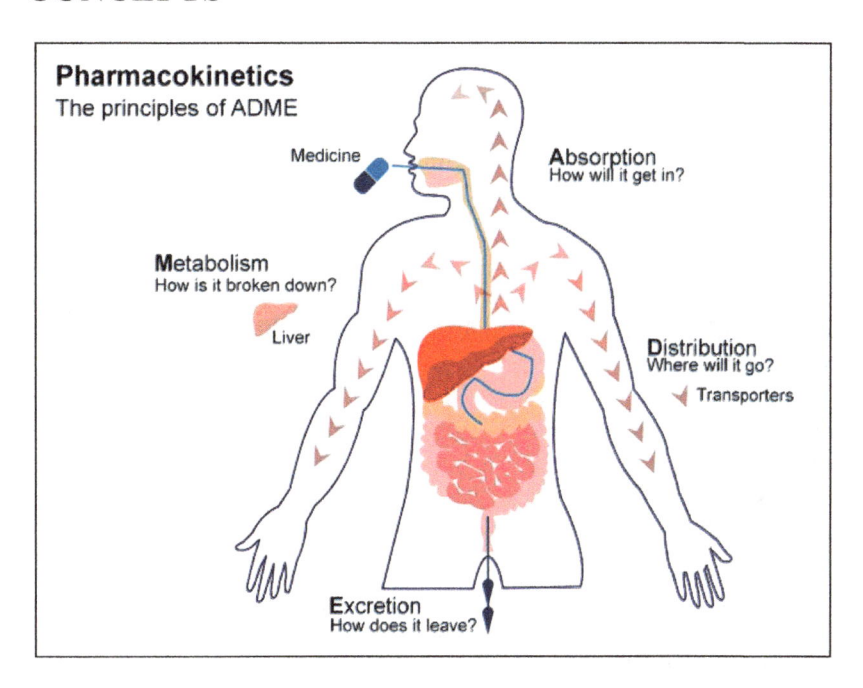

**Pharmacokinetics**
The principles of ADME

- Medicine
- Absorption: How will it get in?
- Metabolism: How is it broken down? — Liver
- Distribution: Where will it go? — Transporters
- Excretion: How does it leave?

Pharmacology, in its most fundamental definition, is the science of studying the chemical effects on biological systems. Psychopharmacology, a specialized area of the pharmacological sciences, is the study of drug effects on the nervous system and how the effects alter behavior. The primary objective of this science is to discover a drug's selective toxicity. That is, how a drug can produce only the desired effect and no others.

The word pharmacology comes from the Greek word, *pharmacon*, which, interestingly, can mean both medicine or "poison", depending on the context in which it is used. The primary effect of a drug is usually its desired effect, or the effect that is intended. A drug's side effects are those effects that are not intended, but take place anyway. Pharmacology is the study of the action and effects of drugs on living systems and the interaction of drugs with living systems. Pharmacology includes the study of prescribed and over-the-counter medications, legal and illegal drugs, natural and synthetic compounds, exogenous (sourced from outside the body) and endogenous (produced inside the body) drugs, and drugs that produce benefit, harm, or both benefit and harm.

**Drugs Have Multiple Effects**
It is almost a truism that every drug has multiple effects. Ideally, a drug would have only one effect, which could be used for a specific therapeutic purpose. More commonly, any given drug may have several major effects and several minor effects. For example, a drug may be given as a muscle relaxant, but have a side effect of producing drowsiness. The same compound may be prescribed for another patient for the purpose of producing drowsiness and lowered anxiety, with a side effect of muscle relaxation. Along with these major effects, several minor side-effects might be common to both prescriptions and include cardiovascular problems, gastrointestinal upset, skin rashes, and so forth. In general, the higher the dosage, the greater the number of different drug effects.

Low doses of epinephrine produce a slight drop in blood pressure, whereas high doses produce a large increase in blood pressure. This curious reversal of effects can be explained as follows: The molecular structure of epinephrine allows it to interact with both alpha and beta receptors. The beta receptors, although fewer in number, are more sensitive than the alpha receptors. With *low* dosages of epinephrine, the *beta* receptors are the only ones effected and they inhibit the smooth muscles of the blood vessels causing a decrease in the pressure through vasodilation.

*High* doses of epinephrine stimulate *alpha* receptors, which cause the constriction of blood vessels and a corresponding increase in blood pressure. The beta receptors are also stimulated, but their influence is overpowered by the effects of the alpha receptors.

Almost exactly the same type of change in blood pressure can be observed with low and high doses of acetylcholine, but for different reasons. *Low* doses of acetylcholine reduce the blood pressure by acting on the muscarinic receptors which inhibit the smooth muscles of the blood vessels to cause vasodilation. *High* doses of acetylcholine produce a large increase in blood pressure by stimulating the nicotinic receptors of the autonomic ganglia. These nicotinic receptors are much less sensitive to circulating levels of acetylcholine, but once stimulated, their effects are much more potent than those of the muscarinic stimulation. Under these conditions, the sympathetic ganglia predominate, and the resulting stimulation of the adrenal gland

and release of norepinephrine from the sympathetic fibers cause an increase in blood pressure. Thus, the large dose of acetylcholine increases blood pressure indirectly via sympathetic arousal.

In these examples, we see the essence of *dose-response interactions.* Two completely different drugs (epinephrine and acetylcholine) produce identical profiles of change in blood pressure (a decrease at low doses and an increase at high doses.) In each instance, the reversal occurs because low doses influence one type of receptor while high doses influence a different type of receptor. Furthermore, in the case of acetylcholine, the final effect is actually due to the indirect activation of an opposing system. This particular set of results makes sense because the underlying mechanisms have already been determined. In many cases of drug and behavior interactions we do not yet enjoy this luxury.

**Individual Differences in Drug Effects**
The effectiveness of specific drugs can also be influenced by a wide range of organismic variables such as species, age, sex, disease status and behavioral history. In many cases, the specific origin of these differences in drug response cannot be identified, but some general comments can be made in relation to the dosage considerations discussed above. The notation of such variables as age, sex, species, and so forth does not describe the underlying cause of differences in drug response, but is rather used as a convenient label for sub-populations that may share some common physiological variable.

One of the most important physiological differences that interact with the behavioral effects of drugs is the status of the brain. There are well documented changes in brain chemistry during the course of development and continuing through senescence. The presence or absence of sex hormones, the environment of the organism, and the behavior that the organism engages in can all modulate these neurochemical changes.

Since most of the behaviorally active drugs produce their effects through interaction with these chemical substrates, the variables that alter neurochemistry interact with drug response. It is simply easier and more convenient to specify some external variable such as age or sex, rather than attempting to outline the more directly relevant neurochemical factors.

Differences in drug response can also occur in the absence of any important differences in the neurochemical substrates. All of the ports of entry into and exit from the bloodstream vary as a function of these external variables. For example, liver function is not fully developed in the very young and no longer fully efficient in the very old.

Differences in behavioral and dietary history will alter liver function, gastrointestinal function, cardiovascular efficiency and general metabolism. Body fat levels vary in response to a wide range of variables. Each of these changes has the capacity to alter the drug response through a simple shift in the time course of effective drug concentration in the bloodstream. The same relative quantity of drug might produce an increase in the behavior of a young organism, no change in adult females, and an impairment of behavior in aging males.

**Generic Drugs**
Generic drugs are chemically identical to the original drug and have similar biological characteristics such as the rate and extent of absorption and elimination. Drugs that are marketed in the United States as generic equivalent are equivalent to the original product and represent an opportunity to save substantial amounts of money compared to the trademarked original product.

In many cases, the generic products are from the same production lines as the original product. There may be many generic versions of a specific drug. Each of them must be similar to the prototype product, but are never tested against each other. This situation can allow one generic to differ from another by more than the accepted tolerance limits. Switching generic brands should be avoided. It is always best to start with one specific brand and not switch to another brand with every refill from the pharmacy. When a change of generic manufacturers cannot be avoided, closer monitoring for adverse effects and loss of efficacy will allow the small dosage adjustments needed to compensate for ay clinically significant differences.

**Pharmaceutical Names**
All drugs have a chemical name that denotes the chemical make-up or composition of the drug. Because chemical names can be quite long and complicated, the drug is usually given a shorter generic name. Also, the drug's manufacturer will typically give the drug a trade name as well. Trade names are always identified by the ® (registered) symbol following the name of the drug, and the first

letter is always capitalized. Thus, it is possible for a substance to be known by several different names.

A drug might have slang or street names by what addicts may call it when distributed and used illegally. A good example of how a single drug will have numerous names is found in the case of amphetamines: the chemical name is *alphamethylphenylethylamine,* the generic name is amphetamine, the trade name is Dexedrine, and the street name is "speed".

**Adverse Effects**
Adverse effects are the unwanted side effects that are caused by the drug that is intended to produce therapeutic benefits. Generally, the more recently developed drugs tend to have fewer and milder adverse effects than older ones. However, it is usually true that any effective intervention will have some adverse effects, even if mild and well tolerated.

The goal of selecting a medication is to achieve high efficacy with minimal adverse effects. Some adverse effects are dose-related and are less common or less severe at lower doses, other adverse effects are not and may be present at any dose. It is important to realize that adverse effects are pharmacologically similar to the therapeutic effects and have a unique dose-effect curve. Use of the lowest possible dose that is effective is the best strategy to minimize adverse effects.

The graph below shows three hypothetical dose-effect curves. Effect A is the desired profile for a drug's therapeutic effect. Between doses of 1 and 10, the effect increases proportional to the dose and approaches the maximum possible effect. Effect B is an example of a dose-limiting adverse effect.

In this case, the benefits of the drug (as shown in Effect A) are limited by adverse effects above doses of 5. Finally, Effect C shows a threshold effect at a dose of 10 that appears so rapidly that there does not appear to be any relationship between dose and the size of the effect. Every drug and effect would have a unique curve in each individual.

The basis of our use of drugs is based on population responses and adverse effects. The inability to predict the exact effect curves in an individual is what causes a lack of response and adverse effects.

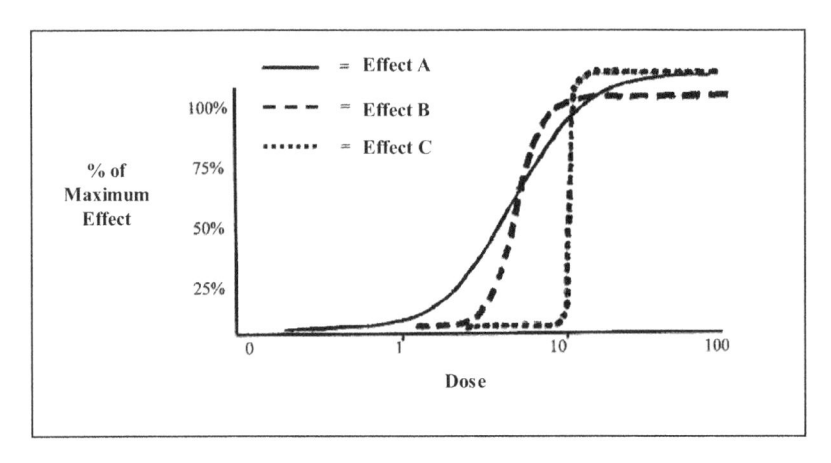

## Dosage Titration

Unfortunately, drug therapy does not work rapidly. This is because of several factors: pharmacokinetics and pharmacodynamics. These cause a delay between a dose adjustment and arriving at the final amount of the drug in then patient's body. After this steady state amount of drug is present, then the effect of the drug can exert its effect. The action of the drug may be indirect and require an intermediate response before the clinical effect can be seen.

An example of this can be seen in the use of an antidepressant. It can take up to two weeks for a clinical response after a dose adjustment. An important consequence of this is that doses are frequently adjusted far too rapidly and may be substantially higher than are needed for the clinical response. The higher dose may increase the chance of the patient having an adverse effect that reduces the clinical benefit. More rapid dose titration has not been shown to increase the rate of response in replicated studies. In general, dosage adjustments should not be made more often than weekly and possibly as infrequently as monthly.

When would the physician make a dose increase? When the adverse effects after reaching pharmacokinetic steady state are acceptable to the patient and physician and the response is still inadequate then the dose might be increased. If the patient has had any improvement at all, it is usually best to wait and see if the improvement will continue without a dose increase. If the adverse effects worsen after a dosage increase, then it may be desirable to decrease the dose to its previous level. Usually the adverse effect will subside and the dose may again be increased if needed for increased response.

It may be possible to increase the dose without unacceptable adverse effects if the dose increment is half of the previous increment and the interval between subsequent increases is twice what it was.

**Drug Interactions Are Not All Bad**
Drug interactions are an important and growing area of research and patient care because more drugs are being used at the same time. There is a common misconception that a drug interaction is inherently bad. Actually, the only bad interactions are those that are not understood and go undetected until a bad outcome occurs. Understanding the mechanism of drug interaction and close monitoring can prevent most bad outcomes.

Lack of knowledge about the patient's total medication and diet regimen can lead to problems, but usually problems occur slowly enough that permanent harm is avoided. Also, if an interaction is well understood, it can actually be used to intentionally to improve the patient. An example would be the addition of a diuretic to a patient on Lithium to decrease urine volume. For the most part, however, drug interactions should be avoided. The easiest way to avoid them is to reduce the number of drugs that a patient is taking and carefully selecting the drugs that they need to take.

Pharmacology has long noted that all psychoactive drugs, legal or otherwise, produce side effects. However, in pharmacology, the noted side effects are not simply unintended aspects to be avoided or minimized. In some cases, a drug's side effects might even be the primary or intended effect.

For example, antihistamines might be used to relieve allergies and may produce side effects of drowsiness and sedation. The same drugs may also be prescribed by a physician to treat anxiety which, when used in this context, would have side effects of allergy suppression. A drug's known side effects can be utilized for various situations, so primary effects have a relative distinction from side effects. It is possible to administer a drug at such a small dosage that no effect occurs. A larger dosage might bring about the intended effect, while an even larger dose might be toxic.

The range between the minimum effective dosage and the maximum dosage where no toxic symptoms occur is the therapeutic index: Psychoactive drugs also have a dose-response relationship. That is, some drugs produce different effects at different dosages. For example, diazepam (Valium) at low doses is a sedative, and at higher doses it induces sleep. Still at higher doses, Valium becomes an anti-convulsant, and with higher levels yet, it can be an anesthetic.

The *potency* of a drug is its ability to produce an intended effect at the lowest dose possible. Many people mistake the word potency for purity levels. However, potency is the specific dose-response relationship the drug can produce. For example, heroin is more "potent" than morphine because it takes less heroin to produce the same level of analgesia as morphine. The route of administration can also produce effects that have nothing to do with its pharmacological aspects; this is called the placebo effect.

## Pharmacodynamics and Pharmacokinetics: Understanding a Drug's Mechanism of Action

*Pharmacodynamics* and *pharmacokinetics* are the two branches of pharmacology, with pharmacodynamics studying the action of the drug on the organism and pharmacokinetics studying the effect the organism has on the drug

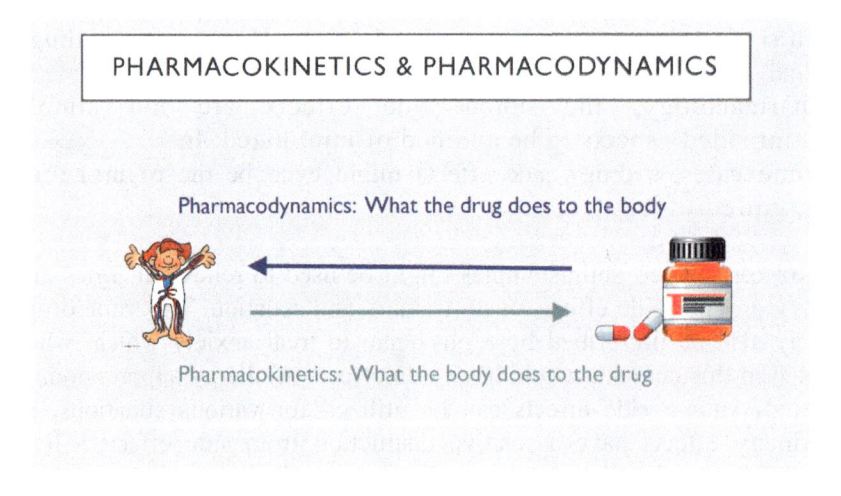

**PHARMACOKINETICS & PHARMACODYNAMICS**

Pharmacodynamics: What the drug does to the body

Pharmacokinetics: What the body does to the drug

Pharmacokinetics is the aspect of pharmacology that seeks to understand how a drug acts after it had been introduced into the body: the drug's *mechanism of action*. It is the study of how a drug is delivered into the body, how it moves throughout the body and brain, and how it eventually gets eliminated. Pharmacokinetics is what the body docs to a drug. It depends on the person's conditions and the chemical characteristics of the drug. Understanding the pharmacokinetic processes is important since it allows prescribers to provide a safe and effective therapeutic management of drugs in their patients.

An example of pharmacodynamics is the binding of morphine to an opioid receptor. Morphine binds with highest affinity to the mu opioid receptor. Additionally, repeated dosage of morphine can lead to tolerance of the drug, often mediated by desensitization
of the receptor. The same example using pharmacokinetics in the context of addiction, would include how the morphine was ingested (administration), much morphine gets to the body (absorption), how fast drug levels rise in the body(distribution and rate of drug onset), how often the drug levels rise and fall (intermittency), how the ingested morphine is deactivated (metabolized) and, how the drug is eliminated (excretion).

The single most important objective in pharmacology is to understand a drug produces its overall effects. In other words, how does morphine suppress pain? How does Cymbalta treat depression? What is the *mechanism of action* of antipsychotic drugs that produce the side effects of impaired movement coordination? Why is it that chemicals like amphetamines or cocaine produce effects of euphoria and inhibit sleep? What are the effects when several drugs are taken in combination (polypharmacy), such as THC and chemotherapy, alcohol and Valium, or morphine and cocaine? What are the mechanisms of action where drug molecules can produce effects and side effects? And how do they work in the brain and body? These are all questions related to a drug's pharmacokinetics - the investigative process of understanding a drug's mechanism of action.

**How Drugs Get Into the Body (Administration)**
Administration of a drug includes the various ways a drug is delivered and released into the body. There are several means by which a drug enters the body. Each route of administration has great bearing on the drug's overall effects.

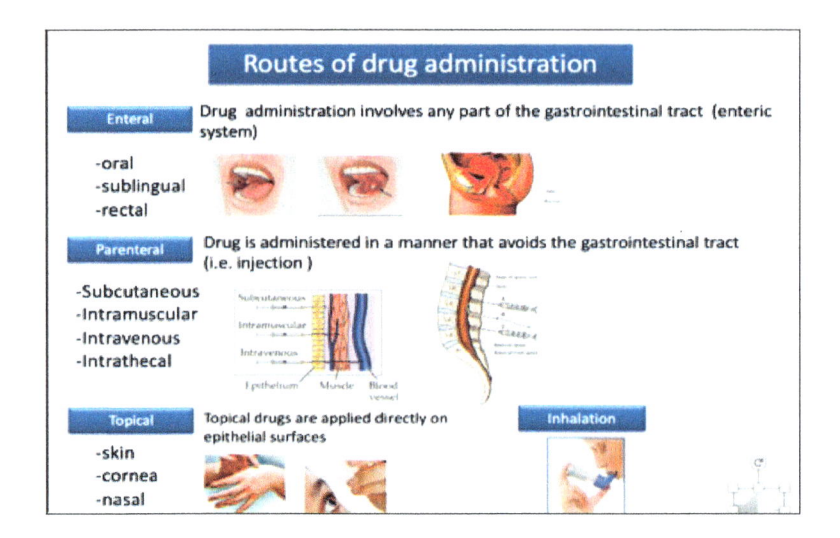

## Routes of drug administration

**Enteral** — Drug administration involves any part of the gastrointestinal tract (enteric system)
- oral
- sublingual
- rectal

**Parenteral** — Drug is administered in a manner that avoids the gastrointestinal tract (i.e. injection)
- Subcutaneous
- Intramuscular
- Intravenous
- Intrathecal

**Topical** — Topical drugs are applied directly on epithelial surfaces
- skin
- cornea
- nasal

**Inhalation**

It is important to understand that drugs do not produce an effect on all body tissues. Most drugs effect only target systems that are fairly specific and limited in their area of influence. This area is referred to as the drug's *site of action.* A drug can enter into the body but unless it reaches its site of action, it will not produce its primary effect.

Thus, it is important to understand how drugs move from their initial route of administration to the final site of action. Some nutritional supplements, foods and medicines may contain large amounts nourishment and healing, but simply putting them into the body (i.e., orally *per os)* is no guarantee that they will produce a desired effect. The route of administration determines whether the drug reaches the site of action and how fast or how much of it gets there.

The major routes of drug administration are *enteral* (through the intestines) or *parenteral* (outside of the intestines), and include several paths into the body where they will enter the bloodstream. The following list details these pathways:

**Enteral:** Taken into the body by way of the intestine
- Oral *(per os):* by way of the mouth, swallowing
- Sublingual: beneath the tongue, sucking
- Rectal: by way of the anus (suppository)

**Parenteral:** Taken into the body or administered in a manner other than through the intestines, as by intravenous or intramuscular injection or inhalation.

- Intracutaneous (IC): within the skin
- Subcutaneous (SC): beneath the skin
- Intramuscular (IM): within the muscles
- Intravenous (IV): within a vein, injection
- Intraperitoneal (IP): within the peritoneal cavity (containing the visceral organs: the liver, the intestines and the spleen)
- Intracardiac: within the heart
- Pulmonary: within the lungs, inhalation
- Transcutaneous: through the skin (patch)

Drugs come in many forms, and the same drugs may be prepared as a pill, a liquid, a suppository, an inhaler, or even an I.V. (injectable) solution. For a drug to produce an effect, it must enter the bloodstream in a way for it to be distributed to its specific target system within the body or brain.

An important factor of the oral *(per os)* route of drug administration is that when the substance has been absorbed into the blood from the gastrointestinal tract, it moves through the liver where a portion of the drug molecule is metabolized or broken down.

The liver prepares substances for elimination by the kidneys by chemically altering them and changing them into what are called metabolites. More on this in the next chapter.

**How Drugs are Absorbed Into the Body.**

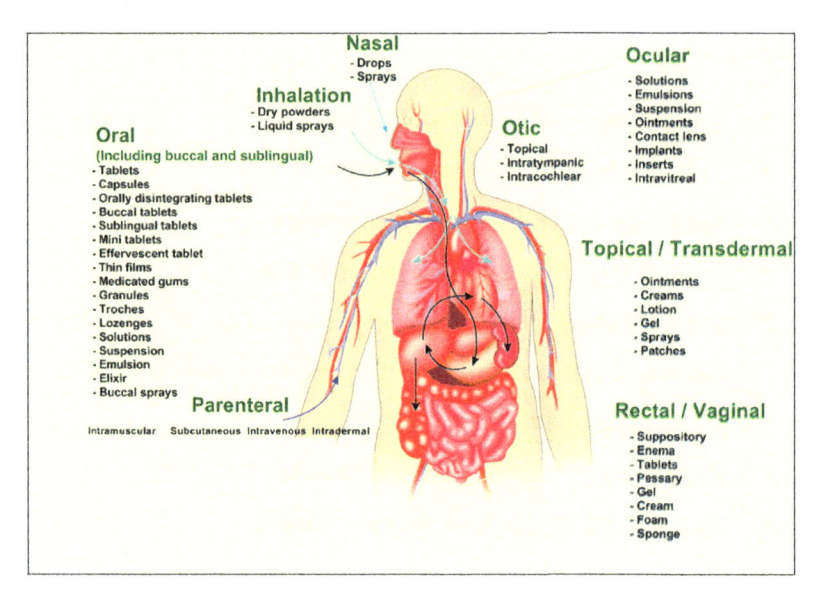

**Nasal**
- Drops
- Sprays

**Inhalation**
- Dry powders
- Liquid sprays

**Oral**
(Including buccal and sublingual)
- Tablets
- Capsules
- Orally disintegrating tablets
- Buccal tablets
- Sublingual tablets
- Mini tablets
- Effervescent tablet
- Thin films
- Medicated gums
- Granules
- Troches
- Lozenges
- Solutions
- Suspension
- Emulsion
- Elixir
- Buccal sprays

**Otic**
- Topical
- Intratympanic
- Intracochlear

**Ocular**
- Solutions
- Emulsions
- Suspension
- Ointments
- Contact lens
- Implants
- Inserts
- Intravitreal

**Topical / Transdermal**
- Ointments
- Creams
- Lotion
- Gel
- Sprays
- Patches

**Parenteral**
Intramuscular  Subcutaneous  Intravenous  Intradermal

**Rectal / Vaginal**
- Suppository
- Enema
- Tablets
- Pessary
- Gel
- Cream
- Foam
- Sponge

Regardless of the route of administration, once a drug has been ingested it must be absorbed by its target system. Following *enteral* administration, the drug must move from the gastrointestinal tract into the circulatory system, where it then is distributed throughout the body. *Parenteral* administration often stimulates faster absorption because of quicker access to the bloodstream.

Membranes are usually made of *lipid* (or fatty) material. For a drug to pass through a wall of cells, such as the lining of the intestines, there must be holes or pores large enough to allow drug molecules to diffuse through. Several factors influence absorption rates, but the primary dynamic is the drug's ability to absorb into fatty tissue.

This rate, called *solubility,* is a central factor in absorption dynamics. In general, the more lipid soluble a drug is, the easier it will absorb into tissue. For enteral administration, absorption is most efficient in the intestines, since intestine walls are lined with capillaries that absorb nutrients from food; they readily absorb drugs as well. All body tissue is made of cells and each cell is surrounded by a membrane. To get to the capillaries, the drug must first pass through the membrane of the intestinal wall.

All drug molecules differ somewhat in their degree of lipid solubility, the ease of which drugs dissolve in and through fatty or lipid tissue. However, when a drug carries an electrical charge, its lipid solubility is significantly reduced. Such a charged molecule is called an *ion*. Ions are not lipid soluble and do not dissolve well in fatty tissue.

When a drug is dissolved in a fluid, some or all of its molecules become ionized. The percentage of ionized molecules in a solution determines its *pH*, which describes the degree to which a solution is either an acid or a base, or its *pKa*, meaning the pH at which half of its molecules are ionized.

The percentage of non-ionized molecules is available for absorption at any given period of time, and therefore determines the rate of absorption. The figure below illustrates the various absorption areas through two different routes of administration

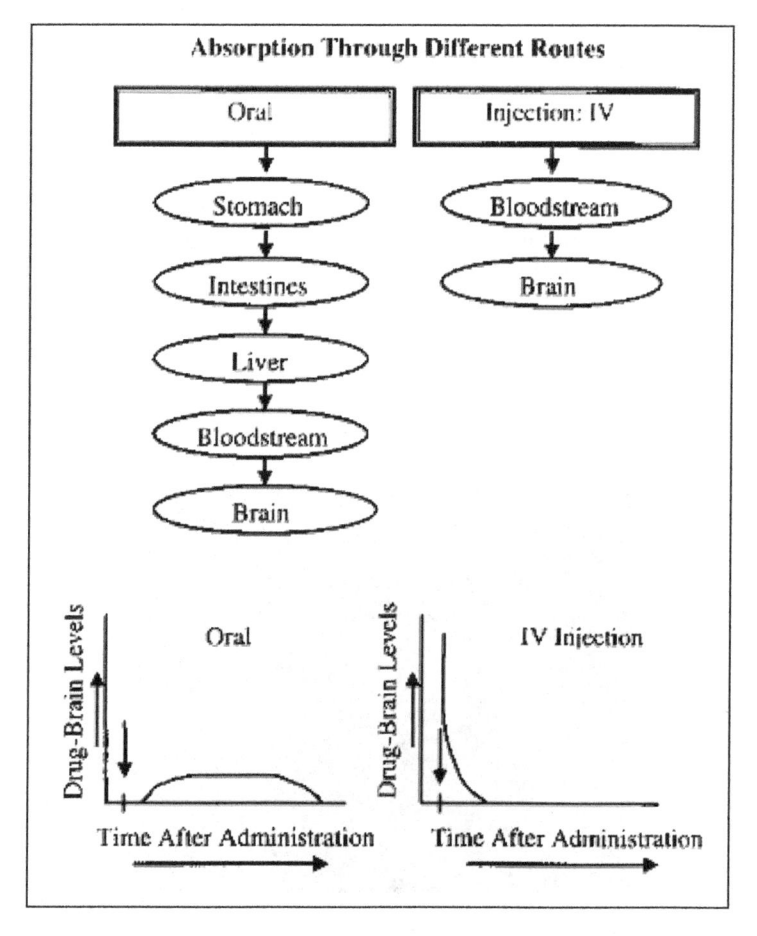

**Absorption Through Different Routes**

Oral → Stomach → Intestines → Liver → Bloodstream → Brain

Injection: IV → Bloodstream → Brain

Oral: Drug-Brain Levels vs. Time After Administration

IV Injection: Drug-Brain Levels vs. Time After Administration

Non-ionized molecules of various drugs have varying degrees of lipid solubility. These ranges of lipid solubility are expressed in terms of the *oil: water partition coefficients,* since testing for solubility involves using olive oil in equal parts with water. The oil and water are put in a container, and a fixed amount of a drug is mixed in. After some time the oil and water separate, and the amount of drug dissolved in each is measured. Drugs that are more lipid soluble have a higher concentration in the oil, and drugs that water soluble concentrate in the water. This test can somewhat predict the degree to which a drug will dissolve in lipid material (fatty tissue) within the body.

The amount of a drug that reaches circulation is called its bioavailability, the percentage of the drug dosage available to the body. Thus, drugs taken intravenously are 100% bioavailable, whereas drugs that are administered by other routes are less bioavailable.

A drug must absorb into a targeted system to produce an effect. In order for a drug to be absorbed and reach the nervous system, it must cross membranes. Drugs cross membranes in different ways, including facilitated diffusion, active transport or passive transport. Most drugs are absorbed by passive transport, where they move across a lipid membrane via a carrier or specialized molecule. A non-lipid soluble drug molecule attaches itself to a "carrier" molecule that diffuses across the membrane, releasing the drug molecule on the other side. In this way, a drug can move from high to low concentration on either side of a membrane.

**The Blood Brain Barrier**

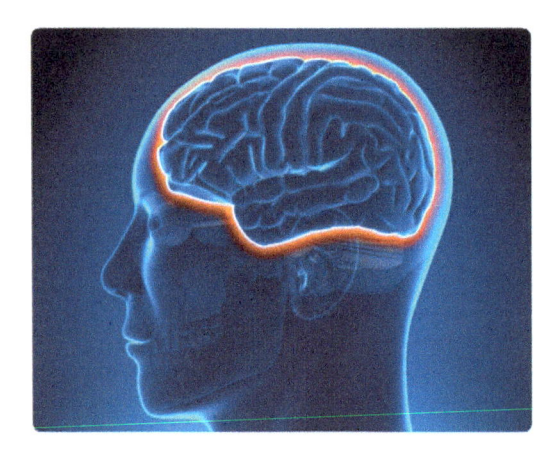

The brain is one of the most richly vascularized (full of blood vessels on which it depends on for nutrients) organs of the body. The two internal carotids and two vertebral arteries (which supply all the blood to the brain) branch out into an extremely dense system of capillaries. Consequently, the brain is responsible for nearly twenty percent of the body's total oxygen consumption, even though it accounts for less than two percent of the body mass. Neurons are particularly vulnerable to ischemia and such a lack of blood flow for as little as four to five minutes can lead to serious brain damage.

The dense capillary system of the brain is very selective in terms of the molecules that will pass through into the surrounding tissue space. Water, oxygen, carbon dioxide pass freely through the endothelial walls. Glucose, which supplies virtually all of the nutritive requirements of brain tissue, also passes through relatively freely. Thus, there is an efficient exchange of molecules that are essential for the high metabolic demands of neural tissue. The capillaries of the brain have two special features that tend to prevent the passage of molecules into the adjacent tissue space. The endothelial cells that form the walls of the capillaries are densely packed, such that only small molecules can pass through the junctions. Additionally, glial cells called astrocytes surround about 85% of the surface of the capillaries, adding a lipid barrier to the system. Thus, large molecules and molecules that are not lipid soluble do not easily penetrate the brain. These special features of the cerebral vascular system have been termed the blood-brain barrier.

Another special feature of the central nervous system is the cerebrospinal fluid (CSF) that fills the ventricles of the brain and central canal of the spinal cord. The CSF is formed by blood vessels within the ventricular system, most notably the concentrated groups in the lateral ventricles which are termed the choroids plexus. The CSF excreted by these vessels is similar to blood plasma, except for very low levels of proteins and cholesterol. It is the extracellular fluid of the brain, which is formed continuously and absorbed at a rate of about 10% per hour. Thus there is a continual flow of the fluid which bathes the brain cells. The capillary walls of the choroid plexus have the same dense epithelial structure as those within the brain tissue proper, hence provide an extension of the blood-brain barrier.

The blood-brain barrier should not be viewed as a system which isolates the brain, but rather as one which buffers it from the changing conditions of the remainder of the body. The critically important ions that determine the electrical excitability of neurons (Na+, K+, Ca+, and Cl-) equilibrate with the brain fluids very slowly, requiring as much as 30 times longer than in other tissues. Relatively small molecules such as urea are exchanged rather freely with muscle tissue and other body organs, but enter the brain very slowly over a period of several hours. Larger molecules such as bile salts and circulating catecholamines (from the adrenal glands and peripheral autonomic nervous system) are essentially blocked from entering the brain. Thus, the brain is protected from fluctuations of chemicals in the plasma compartment, allowing homeostatic processes a considerable margin of time to correct any deviations while the brain's environment remains relatively constant.

The nature of the blood brain barrier poses a number of problems in terms of the behavioral response to drugs. In the most extreme cases, some compounds simply do not enter the brain in significant concentrations. In other cases (e.g., neurotransmitters like dopamine or serotonin), the relevant compound per se does not enter, but the precursor molecules can be administered to facilitate the synthesis of the active form within the brain. The compounds can also be injected directly into the brain or CSF, physically bypassing the barrier, but several compounds have so called paradoxical
effects on brain tissue.

For example, penicillin produces convulsions, epinephrine in the ventricles leads to somnolence, and curare can lead to seizures. Aside from some general guidelines relating to molecular size and lipid solubility, it is difficult to predict with accuracy how easily a drug will penetrate the brain and what the effect will be. In many cases, it is necessary to make an empirical determination. A more subtle aspect of the blood brain barrier is that it is differentially effective in different areas of the brain. The white regions of the brain are composed mainly of fibers, which are surrounded by glial cells to form the myelin sheaths. As a result of this additional lipid barrier, these regions of the brain reach equilibrium with certain drugs much more slowly than the cellular regions of grey cortex. To the extent that these different areas serve different behavioral functions or are differentially sensitive to the drug, the overall response to a drug dosage over time will become increasingly complicated.

### How Drugs are Distributed Throughout the Body
Distribution refers to the delivery of a drug to its site of action. Distribution is of course, greatly influenced by blood flow, since drug

molecules diffuse out of the bloodstream and into the targeted area. The blood-brain-barrier (BBB) impedes the distribution of some molecules into the brain. This is a barrier made of specialized cells called *glial cells* and *astrocytes* that form a tight-knit membrane or matrix that repels water-soluble molecules. The glial cells wrap tightly around capillaries and block pores that molecules would diffuse through. These provide a very strong lipid barrier so that non-lipid soluble molecules have great difficulty getting into the brain.

Because of the BBB, the diffusion of a drug into the brain is inversely proportional to its water solubility. However, psychoactive drugs (which change thought, mood and movement) are lipid soluble and therefore, distribute through the BBB and into the brain quite easily.

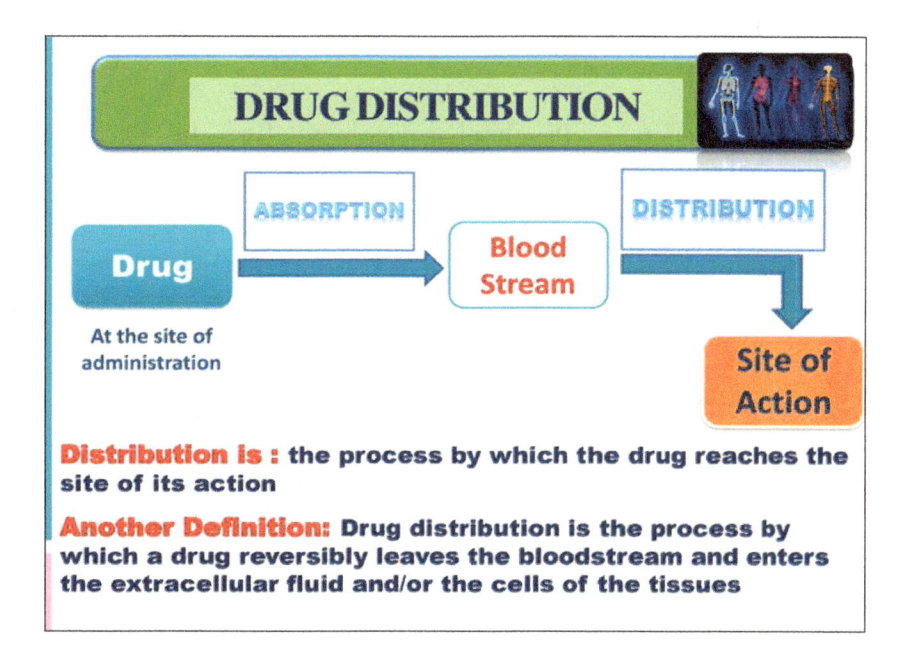

**DRUG DISTRIBUTION**

ABSORPTION → Blood Stream → DISTRIBUTION

Drug (At the site of administration) → Site of Action

**Distribution is :** the process by which the drug reaches the site of its action

**Another Definition:** Drug distribution is the process by which a drug reversibly leaves the bloodstream and enters the extracellular fluid and/or the cells of the tissues

## SUGGESTED READINGS ON THIS TOPIC

1. Goldberg, J. Practical Psychopharmacology. Cambridge University Press; New edition. ISBN-10: 1108450741

2. Preston, JD. Handbook of Clinical Psychopharmacology for Therapists (9th Edition). New Harbinger Publications. ISBN-10: 1684035155.

3. Sinacola RS, Peters-Strickland T, Wyner JD. Basic Psychopharmacology for Mental Health Professional. Pearson; 3rd edition. ISBN-10: 0134893646.

4. Stahl S. Stahl's Essential Psychopharmacology: Neuroscientific Basis and Practical Applications 5th Edition . Cambridge University Press. ISBN-10 : 1108971636

5. Wegmann J. Psychopharmacology: Straight Talk on Mental Health Medications. PESI; Fourth edition. ISBN-10: 1683732987

# CHAPTER 3. HOW THE BODY DEACTIVATES DRUGS (METABOLISM OR "DRUG FATE")

## Key Concepts

| | |
|---|---|
| Conjugation | One of several ways the liver metabolizes by adding a substance to a drug to change it to a form that cannot reabsorb well. |
| Cellular tolerance | Decreasing drug effects as a result of decreasing receptor sites due to repeated drug exposure. |
| Cross tolerance | Reduced potency of one drug because of repeated exposure of another drug of the same category (i.e. alcohol-Valium, heroin-morphine). |
| Cytochrome P-450 | Specialized set of liver enzymes versatile in their metabolizing capacity |
| Direct-acting agonist | A drug that resembles a neurotransmitter and mimics its normal action |
| Direct-acting antagonist | A drug that can bind to a receptor site but inhibits any response. |
| Dose-response | The effects of a drug at varying dosages |
| Drug fate | Metabolism. How a drug is deactivated and eliminated by the body. |
| Drug half-life | The amount of time the body requires to eliminate half of the total drug present in the system. There is an algorithm of the number of half-lives needed prior to achieving steady state. |
| Drug tolerance | The diminished response to a drug, which occurs when the drug is used repeatedly and |

the body adapts to the continued presence of the drug. For instance, when morphine or alcohol is used repeatedly over a period time, larger and larger doses must be taken to produce the same effect. Usually, tolerance develops because metabolism of the drug speeds up (often because the liver enzymes involved in metabolizing drugs become more active) and because the number of sites (cell receptors) that the drug attaches to or the strength of the bond (affinity) between the receptor and drug decrease.

| | |
|---|---|
| Dose-response | The effects of a drug at varying dosages |
| Enzyme Competition | Multiple drugs taken simultaneously compete for a limited number of enzymes. |
| Half-life | This pharmacokinetic principle describes the time it takes for the body to eliminate 50% of a drug's concentration. In other words, once the half-life is reached, the concentration of the drug in the body is half of its starting dose. The concept of half-life helps to determine excretion rates. Different drugs have different half-lives; however, the same rule applies to all of them: after one half-life has passed, 50% of the initial drug amount is eliminated from the body. |
| Indirect-acting agonist | Augments neurotransmitter activity by extending the time they remain in synapse. |
| Indirect-acting antagonist | Reduces neurotransmitter actions by inhibiting their effects |
| Liver | More than 500 vital functions have been identified with the liver. One of the more well-known functions includes how the liver metabolizes drugs into forms that are easier to use for the body or that are nontoxic (aka, metabolism). |

| | |
|---|---|
| Metabolism | The process of how a drug is deactivated or broken down (bio transformed) by the liver. |
| Metabolic tolerance | Drug-induced elevated liver enzyme activity and increased drug metabolism. |
| Oxidation | The most common metabolism process where liver enzymes directly involve oxygen. |

# CHAPTER 3
# HOW THE BODY DEACTIVATES DRUGS
# (metabolism or "drug fate")

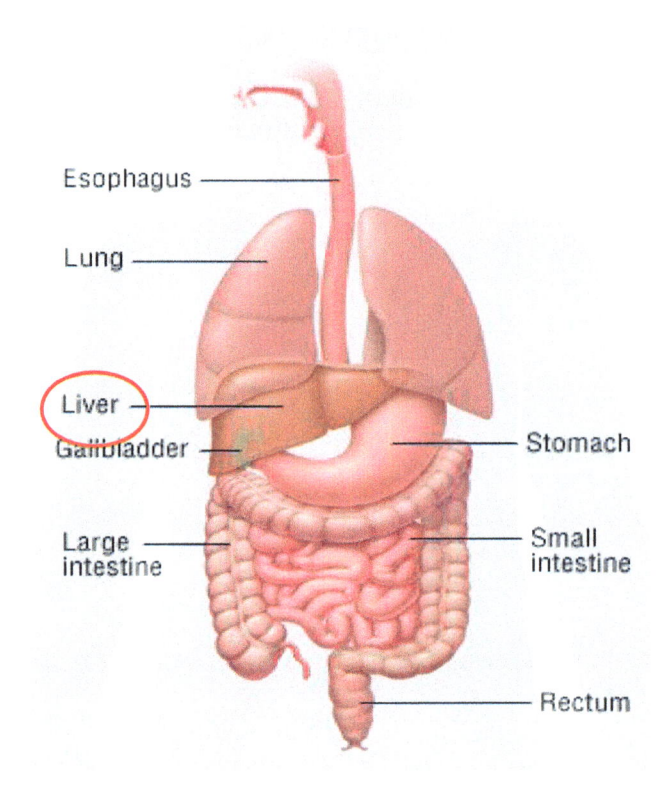

*Esophagus*
*Lung*
*Liver*
*Gallbladder*
*Stomach*
*Large intestine*
*Small intestine*
*Rectum*

When discussing drug ingestion, the primary organ involved is the liver, a large organ located under the diaphragm, up in the abdomen (see illustration above). Its two main functions are to alter substances into forms that are more beneficial to the body (biotransformation), and reduce toxic substances into safer ones (detoxification). These processes are called *metabolism*. Drug metabolism usually refers to chemical breakdown, but metabolism actually describes several biological processes including synthesizing chemicals (anabolism), and producing energy for the body.

Drug fate is how a drug's action is deactivated, so the drug can ultimately be eliminated. In psychopharmacology, *biotransformation* is mostly used in describing drug fate. Most drugs are biotransformed and thus rendered less active by specialized enzymes in the endoplasmic reticulum of the liver, a system usually referred to as the microsomal system.

The microsomal system is also called the mixed-function enzymatic oxidizing system *(MEOS),* and the primary enzyme is Cytochrome P-450. The enzymes in the MEOS are "mixed-function" because they are versatile in what types of substances they act on. Mostly through its specialized P-450 enzymes, the liver transforms substances from one state to another by reducing the drug molecules' lipid solubility so that they cannot absorb well or circulate. P-450 enzymes had probably evolved to digest environmental toxins that might otherwise threaten the body. In general however, biotransformation reduces the effects of many drugs, especially when drugs are ingested orally *(per os)*.

One of the main functions of biotransformation is related to *solubility*. As a general rule, lipid-soluble drugs dissolve and absorb easily into membranes and tissue, whereas water soluble drugs do not. For biotransformation, the liver will reduce the lipid solubility and change the drug into a form that is more water soluble, and hence it will not reabsorb well.

The process of changing a drug molecule's solubility is an essential action of metabolism. The byproducts of metabolism are called *metabolites* (these are usually water soluble). Through biotransformation, the liver essentially alters the potency of a drug by changing its degree of lipid solubility. In this way, a drug will not be able to reabsorb since its lipid solubility is reduced, and in its more water soluble state, it gets trapped by the kidneys and prepared for elimination. Metabolites are usually inactive, but sometimes, the metabolite will have toxic effects on the body as well. Just because a drug gets metabolized does not mean it is necessarily rendered inactive or non-toxic. Drugs such as alcohol, THC and polycyclic hydrocarbons (Benzpyrene and benzanthracene), have active and toxic metabolites that will produce an additive effect with the parent compound. But, metabolites are more likely to get ionized, become unable to reabsorb into the blood, and their action is ended.

The liver utilizes four types of biotransformation to metabolize chemicals; *1) oxidation, 2) conjugation, 3) reduction, and 4) hydrolysis*. Oxidation is the most common form of biotransformation. This is where liver enzymes involve oxygen directly in the metabolism process. A metabolite of oxidation becomes ionized and therefore is unable to reabsorb into the system and will become excreted.

*Conjugation* is where the liver adds a substance to the chemical being metabolized and, as a result, deactivates the chemical or changes it to a form that is too large to reabsorb. *Reduction* is a process where the liver enzymes separate the chemical being metabolized into smaller parts where each part is a simpler compound unable to reabsorb. Since the chemical structure of the substance being metabolized has been "reduced" by this process, it is called reduction.

Finally, *hydrolysis* is where the liver modifies a chemical by adding a water molecule to it. The modification then renders the chemical being metabolized inactive, and is another way to increase water solubility.

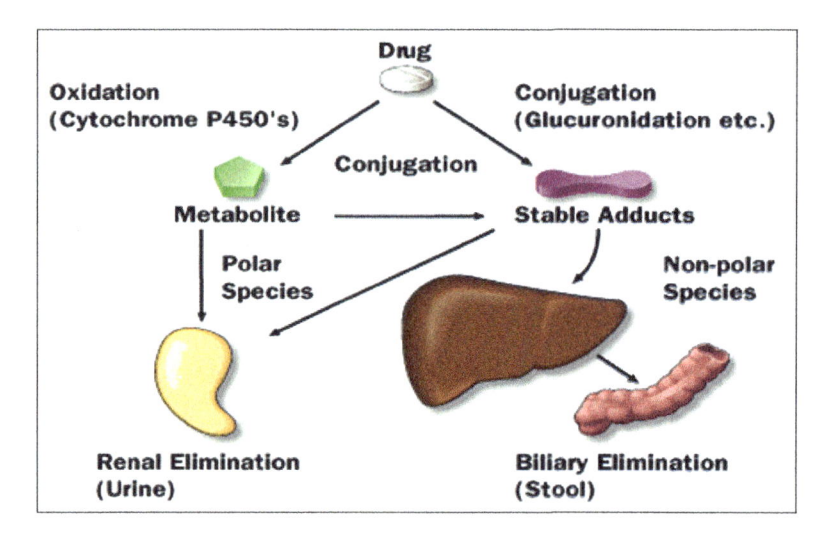

Most biotransformation involves oxidation and conjugation. *Cytochrome P-450* is the principal mixed-function oxidase in the liver. P-450 is the key MEOS responsible for the metabolism of many different drugs including alcohol, anti-anxiety drugs, anti-depressants, and a variety of other drugs.

Several factors influence drug metabolism in the liver and as such, affect each drug's intensity and duration of action. One factor is *liver enzyme induction*, which is an increase in enzyme function from previous exposure to a drug that used that same enzyme for deactivation. Continued exposure to any substance that is oxidized by P-450, for example, will cause the smooth surface of the liver's endoplasmic reticulum to enlarge, and increase production of even more P-450. Remember, it is the liver enzymes that deactivate a drug and render the effects inactive. Thus, the more liver enzymes induced, the more a drug will get deactivated.

When liver enzymes are increased through induction, metabolic tolerance takes place. That is, more of the drug is deactivated by increased liver enzymes which means that less of the drug gets into the brain to produce its effects.

For example, alcoholics will accumulate massive amounts of enzymes, induced by repeated alcohol intake. In the liver, alcohol causes the release of the enzyme alcohol dehydrogenase, which begins the breakdown process of alcohol into alcohol metabolites. Since alcohol induces much more enzyme activity, and since increased enzyme activity means increased metabolism of alcohol, alcoholics build a tolerance to the drug's effects, and are more resistant to intoxication than non-alcoholics. Unfortunately, since more alcohol is deactivated by the liver and therefore never gets to the brain, the person will consume even more in an attempt to stay above the increased enzymes. This can have debilitating effects as we will see in the chapter on alcohol.

Mixed-function oxidases, such as P-450, metabolize many different substances including various drugs, air-born pollutants, pesticides, food preservatives, insecticides and some carcinogens. The concept of *competition* is where molecules from multiple drugs taken simultaneously compete for a limited number of available liver enzymes for their deactivation.

While liver enzyme induction will trigger deactivation of a drug, there are only so many liver enzymes able to be induced. Therefore, when multiple drugs are consumed, they have to compete for available enzymes. If one drug is working on most of the available P-450 then the other substances are forced to wait and will remain active in the bloodstream for a longer period of time than usual.

For example, if an alcoholic who had been drinking the day

of an automobile accident requires a tranquilizer to treat the trauma, the medication will produce its effects too fast, perhaps even fatally. The reason for this is that the alcohol has induced P-450 and there is very little enzyme left to deactivate the tranquilizer. Thus, when the tranquilizer is administered, more of it moves through the liver unchanged and a greater amount reaches the brain.

An opposite example is when a drug has induced liver enzyme activity, but the drug has since left the system while the increase in liver function remains. In our example with the alcoholic, if that person had not been drinking the day of the accident, the liver still has an increase in enzymes but with hardly any drug for those enzymes to work on. When tranquilizers are administered in this scenario, the medication's therapeutic index would be difficult to obtain.

This is due to an abundance of P-450 enzymes with hardly any alcohol to breakdown. When the tranquilizer is administered, much of the drug is readily deactivated by the massive amount of alcohol-induced enzymes, and not enough can get into the brain to produce its sedative effects. Another factor that influences metabolism is a person's age.

Enzyme systems are not fully developed at birth and require time to develop properly to where they are functional for metabolism. Thus, children metabolize drugs much more slowly than their adult counterparts. There is also deficient liver function for elderly people as well. Liver functioning is less efficient in older people, and doses are generally reduced for this population to compensate for decreased liver capacity for drug metabolism.

**Drug Half Life**
Most drugs that are clinically useful have *linear*. The linear refers to dose proportionality where doubling the dose would double the blood level. The drug's pharmacokinetics are usually first-order processes where a fixed-fraction of the dose is processed - absorbed, distributed, metabolized, or eliminated – in a specific length of time which is described by the half-life. A drug's half-life describes the duration of action of psychoactive drugs in the body. Accordingly, a drug's half-life is defined as the time for the plasma level of drug to fall by 50%. It is independent of the absolute level of drug in blood and, a varying

amount of drug is metabolized with each half-life (fewer actual molecules).

Half-lives are measured in hours or in days (recovery from a drug may take a week or more). It takes 4 half-lives for 94% of a drug to be eliminated and 6 half-lives for 98% of a drug to be eliminated. The drug persists in the body at low levels for at least 6 half-lives. For example, if 100 mg of a drug with a 4-hour half-life was administered at 12 noon, then, 50 mg of the drug would remain in the body at 4 pm. If an additional 100 mg of the drug was administered at 4 pm, then 75 mg of drug would remain in the body at 8 pm (25 mg of first dose and 50 mg of second dose). If this administration schedule were continued, the amount of the drug in the body would continue to increase until a plateau (*steady state*) concentration was reached.

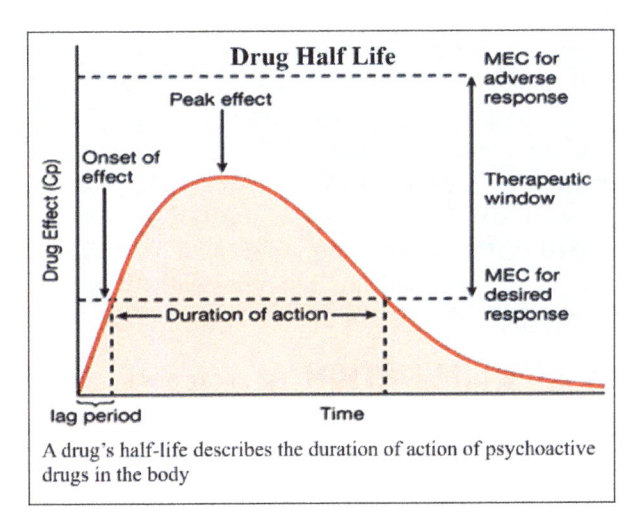

A drug's half-life describes the duration of action of psychoactive drugs in the body

### HALF LIFE AND PERCENT OF DRUG REMOVED (wash out)

| Number of Half-lives | Percent of Drug Remaining | Percent of Drug Removed |
| --- | --- | --- |
| 0 | 100 | 0 |
| 1 | 50 | 50 |
| 2 | 25 | 75 |
| 3 | 12.5 | 87.5 |
| 4 | 6.25 | 93.75 |
| 5 | 3.125 | 96.875 |

**Accumulation and Steady State**
In one half-life, a drug reaches 50% of the concentration that will eventually be achieved. After 2 half-lives, the drug achieves 75% concentration (25% of first dose and 50% of the second dose). After 3 half-lives, the drug achieves 87.5% concentration (12.5 % of the first dose, 25% of the second dose and 50% of third dose. And, after 6 half-lives, the drug achieves 98.4% concentration, essentially at steady state. If the half-life for a drug is known, you can calculate how much will be present at any later time, measured in half-lives.

**Elimination: Metabolism and Excretion**
Drug elimination, which is the removal of the drug from the body, occurs in 2 processes - metabolism and excretion. The primary organ for eliminating a drug from the body is the kidney via metabolism or biotransformation. However, drugs can also be eliminated from the body through the bowels, saliva, sweat glands (tearing), skin (perspiration) and lungs. The associated requirement for drug excretion is the drug's biotransformation into a more water soluble form. The main function of the kidneys is to maintain an optimal balance between water and salt in the body. The functional unit of the kidneys is called the *nephron,* and there are millions of nephrons which work together as a kind of filtering mechanism that physically eliminates certain substances from the body.

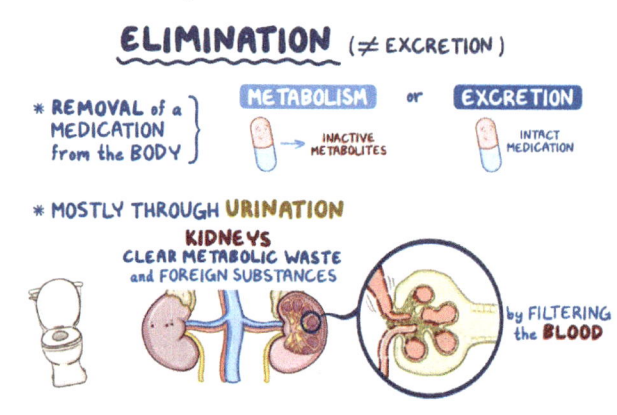

ELIMINATION (≠ EXCRETION)

* REMOVAL of a MEDICATION from the BODY
METABOLISM → INACTIVE METABOLITES
or
EXCRETION → INTACT MEDICATION

* MOSTLY THROUGH **URINATION**
**KIDNEYS** CLEAR METABOLIC WASTE and FOREIGN SUBSTANCES
by FILTERING the **BLOOD**

However, the kidneys do not just filter out impurities from the blood; they seem to filter everything out of the blood and then selectively reabsorb back those substances that are required or needed by the body. The excretion rates of a drug can be influenced by the pH of the urine.

The pH directs the degree of ionization and therefore will influence the degree of reabsorption. Urine is largely acidic, whereas blood tends to be basic. The pH of the urine can be manipulated to be more acidic or more basic.

In general, the acids stay in the blood and the bases tend to stay in urine where they are excreted more easily. Acidifying the urine by administering IV ammonium chloride reduces urinary pH, and thus allows a greater percentage of a weak-base drug to exist in an ionized (excretable) form. For example, acidifying the urine will increase the excretion rate of amphetamines and therefore reduce the duration of an otherwise toxic overdose.

In another example, weak acids like aspirin can be eliminated faster through the administration of sodium bicarbonate, which will alkalinize the urine and reduce the potential overdose of someone who has ingested too much aspirin. In general, the kidneys will excrete excess amount of water from the body (through the urine) and will also excrete molecules of toxins that have been biotransformed by the liver.

In terms of excretion rates, the other factor in determining a drug's fate is its *half-life*. The half-life of a drug is the amount of time the body requires to eliminate half of the total substance present (as measured by its concentration in the blood). Thus, the first half of the substance amount, whether metabolized or not, are then excreted, usually with the urine. Substances can also be excreted with the feces, sweat, saliva, tears, and breast milk. If they are gaseous, they can be excreted by the lungs as well.

**Dosage and Behavior Considerations - Dose-Response Curves**
One of the most important principles of psychopharmacology is the concept of the *dose-response curve*. The most general expectation would be that larger dosages produce larger effects. Indeed, this is almost always true within some range of the drug dosage, but there is usually some level of dosage beyond which this relationship breaks down, and larger dosages produce progressively less of an effect or even an opposite effect.

An example of this type of dose-response relationship can be seen in the Figure below which shows a change in behavior as a function of various dosages of a drug. Using the same behavioral measure, other drugs would show differently shaped curves at different peak plasma levels.

The main point is that the effect of a drug on a behavior cannot be stated in a simple manner: A particular drug may enhance the behavior at low dosages, have no observable effect at some higher dosage, and impair the behavior at still higher dosages.

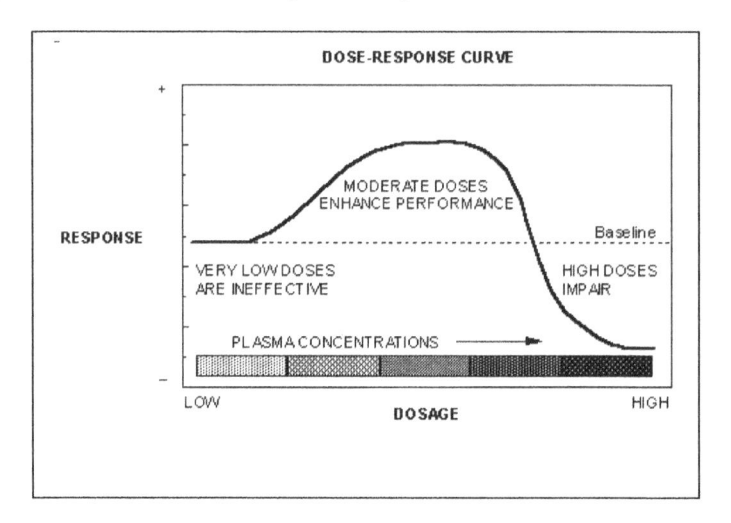

**DOSE-RESPONSE CURVE**

- MODERATE DOSES ENHANCE PERFORMANCE
- VERY LOW DOSES ARE INEFFECTIVE
- HIGH DOSES IMPAIR
- PLASMA CONCENTRATIONS
- RESPONSE
- DOSAGE (LOW to HIGH)
- Baseline

As shown in the Figure below, the plasma concentration of a drug changes continuously over time.

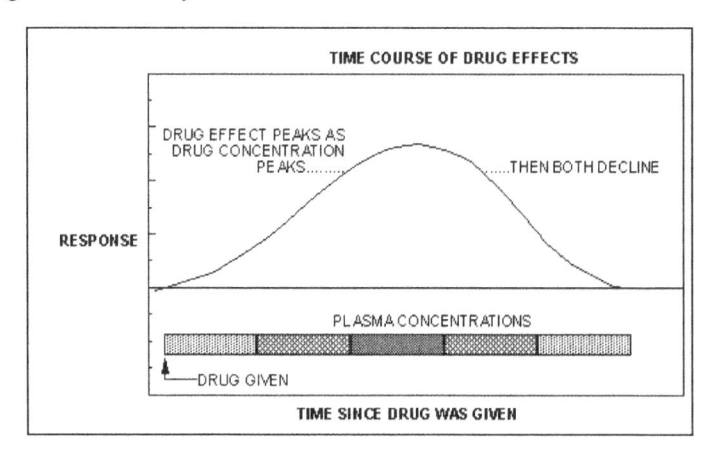

**TIME COURSE OF DRUG EFFECTS**

- DRUG EFFECT PEAKS AS DRUG CONCENTRATION PEAKS........ .......THEN BOTH DECLINE
- RESPONSE
- PLASMA CONCENTRATIONS
- DRUG GIVEN
- TIME SINCE DRUG WAS GIVEN

If one were to transfer sections of this changing concentration curve to the dose response curve in the Figure below, the behavioral effect at any given time would be changing in accordance with the changing concentration curve. In fact, with a single large dosage, it would be possible to show a gradual enhancement of behavior as the drug concentration was increasing, a decline and eventual impairment of behavior as the plasma concentration reached very high levels, a return to enhanced behavior as the drug concentration began to lower, and finally a return to baseline levels as the drug was cleared from the plasma compartment completely. Thus, the effect depends not only on the amount of drug administered, but on the amount of time that has elapsed since the administration.

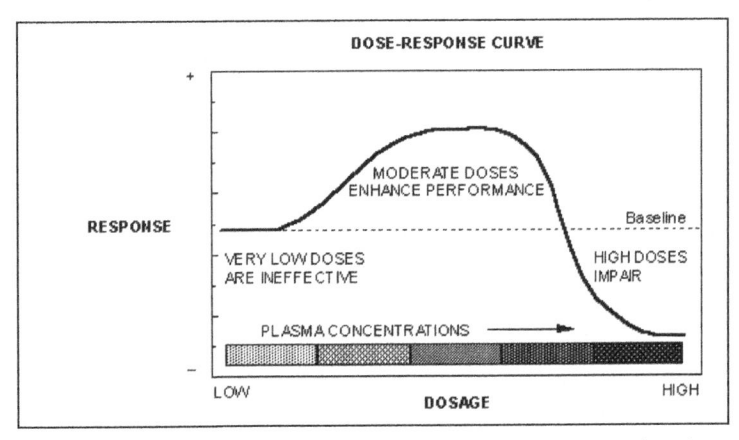

Given the interaction of behavior with drug dosage and the dynamic nature of the drug concentration, about the best one can hope for in terms of a stable effect is that shown in the Figure below. Properly spaced multiple dosages of a drug can lead to a more or less sinusoidal variation in plasma concentrations within the range of dosage that has the desired behavioral effect.

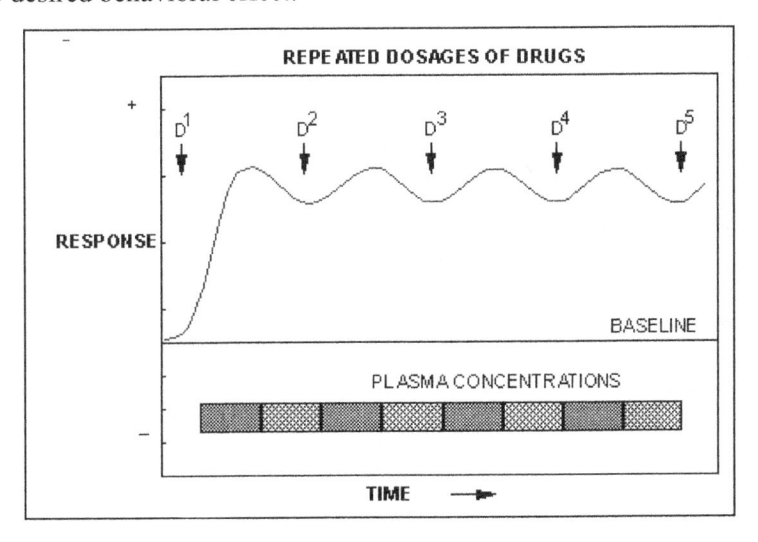

## Drug Tolerance: The body's adaptive response to repeat drug exposure

Chronic administration of a drug can change the drug's potency. As discussed, a drug's potency is defined as the minimal amount necessary to produce a specified effect. In general, tolerance is the decreased potency of a drug as a result of over-exposure. However, there are actually six different types of tolerance that result from different systems affected by repeat exposure to many drugs: *cellular tolerance, metabolic tolerance, cross tolerance, rapid tolerance* (tachyphylaxis), *behavioral tolerance,* and *reverse tolerance* (sensitization).

Cellular tolerance is when the potency of a drug is decreased as a result of a reduction in the drug's mechanism of action. The compromised action is caused by a reduced number of neurotransmitter receptors where the drug molecule binds. If a drug molecule requires binding at a neurotransmitter receptor site to produce its effects, and the system adapts to this activity by decreasing the number of available receptor sites, more drug will be required to produce the same level of effect.

Cellular tolerance is related to a process called *down regulation.* This is a condition where neurons have decreased their receptor site sensitivity to a drug when there is an excess of chemical activity causing over stimulation. For example, if a person over stimulates neurons with methamphetamine, the neurons might counter the response by decreasing the number of available receptor site "entry points" used for the stimulating effects. The reduction of receptor sites by neurons seems to act in a compensatory function for the system to exert some control on the level of its own sensitivity to stimulation.

Metabolic tolerance, described earlier, is where repeat drug exposure increases the liver function, causing an increase of available liver enzymes to deactivate a greater portion of the drug. Since more of the drug is deactivated prior to it getting into the brain, the drug's mechanism of action is reduced because of an increase in metabolism.

Cross tolerance is the reduction of potency of one drug because of chronic exposure to another one, usually in the same drug category. For example, tolerance to heroin produces cross tolerance to morphine or codeine. Tolerance to alcohol produces cross-tolerance to barbiturates and benzodiazepines. Following chronic use of diazepam (Valium) to induce sleep, a tolerance to the drug's sedative effects will develop. Switching to another benzodiazepine to produce sedation will not work because the person is equally as tolerant to that drug as well.

A rather interesting type of tolerance can develop very quickly (between 2 and 24 hours) with certain types of drugs. This is called rapid tolerance, commonly known as *tachyphylaxis* (pronounced, "tacky filaxis"). The effects of drugs such as LSD can produce a fast reduction in potency even *after* the first dose.

Some drugs, which are normally not tachyphylactic produce rapid tolerance, when smoked or inhaled. Such drugs include crack cocaine and smokable methamphetamine, called *crystal*, ice, or *shabu*. Second day administration of the drug requires a marked increase in dose to achieve an equivalent effect. For smokable cocaine and methamphetamine there is the rapid depletion of both norepinephrine and dopamine. The rapid tolerance produced by LSD is still unknown.

Behavioral tolerance is where a deliberate change in behavior offsets the potency of the drug. The behavioral change is usually a response to anticipated adverse consequences of being discovered by others for being under the influence. For example, heavy alcohol intake impairs motor coordination, so the alcoholic learns to behave in ways as to not draw attention to themselves, like not standing up too fast (to avoid falling down). Alcoholics will often walk close to stationary objects and use their hands to coordinate quick adjustments of vertical posture. Marijuana users avoid bending over due to orthostatic hypotension (dizziness and vertigo). Heroin addicts learn to inject their drug of choice in a comfortable location so they can sit or lie down during the initial drug "rush" which could cause them to lose their balance. In other words, addicts and alcoholics often adapt behaviors so that the effects of the drug are less pronounced.

As we are discussing, tolerance is where the potency of a drug is reduced as a result of chronic exposure. Reverse tolerance (sensitization) is the opposite, where there is an increase in potency as a result of continuous exposure to a drug. Cocaine, for example, will increase motor activity when administered to an animal. However, after several exposures to the drug, the original dose level actually produces a greater motor response. Drug dose-response studies of chronic cocaine exposure show that the same level of motor activity can be achieved with a lower dose of cocaine. The animal has, in a sense, been sensitized to the drug. This is somewhat different than "priming", which is where several exposures of a drug are required before a desired specific effect takes place.

Reverse tolerance can also be a sign of pathological development in target organs as a result of chronic exposure. For example, chronic alcoholics can show a marked decrease in their ability to metabolize alcohol, and so the effects of very small amounts will produce intoxication. In this case, potency has been radically altered. Reverse tolerance such as this is usually an indication that the liver is so damaged it cannot induce sufficient levels of enzymes to metabolize alcohol. This can be an important medical concern because if the person's liver can no longer produce enough enzymes to deactivate alcohol, it will not be able to respond to a host of other toxins, since the same enzymes work on many different substances.

**Dose Response Relationships**
Science uses the metric system to describe amounts, specifically drug doses which are usually described in milligrams (mg). A milligram is 1/1000 of a gram, and there are over 28 grams in an ounce. In research, doses are generally illustrated in terms of the amount (mg) per body weight (kilograms or kg). A kilogram is equal to about 2.2 pounds. Even though the overall effects of a drug are certainly related to the amount ingested by an individual, the effects are also related to the drug's concentration in the body. Thus in research science, measuring a drug's effects is described in mg/kg (like the amount of the drug being studied in a specified body weight).

In order to determine the various effects of a drug, science needs to know the possible range of effects and their intensities. In this way, we can determine what dose level produces a predictable response in a given group of animals or humans. The range of responses can be observed, studied and plotted along a graph called a *dose-response curve* (DRC). There are many ways to show a DRC. One way generally used in pharmacology, is to plot the frequency distribution of certain responses to different drug doses, then chart the cumulative percentage of subjects who show the particular drug effects. This type of DRC will also show variance of responses to a drug in a given group of subjects.

In DRC's that use cumulative percentiles, it is common to describe curves and compare effectiveness of different drugs by using the ED50 notation. ED50 is the median effective dose, or the dose that is effective in 50% of the individuals studied. If, for example, a dose of a drug being tested produced an ED10, it would mean that the dose was deemed effective in 10% of the subjects being tested.

If, in the continued DRC testing, a larger dose produced an ED85, it would mean that the dose was effective in 85% of the population being tested. This way of illustrating the DRC in populations is used to calculate the relative safety of drugs.
All psychoactive drugs produce side effects. Since drugs will produce multiple effects, DRC's can measure the side effects in determining a drug's safety as well. For instance, a drug being tested may have an ED95 for one effect and also show an ED10 for side effects.

This would mean that the effective dose worked in 95% of the population studied and that about 10% showed side effects to the drug dose. Another factor in DRC's is the lethal dose range (expressed by the letters LD). So, a drug's LD50 would be the dose that causes death in 50% of the population being studied. Obviously, in drug testing during clinical trials, the DRC range is important to know in order to stay in or above the ED90 range. And, of course, the further away the LD is from the ED, the safer the drug being studied. The relationship between the LD and the ED is reflected in the therapeutic index (TI). The TI is the ratio of the LD50 to the ED50 and can be expressed by the formula; TI = LD50/ED50. By utilizing the TI, scientists will note that the higher the index, the safer the drug will be. Drug safety can also be described as the ratio of ED99 and LD1.

**Agonists and Antagonists**
Drugs are administered for the effects they can produce as related to the drug's overall mechanism of action. Generally speaking, drugs can be divided into groups as to whether they cause an increase in neural activity (agonist) or cause a decrease in activity (antagonist). The drugs that affect receptor site systems can be classified into one of four groups which describe its overall mechanism of action: direct-acting agonists, indirect-acting agonists, direct-acting antagonists and indirect-acting antagonists.

# Agonist VS Antagonist

The words agonist and antagonist can be used in different contexts but you'll hear them when talking about the medical treatment of drug addiction more often than anywhere else. Though these two words sound very similar, there is a big difference between them.

## DEFINITION

- An AGONIST creates a certain action.
- If a drug is an agonist, it produces a chemical reaction after being attached to the receptors of the brain.

## DEFINITION

- An ANTAGONIST opposes a certain action.
- When an antagonist drug is given to a patient, it blocks the addictive drug from activating the receptors of the brain.

## EXAMPLES

- This drug is the only dopamine agonist generally available.
- Inverse agonist is a new type of classification.
- When bending the elbow the biceps are the agonist.
- The M receptor agonist pilocarpine was similar to the effects of ACh.

## EXAMPLES

- A specific leukotriene receptor antagonist awaits development.
- Naltrexone hydrochloride is a new morphine - like antagonist in our country now.
- When bending the elbow the triceps are the antagonist.
- This drug is both a histamine and a serotonin antagonist, and it also has anti cholinergic properties.

💡 An example of an agonist drug is methadone, while naltrexone is an antagonist drug. Both of them are used to treat opioid addiction.

### Direct-Acting Agonists

A direct-acting agonist drug is one that resembles a chemical messenger on a receptor site and will mimic the normal chemical action by neurotransmitters at synapse. Heroin, for example, is a direct-acting agonist in that it binds directly at opioid receptor sites just like endorphins normally do.

### Indirect-Acting Agonists

Indirect-acting agonists will augment the activity of neurotransmitters by extending the amount of time they remain in synapse. The antidepressant Prozac, for example, disallows the neurotransmitter from going back into the cell and therefore prolongs its activity in synapse. Note that indirect-acting drugs usually do not mimic a neurotransmitter by direct binding released at a receptor site.

### Direct-Acting Antagonists

Direct-acting antagonist drugs can bind at a receptor site but disallow any response. As a receptor site blocker, for example, a direct-acting antagonist will inhibit neural activity. When such a drug blocks a receptor site, it will interfere with the neurotransmitter's ability to occupy the receptor and therefore reduce the effect. An example of such a drug is naloxone (Narcan) which blocks the effects of morphine-like drugs (including heroin) by taking up all of the receptor site entry points where the neurotransmitter or the drug itself would otherwise bind and stimulate.

### *Indirect-Acting Antagonists*
An indirect-acting antagonist will reduce neurotransmitter actions usually by causing a depletion of neurotransmitter storage in neurons. Depleting these yet-to-be released neurotransmitters results in the unavailability of enough substance to produce any action once they are released into the synapse. A drug called Reserpine, for example, is an indirect-acting antagonist in that it works by causing stored neurotransmitters to get destroyed prior to their release into synapse. In general, knowing about these different agonist and antagonist strategies can be very helpful in understanding the pharmacological actions of most drugs.

The overall functions of the liver:

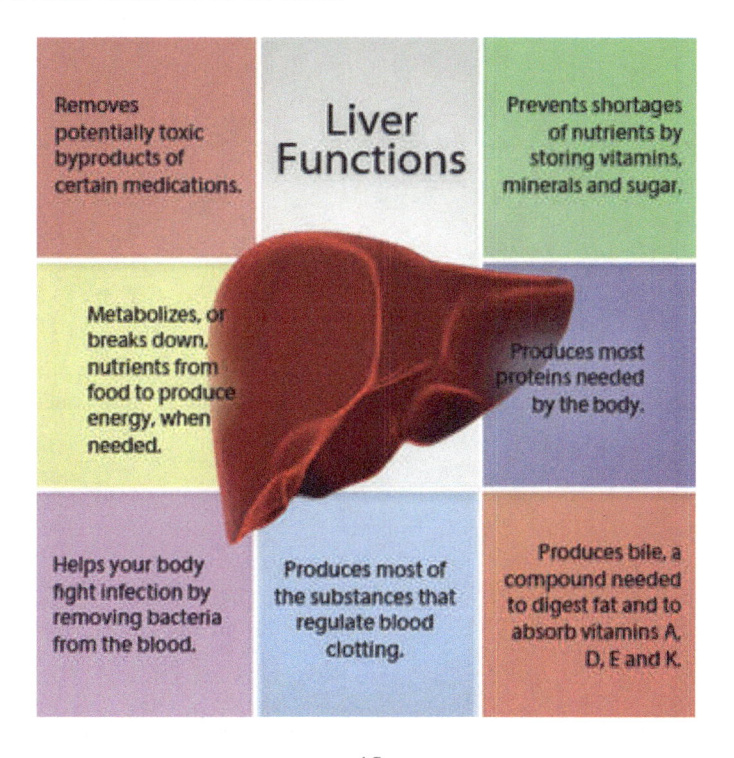

**Liver Functions**

- Removes potentially toxic byproducts of certain medications.
- Prevents shortages of nutrients by storing vitamins, minerals and sugar.
- Metabolizes, or breaks down, nutrients from food to produce energy, when needed.
- Produces most proteins needed by the body.
- Helps your body fight infection by removing bacteria from the blood.
- Produces most of the substances that regulate blood clotting.
- Produces bile, a compound needed to digest fat and to absorb vitamins A, D, E and K.

## SUGGESTED READINGS ON THIS TOPIC

Arias, IM. The Liver Biology And Pathobiology. Wiley Blackwell. 6th Edition. ISBN-13: 9781119436836.

Chopra, S. The Liver Book: A Comprehensive Guide to Diagnosis, Treatment, and Recovery. Atria; 1st edition. ISBN-10: 0743405846.

Manouni, C. The main functions of the liver: hepatic anatomy physiology.
Our Knowledge Publishing. ISBN-10: 6202619791.

Wright., KB. Know More About Your Liver: The greatest guide to diagnosing, treating, and preventing all liver diseases. Independently Published. ISBN-13: 9798867951795.

# CHAPTER 4. THE NERVOUS SYSTEM & HOW IT WORKS

## Key Concepts

| | |
|---|---|
| Afferent nerves | Specialized sensory fibers that carry information into the CNS from sense organs. |
| Amygdala | Located in the Limbic system, it is important for emotional or affective behaviors. Emotional memory seems to be stored there as well. |
| ANS | The autonomic nervous system (ANS) regulates unconscious rates and temperatures. |
| Basal ganglia | Coordinates muscle movement, and located on the left and right of the thalamus. |
| Broca's area | Located in the inferior frontal gyrus of the left frontal lobe, an area critical for human language production. |
| Cerebellum | Aka, "Little brain", is an important hind-brain section that coordinates movement and learning. |
| Cerebral Cortex | The most recently developed and most complicated area of the brain involved in higher functioning. |
| CNS | The central nervous system, including the brain and the spinal cord. |
| Efferent nerves | Specialized motor fibers that carry information away from the CNS to muscles. |
| Fissures | Large grooves or convolutions of the cerebral cortex. |

| | |
|---|---|
| Frontal lobe | The frontal lobes are considered our emotional control center and home to our personality. They are involved in the ability to recognize future consequences resulting from current actions, to choose between good and bad actions (or better and best), override and suppress unacceptable social responses, and determine similarities and differences between things or events. |
| Ganglia | The name for a collection of neurons specifically in the PNS. |
| Gonads | Sexual glands including the ovaries and testes, that secrete sex hormones. |
| Gray matter | Cells that predominate and give the cerebral cortex a grayish brown color. |
| Hippocampus | The limbic structure that plays an important role in short-term, or recent memory. |
| Hypothalamus | Controls autonomic functions and the hormone system from the base of the brain. |
| Limbic system | Contains an interconnecting circular route between the cortex and hypothalamus. |
| Meninges | Three layers of special membranes that protect the brain and spinal cord. |
| Nucleus accumbens | A primary area of the reward circuitry involved in pleasure and reinforcing behaviors. |
| Occipital lobe | The main region where thalamus axons innervate from the visual pathways. |
| Parietal lobe | Monitors touch, stretch and joints from between occipital lobe and central sulcus. |
| Pituitary gland | Releases hormones into the bloodstream that regulate activities of other glands. |

| | |
|---|---|
| PNS | The peripheral nervous system, nerves that extend away from the CNS. |
| Pons | Meaning, "bridge", the Pons are large bulging structures in brain stem that regulate sleep or arousal. |
| Reticular formation | Receives sensory information and projects axons into the spinal cord. |
| Satiation point | The cutoff when behavioral release from tension is no longer rewarding. |
| Temporal lobes | Located near both temples, primary target for hearing. |
| Thalamus | Referred to as the "sensory way-station" of information on its way to the cortex. |
| Wernicke's area | The area responsible for the comprehension of language in the left temporal lobe. |
| White matter | Large concentration of myelin that gives the sub-cortex an opaque appearance. |

# CHAPTER 4

## THE NERVOUS SYSTEM & HOW IT WORKS

The primary target organ for psychoactive drugs is the brain. Psychoactive drugs are those substances that alter thought, affect (mood) and movement. Since psychoactive drugs alter behavior, and behaviors are facilitated by the nervous system, it is important to understand the basics of how the human nervous system works.

The nervous system consists of two subdivisions: the *central nervous system* (CNS), which refers to the brain, and the spinal cord, and the *peripheral nervous system* (PNS) that part of the system outside of the CNS which consists of nerves that extend from the CNS. The PNS contains those nerves that link the periphery of the body, including the smooth muscles and internal organs, to the CNS. Notice in the chart below how the PNS and CNS contain various sub-systems, which they govern, to facilitate behavior. The illustration below shows the physical relationship between the CNS and PNS in the body.

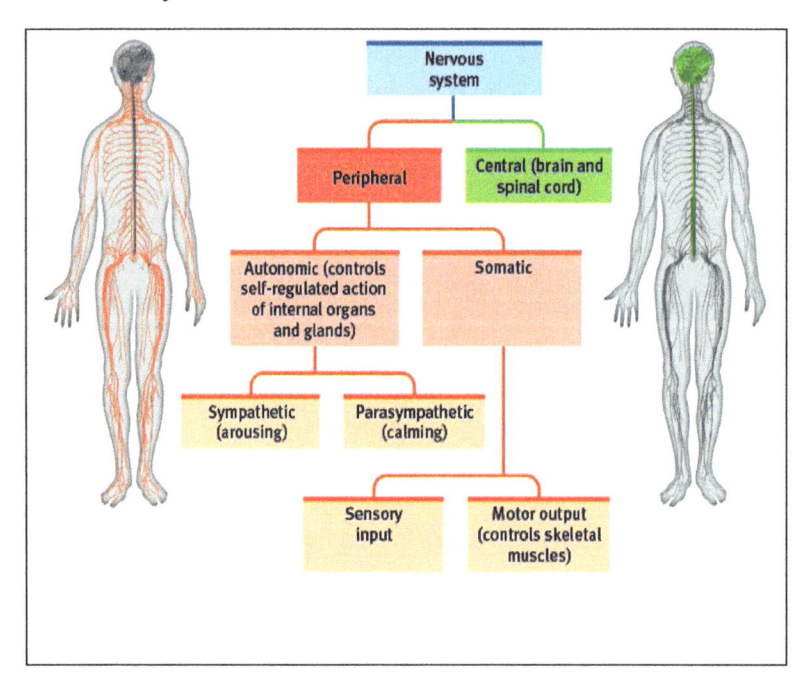

**The Peripheral Nervous System (PNS)**
The PNS is divided into two areas: the somatic nervous system facilitates voluntary muscle movement and allows conscious control over the skeletal muscles, and the autonomic nervous system (ANS) regulates all unconscious events such as heart rate, digestion, respiration, blood pressure and body temperature. The peripheral nervous system (PNS) consists of all the nerve fibers that transmit data to and from the central nervous system (CNS) as well as those that lie outside of the CNS.

Specialized nerve fibers, called *afferent* (sensory) nerves, carry information into the CNS from the various sense organs and therefore aid sensations of pain, temperature and touch. Other specialized nerve fibers within the PNS, called efferent (motor) nerves, carry information away from the CNS for muscle control, movement and specific body functions.

*Efferent* nerves are divided into two categories: somatic fibers that control the function of skeletal muscles, and autonomic fibers, which control activities of the viscera (smooth muscles), heart muscle and the exocrine (secretory) glands. Somatic nerve fibers leave the spinal cord as a continuous uninterrupted unit from their originating site (via a motor neuron) and attach to the skeletal muscles.

The ANS is again divided into three areas: 1) the sympathetic nervous system (SNS), 2) the parasympathetic nervous system (PNS) and 3) the enteric nervous system (ENS). Sympathetic nerve fibers leave from the thoracic and lumbar sections in the middle of the spinal cord. The parasympathetic nerves leave from the upper cranium and lower sacral parts of the spinal cord. There is both a physiological and biochemical difference in these two divisions of the ANS.

The enteric nervous system, not discussed much, is a meshwork of nerve fibers that connects and coordinates actions of the viscera including the gastrointestinal tract, pancreas and gall bladder. As you see in the chart below, the SNS activates the system for the fight-fright because it prepares the body for high level activity and rapid response. The PNS, which controls subconscious activity during periods of relaxation, activates those physiological factors related to the deceleration or slowing down of various bodily processes including heart rate. Since the PNS, when activated, increases food digestion, it is sometimes referred to as the "feed and breed" system.

## Autonomic Nervous System

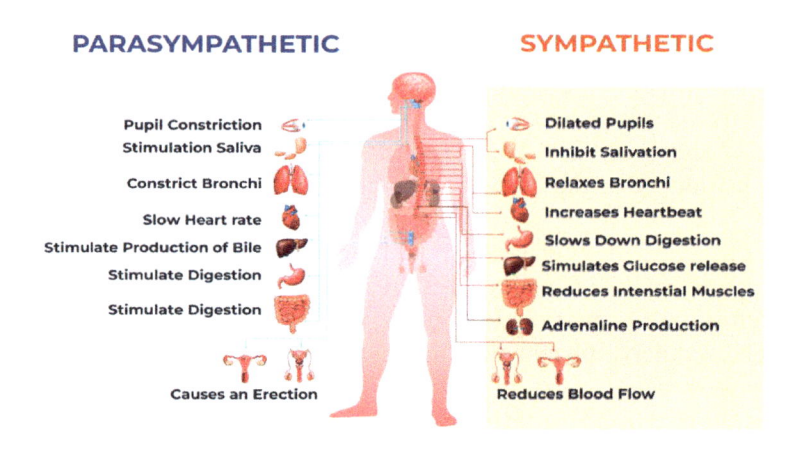

**PARASYMPATHETIC**

- Pupil Constriction
- Stimulation Saliva
- Constrict Bronchi
- Slow Heart rate
- Stimulate Production of Bile
- Stimulate Digestion
- Stimulate Digestion
- Causes an Erection

**SYMPATHETIC**

- Dilated Pupils
- Inhibit Salivation
- Relaxes Bronchi
- Increases Heartbeat
- Slows Down Digestion
- Simulates Glucose release
- Reduces Intenstial Muscles
- Adrenaline Production
- Reduces Blood Flow

Drugs act both centrally (within the CNS) and peripherally (within the PNS). For example, methamphetamine acts centrally by altering thought and mood, producing effects of euphoria, sleep and appetite suppression, perhaps causing paranoia and severe depression. Its peripheral actions affect target organs and peripheral muscles, including tachycardia (racing heart), arteriole constriction and elevated blood pressure. NOTE: In the PNS, a collection of neurons is called ganglia, and axons are called nerves. In the CNS, a collection of neurons is called a nuclei, and axons are called tracts.

**The Central Nervous System (CNS)**
The brain receives signals from both inside and outside the body. It maintains basic bodily functions like heart rate, breathing rate and body temperature without us having to be conscious of these behaviors happening. CNS also initiates conscious decisions to do things like running, walking, playing a musical instrument and many more complex motor tasks. Although the CNS creates our personalities, moods and emotions come from, the human brain only makes up about one-fiftieth (1/50) of the body's weight.

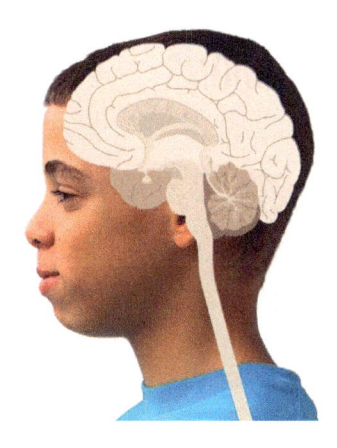

Three layers of special membranes called meninges cover the brain and spinal cord where they serve as a protective covering. The space between the middle and inner layers contains cerebrospinal fluid, a clear, watery solution similar to blood plasma. It circulates over the entire surface of the brain and spinal cord and provides a protective cushion as well as a source of nourishment for these structures. The cerebrospinal fluid is continuously being formed by a plexus (network) of blood vessels in the brain. As it forms, a like amount is continuously reabsorbed.

The human brain is a complex organ that controls thought, memory, emotion, touch, motor skills, vision, breathing, temperature, hunger and every process that regulates our body. Together, the brain and spinal cord that extends from it make up the central nervous system, or CNS. Weighing about 3 pounds in the average adult, the brain is about 60% fat. The remaining 40% is a combination of water, protein, carbohydrates and salts. The brain itself is a not a muscle. It contains blood vessels and nerves, including neurons and glial cells. The brain is thought to contain 100 billion neurons - about the same number as the stars in our Galaxy. Each neuron may be in contact with a thousand other cells, providing the possibility for over a trillion different types of communication routes. The human brain is truly an amazing organ.

The major divisions of the brain are the **hindbrain, midbrain** and **forebrain,** resulting from its own evolutionary development. Each division, or region, contains some principal structures as described below.

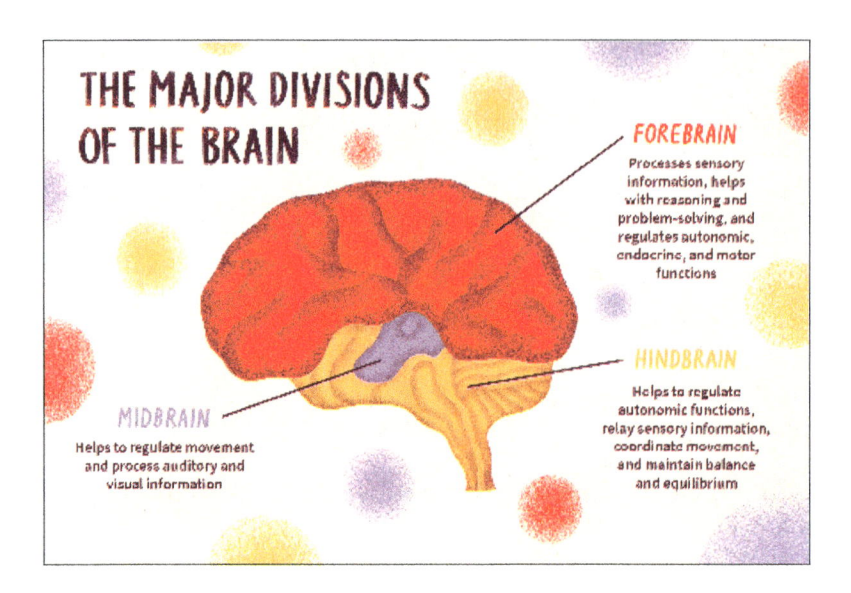

**THE MAJOR DIVISIONS OF THE BRAIN**

**FOREBRAIN**
Processes sensory information, helps with reasoning and problem-solving, and regulates autonomic, endocrine, and motor functions

**MIDBRAIN**
Helps to regulate movement and process auditory and visual information

**HINDBRAIN**
Helps to regulate autonomic functions, relay sensory information, coordinate movement, and maintain balance and equilibrium

## HINDBRAIN STRUCTURES

### Spinal Cord
The simplest part of the nervous system is the spinal cord. Many behaviors can be regulated within the spinal cord and signals do not have to travel into the brain for analysis and action commands. For example, the knee-jerk reflex, sneezing, and eye blink reflex are some reflex behaviors that originate in the spinal cord

The spinal cord is basically the "information super-highway" for nerve impulses traveling into and out of the brain. In fact, all communication with the brain travels through the spinal cord. The two principal functions of the spinal cord are to distribute motor fibers to effecter organs of the body (glands and muscles), and to collect sensory information to be processed by the brain.

The spinal cord, like the brain, consists of white and gray matter. Unlike the brain, its white matter (ascending and descending bundles of myelinated axons) is on the outside, and the gray matter (neural cell bodies and short unmyelinated axons) is on the inside. The spinal cord contains 31 pairs of spinal nerves, with both sensory and motor fibers, that lead from the cord to all parts of the body. The spinal cord is protected by the vertebrae structures.

**Cerebellum** (Balance and Coordination)
The *cerebellum* (meaning "little brain") plays an important role in coordination and movement. Complicated movements are initiated, coordinated and stored as fixed behavioral patterns within the cerebellum. The cerebellum is present even in primitive animals, and its importance increases along the evolutionary scale. The more complicated the motor activity of an animal, the larger the cerebellum. Damage to the cerebellum impairs standing, walking or performing coordinated movements. The cerebellum is also involved in learning.

**Pons**
The *pons* are large bulge-like structures in the brain stem. Pons, meaning "bridge", play a role in the regulation of sleep and arousal as well as coordination of movement patterns.

**Medulla** (Autonomic Reflexes)
The *medulla* is located just above the spinal cord and is involved in the regulation of respiration (breathing), cardiovascular function (heart rate), coughing, sneezing, salivation and other reflex behaviors.

**Reticular Formation** (Alertness)
The reticular formation receives the sensory information from neural pathways and projects axons into the cerebral cortex, thalamus and spinal cord. It plays an important role in the coordination of sleep and arousal (the sleep-wake cycle), attention, muscle tone, movement and various vital reflex behaviors including the startle reaction.

**MIDBRAIN STRUCTURES (Sight and Movement)**

**Tectum** (Hearing and Vision)
The tectum contains two substructures involved with hearing and vision. The first substructure, called the inferior colliculus, is involved in the perception and conveying of auditory information. The other substructure within the tectum, called the superior colliculus, is a part of the visual system, and in mammals is primarily involved in visual reflexes and reactions to moving stimuli.

**Tegmentum** (Movement Coordination)
The tegmentum is located beneath the tectum and is part of the motor system that coordinates nerve signals down the spinal cord or up to the basal ganglia. The tegmentum contains two primary substructures involved in coordinating gross body movements; the substantia nigras and the ventral tegmental area (VTA).

The **substantia nigras** contains dopamine-secreting neurons and plays a critical role in movement and muscle coordination. Degeneration of neurons within the substantia nigras causes Parkinson's disease. The *VTA* also contains dopamine-secreting neurons that project to the basal forebrain and cerebral cortex and have been implicated in the behaviors of learning and motivation.

## FOREBRAIN STRUCTURES

**Limbic System** (Emotion)
The limbic system contains interconnecting areas that run in a circular route between the cortex and hypothalamus. The limbic system actually includes parts of the frontal cortex, thalamus, hypothalamus, amygdala and hippocampus. Functioning together in a complex neural group, all of these areas contribute to the control of emotional behavior and memory. Substructures within the limbic system include the amygdala, hippocampus and the septum.

The amygdala is a structure that governs aggressive behaviors, fear and territoriality. In addition to aggression, the amygdala has some of the circuitry for sexual behavior. Studies have shown that stimulation of certain parts of the amygdala in primates will induce aggressive, assaultive behaviors, stimulation in adjacent areas can even produce fear responses and amnesia.

The hippocampus plays an important role in memory. One interesting case history that shows the effects of a damaged hippocampus is where a man had a severe form of viral encephalitis. This caused a destruction of brain hippocampal areas, and his ability to retain new information was greatly impaired. For example, each time he saw his wife, even after only a few minutes, his reaction was as if he had just seen her for after she had been gone for a long period of time. The man's condition did not allow him to retain new information for any longer than a few *minutes*. It was as if his memory storage could not hold any information. Every time he would turn away from an interaction, any memory of the event disappeared ( this is the case study of Clive Wearing, one of the most famous in cognitive psychology).

Interestingly in this case history of damage to the hippocampus, memories stored prior to the illness remained intact. In fact, this man was a rather popular musician and could retain his musical abilities both as a performer and conductor. However, when he was out of this context, his memory abilities were observably deteriorated. This case, as well as many others, has told us something about the hippocampus and its role in memory processing.

The septum is involved with inhibition. It seems that the septum is the "checks and balances" to the amygdala. That is, where the amygdala becomes active during times of fight-flight and is associated with immediate survival modes of behavior, the septum governs more nurturing behavioral aspects including mating rituals, grooming and hygiene, caring for offspring and sexual arousal.

**Basal Ganglia** (Posture and Movement)
The basal ganglia is located to the left and right of the thalamus and in general, coordinates muscle movement. However, the basal ganglia does not control movement directly, and there are no axons that extend directly into the medulla or spinal cord. Rather, they send signals to the thalamus and the midbrain, which in turn relay the information to the cerebral cortex which then sends messages to the medulla and spinal cord.

**Thalamus** (Sensory Processing)
Much of the surface of the cerebral cortex is divided into regions that receive neural projections from parts of the thalamus. Practically all sensory information projects first to the thalamus in the center of the forebrain, and then to the cerebral cortex, with the exception of the sense of smell which enters the olfactory bulb. The thalamus, based on its functioning, is sometimes referred to as the "sensory way-station" of information on its way to the cortex.

**Hypothalamus** (Neurohumors and Hormones)
The hypothalamus lies at the base of the brain beneath the thalamus. Although a small structure, its functions are enormous. Basically, the hypothalamus controls autonomic functions and the endocrine (hormone) system, through its connections with the pituitary gland. It also coordinates those behaviors related for the survival of the species — fighting, feeding and mating. The hypothalamus has wide-spread connections into the forebrain and midbrain areas and plays a critical role in the behaviors of eating, drinking (body water fluid level), body temperature regulation, sexual behavior, aggression and energy levels.

The hypothalamus has direct control over the pituitary gland and thus regulates the hormone secretion. The hypothalamus contains special receptors for specific hormones. In response to changes in the levels of certain hormones, the hypothalamus will signal chemical messages to the pituitary gland and stimulate it to release hormones. Damage to one of the hypothalamic nuclei causes abnormalities in eating, drinking, temperature, aggression and sexual arousal.

**Pituitary and Endocrine Glands** (Hormones)
Attached to the base of the hypothalamus is the pituitary gland, which is divided into two sections: the anterior and posterior. The anterior part of the pituitary gland releases hormones into the bloodstream that regulate the activities of the other glands. The hypothalamus actually only controls the anterior part of the pituitary gland. There is a chemical interplay between the hypothalamus and the anterior pituitary that regulates many of the body's hormonal levels. Basically this starts with the hypothalamus detecting some hormone level decrease which is beginning to adversely affect the system.

The hypothalamus releases a chemical known as a releasing factor, that acts on the anterior pituitary. The anterior pituitary, in response, releases a hormone that is delivered to the target gland and stimulates it to release more of its own hormone. Target glands are specialized cells that have the ability to produce and release various hormones. The target glands controlled by the anterior pituitary include the *thyroid, adrenal cortex* and the *gonads.* The thyroid releases the hormone called thyroxine, which regulates a substance called adenosine triphosphate (ATP) and has potential energy for behavior. ATP augments energy and distributes it through cells. A deficiency in thyroxine (hypothyroidism) includes symptoms of fatigue and energy drain.

The adrenal cortex produces over forty different hormones known collectively as *steroids.* Steroids generally have a four-fold function: they regulate metabolism and blood pressure, and control sexual appearance and sexual behavior. The gonads include the ovaries and testes and secrete steroidal sex hormones. In males they secrete testosterone, and in females they secrete estrogen and progesterone. These hormones control the development of sexual appearance and maintain reproductive organs as well as sexual behavior in adults. Not all hormones are controlled by the hypothalamus-pituitary axis (also called the hypax). Insulin is one example.

**Medial Forebrain Bundle** (Pleasure, Learning and Motivation)
Within the medial forebrain bundle (MFB) are the neural communication systems between the brain stem, the limbic system and the cerebral cortex. Of particular importance within this communication system is an area called the nucleus accumbens.

**Nucleus Accumbens** (Reward Circuitry)
Over the last twenty years, research has demonstrated the role of the nucleus accumbens in brain stimulation-reward experiments. These widely published studies show convincingly that the brain's reward circuitry includes the nucleus accumbens as a major area involved in pleasure and reinforcement in learning behaviors. For example, laboratory animals with electrode implantations in the nucleus accumbens will learn to press to gain pleasurable stimulation from the electrode. The animal will continue pressing the lever until it becomes exhausted. In fact, the reinforcing effects of brain stimulation-reward in the nucleus accumbens is so strong that the animal will prefer this type of brain stimulation over the intake of food and water.

Studies with humans have also shown that brain stimulation-reward in the nucleus accumbens reinforces those behaviors that had the effect on that brain area. It seems that the nucleus accumbens coordinates pleasure responses that normal reinforce behaviors of eating, sleeping and procreating, and the desire to repeat these behaviors is strengthened. Psychoactive drugs of abuse apparently act on this area of the brain and therefore can become powerfully reinforcing.

Indeed, all experiences of relief from biological tensions will include the activation of the nucleus accumbens. In terms of the normal tension-release patterns of hunger, thirst, and sexual drive, there is a *satiation point* when behavioral release from tension is no longer rewarding. It seems that for these types of sensations, animals will *satiate* and stop trying to relieve biological tension. The feeling of fullness or contentment will ultimately override the need or desire to reduce the biological tension. Animals will stops eating when full, stop drinking when no longer thirsty and stop sexual activity after orgasm.

Interestingly, for drug abuse behavior, there is no apparent satiation point. That is, animals will continue to act in ways to receive drug reward to the point of sheer exhaustion. One study showed that animals will even exceed pain thresholds for drug reward beyond those for food and water. In other words, the animal is apparently willing to pay a very high price with adverse consequences for drug induced brain stimulation.

For some time now, research has confirmed the role of the nucleus accumbens in the brain's reward circuitry during substance use disorders. When the nucleus accumbens is removed in animals that have become addicted to drugs, there no longer is any interest in the self-administration of those drugs. It is as if the reinforcing actions of the drug have disappeared and the animal loses interest in pursuing more of the drug (Phillips AG, Fibiger HC. 1978). More will be discussed on the nucleus accumbens and its role within the brain-reward circuitry of the *mesolimbic pathway* (MLP) in chapter 7 on the Neurobiology of Substance Use Disorders. But for now, however, suffice it to say that if a drug has any potential for abuse, it is because it targets and acts on the brain's MLP.

**Cerebral Cortex** (Higher Functioning)
The *cerebral cortex* is the most complicated region of the nervous system. In humans, the cerebral cortex is greatly convoluted. These convolutions, consisting of sulci (small grooves), fissures (large grooves) and *gyri* (bulges between adjacent sulci or fissures), greatly enlarge the surface area of the cortex, compared with a smooth mass. The cerebral cortex is made of glial cells and neurons. Because cells predominate, giving the cerebral cortex a grayish brown color, it is referred to as gray matter. Beneath the cerebral cortex are millions of neuronal axons that connect the neurons in the cerebral cortex with those located elsewhere in the brain. The large concentration of myelin gives this tissue an opaque white appearance and therefore the term white matter. The cerebral cortex is divided into four parts, called lobes, named after the bones of the skull that overlie them; the *parietal lobe,* the *temporal lobes,* the *occipital lobe* and the *frontal lobe.* All sensory perceptions are projected onto the cerebral cortex, and the outside world is represented by these projection fields.

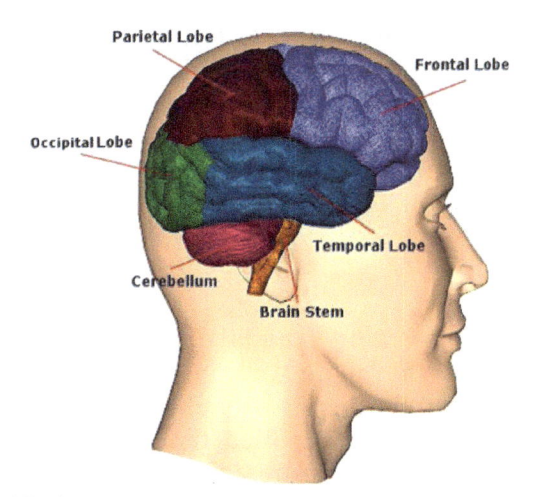

## The Parietal Lobe

The *parietal lobe* lies between the occipital lobe and the central sulcus, one of the deepest grooves in the surface of the cerebral cortex. The parietal lobe is specialized for dealing with the sensory information of touch, muscle-stretch and joint receptors. It is the brain's primary somatosensory area where the integration of many incoming sensations are processed and experienced. The parietal lobe is also important for relating visual information to spatial information. For example, you know you are looking at the same object even if you alter your perspective (i.e. looking at this page and then tilting your head to view it sideways, you know it is still the same page).

Damage to the parietal lobes can result in symptoms where the person has great difficulty interpreting information from touch and using it to control movement. Such symptoms from damage to the parietal lobes might include: impairment of identifying objects by touch, lack of coordination on the opposite side of the body where the brain damage took place, inability to draw or use maps, difficulty giving directions, or problems recognizing different angles of view.

## The Temporal Lobes

The temporal lobes are located in both left and right hemispheres near the temples, on each side of the head. They are the primary target for auditory information (hearing) and coordinate with the vestibular organs (the inner ear that deals with equilibrium and balance). The temporal lobes also contribute to the complexities of vision and perception, such as recognition of patterns that make up faces. In humans, the left temporal lobe contain the area called *Wernicke's area*, which is the brain area responsible for the comprehension of language. The temporal lobes may also play a role in some emotional and motivational behaviors. Damage to the temporal lobes can lead to unprovoked laughter, joy, anxiety, depression or violent behaviors.

**The Occipital Lobe**
Located at the posterior (caudal) end of the cortex, the occipital lobe is the main region where axons from the thalamus innervate from the visual pathways. The very posterior pole of the occipital lobe is called the primary visual cortex. Complete destruction in this area can lead to blindness. In addition to vision, the occipital lobe is responsible for types of learning as well.

**The Frontal Lobe**
The frontal lobe extends from the central sulcus to the anterior part of the brain. The posterior area of the frontal lobe controls fine movements, such as moving one finger at a time. The left frontal lobe, in humans, is an area critical for language production called *Broca's area*. The anterior area of the frontal lobe is called the prefrontal cortex which is the only area of the cortex that receives input from all sensory modalities including olfaction (smell). The prefrontal cortex is critical for memory, emotional expression, and social inhibitions. The illustration below provides a view of the relative location of the four lobes of the brain.

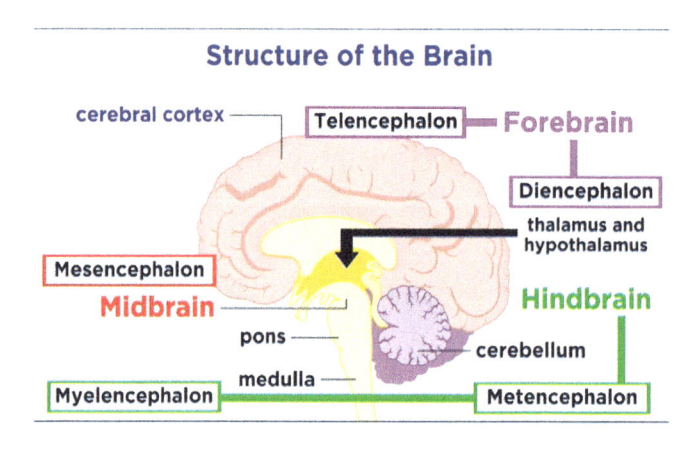

**Structure of the Brain**

## SUGGESTED READINGS ON THIS TOPIC

Bradshaw, K. The Human Brain: "Over 100 Billion Neurons and 1 Quadrillion Synapses". CreateSpace Independent Publishing Platform. ISBN-10 : 1976228972 .

Carter, R. The Human Brain Book: An Illustrated Guide to its Structure, Function, and Disorders. DK. ISBN-10 : 1465479546.

Glass, S. The Nervous System. Perfection Learning. ISBN-13: 9780756998721.

Mai, JM. The Human Central Nervous System. Elsevier Science. Edition 3. ISBN-10: 0123742366.

Phillips AG, Fibiger HC. The role of dopamine in maintaining intracranial self-stimulation in the ventral tegmentum, nucleus accumbens, and medial prefrontal cortex. Can J Psychol. 1978 Jun;32(2):58-66.

Taussig, M. The Nervous System. Routledge Publishers. ISBN-10: 0415904455

Vanderah, TW. Nolte's The Human Brain: An Introduction to its Functional Anatomy. Elsevier; 8th edition. ISBN-10: 0323653987.

# CHAPTER 5. FUNCTIONAL NEUROANATOMY: THE INNER WORKINGS OF THE BRAIN

## Key Concepts

| | |
|---|---|
| Action potential | A change in electrical potential on the surface of a cell that occurs when it is stimulated, resulting in the transmission of an electrical impulse. |
| All-or-none law | Basic principal that states that the action potential either fully occurs or not. |
| Autoreceptors | Specialized to inform presynaptic neurons about the chemical levels in the areas of the synapse. |
| Axon | The part of the cell that transmits a signal away from the soma to the axon endings. |
| Dendrites | Greek for "tree", the part of the neuron that receives neurochemical info to the soma for potential processing. |
| Depolarization | An action potential, an impulse created by a neuron stimulated beyond its threshold. |
| Glial cells | Forms a connective tissue which bind bundle of cells together. |
| Graded potential | Varied signal from dendrites in proportion to the magnitude of the stimulation. |
| Homeostasis | The ability or tendency to maintain internal balance by adjusting physiological processes. |
| Mechanism of action | How a drug works to provide an effect either as an agonist, an antagonist or a combination of the two. |

| | |
|---|---|
| Membrane | Cell wall that limits the flow of materials inside the cell to outside environments. |
| Mitochondria | The part of the cell that performs metabolic activities to make energy for other activities. |
| Myelin | Cells that wrap themselves around the axon to create directional flow during an action potential. |
| Nodes of Ranvier | Bare unmyelinated points along the axon that speed the signal transfer of information. |
| Nucleus | Inside the soma, a structure that converts amino acids into neurotransmitters needed for neural communication. |
| Polarization | Also called resting potential, this is where neurons that have the potential for energy release are not activated and are" at rest" until a biochemical event causes an action potential. |

# CHAPTER 5

## Functional Neuroanatomy: The Inner Workings of the Brain

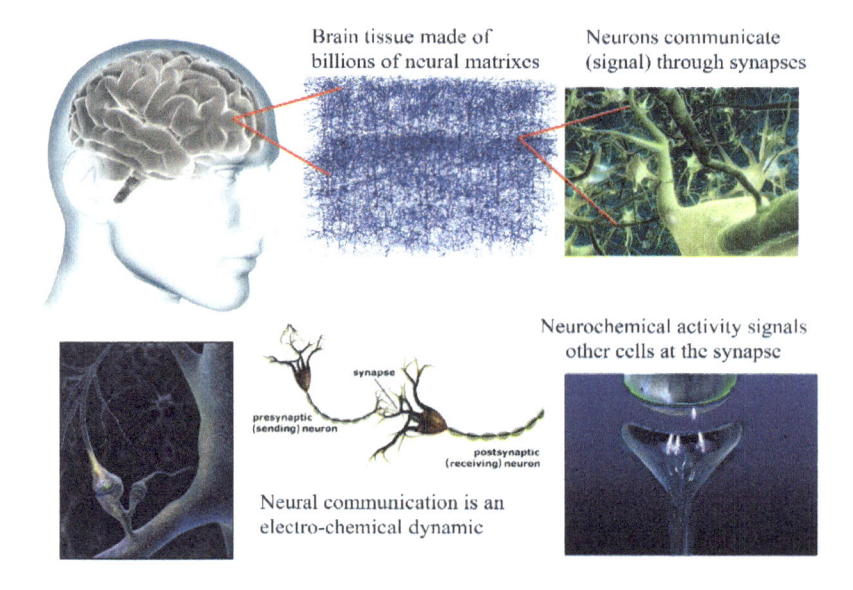

Brain tissue made of billions of neural matrixes

Neurons communicate (signal) through synapses

Neurochemical activity signals other cells at the synapse

presynaptic (sending) neuron
synapse
postsynaptic (receiving) neuron

Neural communication is an electro-chemical dynamic

The fundamental unit of messaging activity in the nervous system

> The illustration above shows the brain, the vast and intricate complex matrix neural networks, the individual neuronal synapses signaling other cells, and the actual synapse itself where neurotransmitters are the

is the *neuron*. The ability of the neuron to transmit information is a function of both its ability to send electrical charges as well as its capacity to synthesize, store and release very specific chemicals from its axon endings.

The basic function of electrical activity within a neuron is to transfer signals to other nerve cells. The critical operation of the brain, processing sensory information, programming movement and emotions, learning and memory - all are carried out by individual neurons. To create a behavior, each sensory or motor neuron involved carries out a sequence of responses. For each neuron – regardless of size, shape, dedicated neurotransmitter substance or behavioral function – most neurons can be described functionally by four components; an integrative component *(signaling)*, a local input component *(receiving)*, a conductile component *(triggering)* and an output component *(chemical release)*. One or more of these four components can become impaired with substance use. Furthermore, behavioral neuroscience has discovered that imbalances in neural components contribute to many psychiatric disorders that will be discussed later. For now, it is important to understand how neurons communicate, since this is the common *lingua franca* of the neurobiology of behavior.

The brain is composed of two classes of cells: *nerve cells* (neuron) and *glial cells*. The glial cells are basically a connective tissue which bind bundle of cells together. Neurons, however, are cells that transfer information within the nervous system, and process it to form behavior. The network between neurons increases dramatically during the first years of life, when new connections are constantly developing. Neurons can alter their shape even after maturity. An enriched environment can lead to longer and more widely branched dendrites which produce more routes that did not previously exist. However, adverse neural effects can be caused by deficient environments, including alcohol abuse which can shrink dendrites. Healthy and alert elderly people seem to have an increased proliferation of dendritic branches, whereas senile persons have slightly shrunken dendrites. Neurons come in many shapes and varieties according to the type of function they perform (see Figure below).

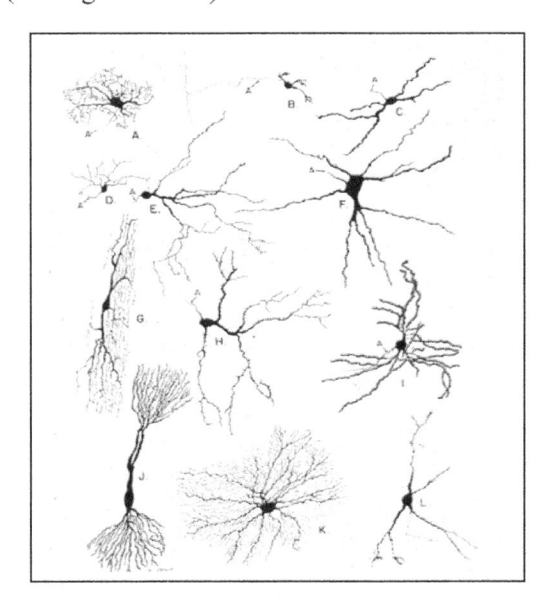

Regardless of the type of neuron, they all possess the same basic anatomy (see Figure below). The neuron is composed of four major structures: the soma (cell body), the dendrites, the axon and the axon endings (presynaptic terminals).

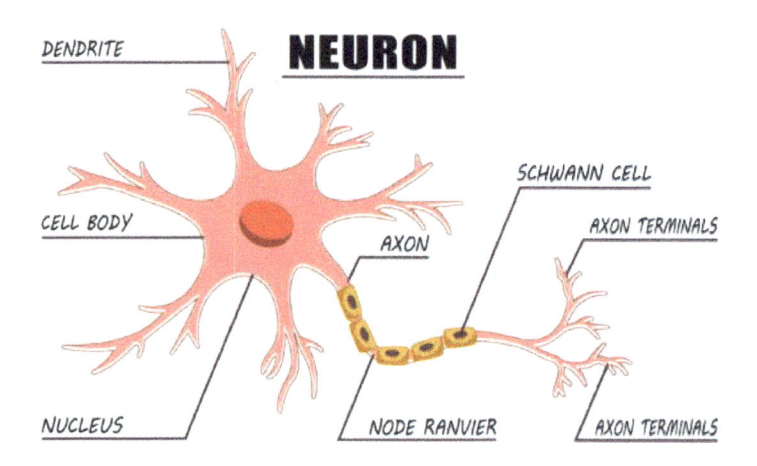

**The Soma** (aka, cell body) - Integrative Component / Signaling other neuron cells. The *soma,* or cell body, is essentially the heart of the neuron. Inside the soma is the *nucleus,* a structure that contains the chromosomes. The nucleus is also the part of the neuron that makes specific neurotransmitters, chemicals that are used to convey information from cell to cell. The soma also contains much of the biological "machinery" that sustains and nurtures the cell as a whole. One of the "machines" in this regard is the *mitochondria,* where the cell performs all of its metabolic activities that provide energy for the cell's other activities, including transmitting data to other neurons.

**The Dendrites** - Local Input Component / Receiving
Dendrites (Greek for "tree") carry neurological information to the soma for interpretation and potential processing. As neurons communicate with each other, the dendrites serve as important recipients of these messages. The dendrite's surface is lined with specialized junctions at which the dendrite receives information from other neurons. In general, the larger the surface area of the dendrite, the greater the amount of information it can receive.\

**The Axon** - Conductile Component / Triggering
The axon is a long slender tube that carries information away from

the soma to the axon endings. The message is electrical in nature until it reaches the axon endings where the message is converted to a chemical one. Some neurons have very small axons, while others have axons that are very long. There are also some types of neurons with more than one axon.

The end of the neuron's axon does not actually touch the adjoining neurons. Thus, between each neuron there is a small space called the *synapse*. The neuron that transfers information into the synapse is called the *presynaptic neuron* and the neuron that is on the other end of the synapse, and receives information is called the *postsynaptic neuron.*

A difference between axons and dendrites is the material surrounding them. Most axons are covered with a fatty 'sheath, known as myelin, which gives axons a white appearance, but no such sheath surrounds dendrites. Myelin is made of special non-neural cells that literally wrap themselves around the axon in layers. In the peripheral nervous system, they are *Schwann cells,* and in the central nervous system they are called *oligodendrocytes.,* but both are glial cells. They prevent nerve signals of adjacent neurons from interfering with one another.

Myelin also insures that nerve impulses during depolarization are directional. A disease related to the *demyelination* (destruction of myelin) is Multiple Sclerosis (MS). As one might imagine, symptoms of MS caused by poor coordination of nerve impulse result in tremors and postural rigidity. Myelin destruction eliminates the insulation between adjacent neurons and results in the scrambling of neural messages.

The myelin sheath itself is divided into segments that leave bare unmyelinated points along the surface. These points are the *nodes of Ranvier,* which speed the process of the myelin sheath conducting information through the nervous system. Nerve cell activity, called depolarization or "firing", is triggered at each node of Ranvier, and is passed along the myelinated area to the next node. This jumping from one node to the next is called saltatory conduction (from the Latin *saltare,* "to dance").

**Axon Endings -** Output Component /Neurochemical Release
The axon divides and branches several times. At the ends of the axons are tiny bulbs, called axon endings (sometimes also called

*terminal buttons*) which have a specialized function. The axon endings release chemicals that cross through the synapse, the junction between each neuron. When a message is transmitted down the axon to the axon endings, a chemical messenger, called a *neurotransmitter,* is released. According to the National Institutes Health (NIH), there are over 100 different types of neurotransmitters which either excite or inhibit further action in receiving cells.

**The Nerve Impulse**
The nerve impulse is an *electro-chemical* event. That is, the information moves as an electrical pulse (from dendrite to the soma and along the axon) and then becomes transferred to a chemical transmission (the neurotransmitter that crosses the synapse and affects the postsynaptic neuron).

Every cell *is* surrounded by a *membrane* that *limits* the flow of materials between the inside of the cell and the outside environment. A few chemicals like water, oxygen and carbon dioxide, flow freely across the membrane, while other chemicals, such as large molecules, do not. The neuron's membrane is *selectively permeable* to chemical passage, which means it will allow some molecules to pass through but not others. Several important ions such as sodium, potassium and chloride enter the cell through pores or channels in special proteins that are embedded in the membrane.

The neuron, like an electrical wire, is a conductor of electricity. Neurons maintain a difference in electrical charge (measured in millivolts or mV) across their external membrane. This difference is the resting potential, also called *polarization* since positive and negative charges are polarized, and kept separate by the cell membrane. Thus, the difference in electrical charge is determined by the distribution of ions outside versus inside the neuron. The resting potential is caused by unequal distribution of sodium (Na+), potassium (K+), and chloride (Cl-) ions, and organic protein anions (A-) across the cell membrane. Changes in the neuron's membrane permeability to Na+ and K+ will produce the electrical message that will ultimately be transmitted down the axon.

During resting potential, there is an accumulation of Na+ ions outside the cell, producing a more positive charge than the inside negative charge created by the amount of organic anions (A-). The distribution of ions this way establishes the potential for energy release by the neuron, but unless an event happens to allow Na+ ions to permeate the membrane, the cell remains in a state of polarization.

It is important to remember that during resting potential, where there is the potential for energy release but none is taking place, the membrane permeability to K+ is high and to Na+ is low. Neurons are able to maintain a resting potential by means of a hypothetical energy driven sodium-potassium "pump" which controls the flow of ions in and out of the neuron in such a way as to keep the outside of neuron slightly more positive than inside. The resting potential will remain stable until the neuron is stimulated.

When the neuron is stimulated beyond a certain threshold, it will generate a nerve impulse, called the action potential. When an action potential occurs, its size (amplitude) is independent of the intensity of the stimulus that initiated it.

This *all-or-none law* basically states that the action potential either occurs or it does not. Once triggered, it is transmitted down the axon to the axon endings. All action potentials take place in the axon and are equal in size. In contrast, dendrites will produce what are called *graded potentials* which will be proportional to the magnitude of the stimulation. So as the strength of the stimuli decreases, so will the intensity of the graded potential.

The action potential is related to the movement and distribution of ions across the cell membrane. When the stimulation reaches the threshold, it causes a change in the permeability of the membrane.

The channels along the membrane previously too small to accommodate Na+ molecules are now opened wider. As Na+ now moves inside the cell, there is a reversal of charge to where the inside is more positive and the outside is more negatively charged.

When this occurs, the neuron has depolarized or "fired", meaning that it has released energy for the neural communication process.

**ACTION POTENTIAL**

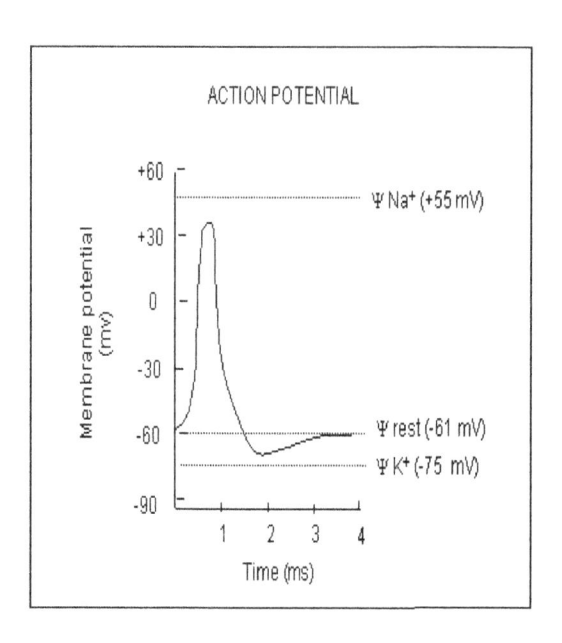

$\Psi\,Na^+\,(+55\,mV)$
$\Psi\,rest\,(-61\,mV)$
$\Psi\,K^+\,(-75\,mV)$

After depolarization, the neuron apparently requires a brief period when it is resistant to re-excitation. For 1 millisecond after an action potential, the cell is in a *refractory period*. The first part of this period is called the *absolute refractory period* because no matter how strong the intensity of a new stimulus is, the cell will not produce an action potential. The second part of the period is called the *relative refractory period,* during which a stimulus must exceed the usual threshold in order to produce an action potential. The time span during refraction is apparently required for the sodium channels to recover after depolarization.

Stimulation of the neuron inverses the membrane potential from negatively charged (at rest) to positive (action potential). This transformation occurs only at the point of stimulation. The positive charges inside the membrane attract neighboring negative charges and travel towards them. A similar process occurs outside the membrane as well. This results in positive charges transferring along the axon towards the synapse, and negative charges towards the soma. Sodium channels open when the membrane potential is positive. Indeed, the open sodium channels allow in sodium which leads to the action potential. The new action potential attracts nearby ions and produces a new action potential further along the axon.

It is now apparent that the nerve impulse is an electro-chemical event as the distribution and movement of ions across the cell membrane addresses the electrical part of the nerve impulse, and the chemical neurotransmitter messengers released into synapse address the chemical aspects.

**The Synapse**
The electrical action potential travels from the soma to the end of the axon, but cannot continue to the next cell in its electrical form due to a gap between the cells called the synapse. Synapses are fluid-filled spaces between the axon endings of one neuron and the somatic or dendritic membranes of another (see Figure below). A synapse, while varying in size, averages to about 200 angstroms wide. An *angstrom unit* is one ten-millionth of a millimeter, so the synaptic gap is quite small indeed.

Because a message only travels one direction, the membranes on the two sides of the synapse are named accordingly: the transmitting neuron is called the presynaptic membrane, and that of the receiving neuron is the postsynaptic membrane. The postsynaptic membrane contains specialized protein molecules that act as "receptors" which can detect the presence of neurotransmitters in the synapse. When the released neurotransmitters diffuse across the synapse and bind at these postsynaptic receptors, the receiving neuron can initiate changes along its own membrane that will either excite or inhibit the rate of depolarization of the neuron's axon.

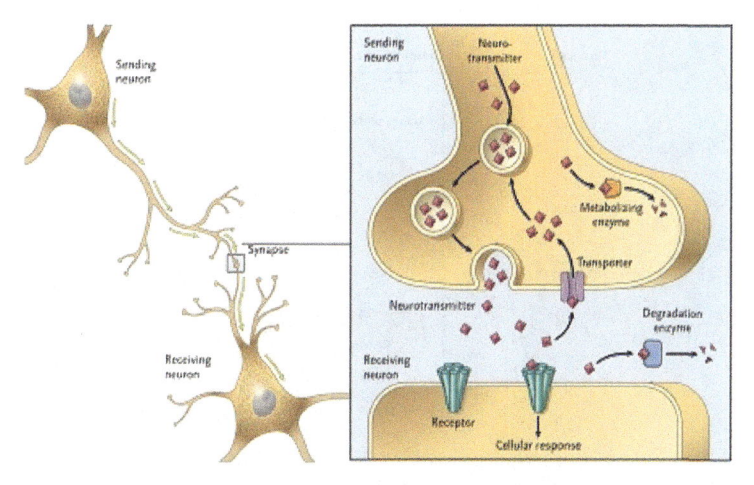

In order for electrical pulses generated by the action potential to cross a synapse, a neurotransmitter is released from one axon ending to travel across the synapse and stimulate receptors of the postsynaptic nerve. As a rule, the synthesis of neurotransmitters occurs within presynaptic terminals of the neuron. The chemical reactions that produce these transmitter substances are called *enzymes* and are themselves made in the cell body (soma). Neurotransmitter substances are stored in tiny sacs, called synaptic vesicles, after they have been produced.

When a neuron "fires" (producing an action potential), a number of synaptic vesicles filled with a neurotransmitter migrate to the presynaptic membrane, fasten to it, and then burst forth spilling their contents into the synapse. The whole process of synaptic transmission begins with the nerve impulse, traveling down the axon, reaching the axon endings, and triggering the vesicles' release of the neurotransmitter into the synapse. This release process occurs rather indirectly; the nerve impulse causes calcium (Ca+) ions to enter into the axon endings, and it is actually the Ca+ that triggers the release. When Ca+ enters the axon endings and facilitates the releasing process, it "primes" the vesicle to rupture and disperse the neurotransmitters into the synapse. The importance of Ca+ to synaptic transmission cannot be emphasized enough, because without it the synapse is rendered inoperative. As a released neurotransmitter diffuses across the synapse and meets with the postsynaptic membrane, it attaches to the membrane. The postsynaptic membrane contains structural "slots" that relate to the molecular shape of the neurotransmitter (see Figure below).

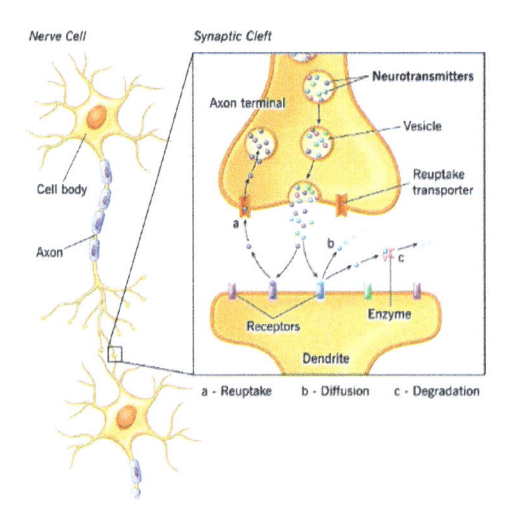

These slots, called *receptor sites,* are specialized protein molecules embedded in the postsynaptic membrane. The process of the neurotransmitter attaching to a receptor is called *binding*. Once it binds, the postsynaptic receptor opens a neurotransmitter-dependent ion channel which then allows particular ions to pass through the membrane, changing the local membrane potential. Stating it another way, the neurotransmitter will bind at a receptor site and produce a change in the postsynaptic membrane's permeability to a certain type of ion, that either excites or inhibits a nerve impulse.

Unlike the membrane along the neuron's axon that is controlled by the electrical charge across its membrane, the postsynaptic nerve is controlled by chemical neurotransmitters that interact with the membrane. When neurotransmitters bind to receptors, they literally change the shape of the protein-molecule receptor site, opening ion channels and inhibiting the receiving neuron.

Neurotransmitters open ion channels in two ways. The primary way is where the neurotransmitter (known as the *first messenger*) binds directly at the receptor site producing changes. Some receptors cannot open ion channels directly from the neurotransmitter but instead produce the so called *second messenger,* composed of cyclic nucleotides. Attached to the receptors of the postsynaptic membrane at some synapses are molecules of an enzyme called *adenylate cyclase.*

When this receptor binds with a certain type of neurotransmitter, *adenylate cylcase* activate causing *adenosine triphosphate* (ATP) to be converted into *cyclic AMP* (cyclic adenosine monophosphate). After the cyclic AMP triggers the opening of ion channels, it is destroyed by the enzyme *phosphodiesterase*. Most drugs of abuse act on second messenger systems and thus impair the nerve impulse.

The two types of binding produce different changes in neuron membrane permeability that apparently mediates different types of behavior. The direct first messenger system initiates a rapid, brief change in the membrane causing rapid behaviors such as muscle contractions and quick response movements. Second messenger systems produce slow and relatively long-lasting changes in the membrane (from minutes to hours) causing long-term alterations in behavior such as learning and memory.

**Synaptic Defenses (**Keys to a drug's *Mechanism of Action*)
Whether an interaction in synapse is direct or indirect, the duration

of that action and the impact it has on the postsynaptic membrane is very brief. Soon after the process initiates, the neurotransmitter is eliminated from the synaptic environment. Apparently, the human brain is extremely conservative in its chemical interactions within the synapse. That is, almost as soon as the neurotransmitter is released into synapse, it is removed or eliminated.

*Behavioral homeostasis,* the person's maximum capacity defined by his or her genetics and environment, is maintained by four neurological dynamics or "defenses" that take place in the synapse: *binding, reuptake, enzymatic degradation* and *autoreceptor* functions.

The biological objective, an internal biological imperative which seeks to maintain homeostasis, is to keep the synapse chemically stabilized. Therefore, postsynaptic membrane activation cannot be too long or too short in intensity and duration. The four synaptic defenses work in concert with each other to accommodate the biological objective for behavioral homeostasis. When the synaptic environment becomes hyperactive (too active) or hypoactive (under active), because of too much or too little neurotransmitter release, behavioral homeostasis becomes compromised.

Binding serves two primary functions. As mentioned, binding is where the neurotransmitter diffuses across the synapse and occupies a receptor site on the postsynaptic membrane where it will excite or inhibit an action potential. The second function of binding involves its role as a synaptic defense. Binding can be viewed as a process by which the neurotransmitter is removed from the synaptic environment. When a neurotransmitter binds at a receptor site, it is cleared from synapse. Thus, binding also maintains chemical stability within the synapse to further assist in maintaining homeostasis.

The postsynaptic changes induced by neurotransmitters at receptor sites are kept brief primarily through the process called *reuptake*. This is the rapid removal of the neurotransmitter from the synapse by the axon endings. When an action potential arrives, the axon endings release a small amount of neurotransmitter substance into the synapse and then take it back, giving the postsynaptic membranes only a brief exposure of the substance. Thus, reuptake essentially removes the neurotransmitter from synapse and thereby helps to maintain chemical stability.

*Enzymatic Degradation* is the synaptic defense where an enzyme destroys the neurotransmitter molecule. Enzymatic degradation can take place in the fluid inside of the cell (called cytoplasm or intracellular fluid) and outside of the cell within the synapse area (called extracellular fluid). Enzymatic degradation changes the structure of a neurotransmitter rendering it useless, where it eventually gets "washed out" of the synapse.

For example, neurotransmission at synapses on muscle fibers and at some points between neurons is mediated by the neurotransmitter called acetylcholine (ACh). ACh is destroyed by an enzyme called *acetylcholine esterase* (AChE) where it cleaves the ACh into its constituents of choline and acetate. Because neither of these constituents is capable of binding at receptors along the postsynaptic membrane, they are removed from the synapse. Many types of neurotransmitters have specific enzymes responsible for their degradation as well, although the type of degradation process will vary. However the manner of enzymatic degradation, the process itself is yet another way of removing neurotransmitters from synapse and thus serves to help maintain the chemical stability to insure homeostasis.

The amount of neurotransmitter released by a neuron seems to be controlled by a kind of biochemical "feedback" mechanism. Generally, after a neurotransmitter is released, it not only diffuses across the synapse and acts on postsynaptic membranes, but it also chemically "informs" the presynaptic neuron about the relative level of its own presence. In other words, presynaptic neurons have specialized receptors called *autoreceptors,* that keep the presynaptic neuron informed about the level of its own neurotransmitter in the synapse. The presynaptic receptors essentially respond to the transmitter substance that they release.

Autoreceptors can be found on the membrane of any part of the cell including the axon ending, soma or dendrite. Autoreceptors regulate internal processes of the neuron. So if there is too little or too much, the production of neurotransmitters is adjusted accordingly. When neurotransmitters are removed from the synapse by autoreceptors, the synaptic environment is helped to maintain chemical stability. Thus, in addition to the feedback function, autoreceptors are also a synaptic defense.

It is important to understand events at synapse because most psychoactive drugs act there to produce their effects. That is, drugs alter various events taking place in the synapse. Actually, *psychoactive drugs produce their effects on the nervous system by interrupting one or more of the synaptic defenses.*

The action of psychoactive drugs depends on what synaptic defense they alter; antipsychotic drugs prevent binding by blocking receptors, methamphetamines increase production of newly synthesized neurotransmitter and blocks reuptake as well as enzymatic degradation. Some of the new antidepressants (such as mitrazepine) also affect autoreceptor function. Drugs affect one or more synaptic defenses, causing their mechanism of action as either an agonist or antagonist and also the drug's side effects.

**Pharmacology of synapses**

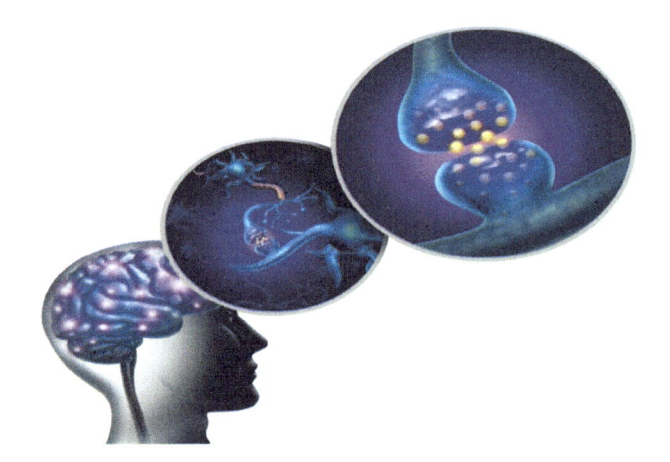

In psychopharmacology, scientists have discovered many drugs that affect the production, storage, release, deactivation, or re-uptake of neurotransmitters or that stimulate or block postsynaptic receptor sites. Many of these drugs are developed to study the functions of the nervous system and others are used to treat mental illness.

A drug's *mechanism of action* is how it has the ability to produce its effects. Drugs have a very general mechanism of action as either a direct-acting or indirect-acting agonist or antagonist or a combination of the two, known as a partial agonist-antagonist. As you recall from previous sections, an agonist is a drug that facilitates the effects of a particular neurotransmitter on the postsynaptic neuron, meaning that it will stimulate a receptor. An antagonist drug counteracts or inhibits the effects of a particular neurotransmitter on the postsynaptic neuron.

There are a variety of ways that drugs can act as agonists and/or antagonists. First, a neurotransmitter substance must be synthesized from its precursor (usually an amino acid). It has been noted in some cases, that the rate of neurotransmitter production and release can be affected when a precursor is administered. In these cases, the precursor itself acts as an agonist (i.e. the substance, *L-DOPA)*.

The process of converting an amino acid precursor into a neurotransmitter is controlled by enzymes. Thus, if a drug deactivates one of these enzymes, it prevents the neurotransmitter from being manufactured. The drug, *a-methyl-p-tyrosine* (AMPT) blocks the enzyme tyrosine hydroxylase and therefore prevents the synthesis of the catecholamine neurotransmitters (norepinephrine and dopamine). AMPT would thus be considered an antagonist

Neurotransmitters, when synthesized are placed in synaptic vesicles and stored until they are needed in synapse. A drug called *reserpine* deteriorates the membrane of those vesicles containing the monoamine neurotransmitters (norepinephrine, dopamine and serotonin). When the vesicle is "eaten away" by the drug, the neurotransmitters spill out of the vesicle into the cytoplasm of the presynaptic membrane where they are destroyed by enzymes. As this occurs, the neurotransmitter is eliminated before it gets placed into synapse. Resperpine, then, is considered a monoamine antagonist drug.

Other drugs act as antagonists by preventing the release of neurotransmitters from the axon endings. *Botulinum* toxin, produced by bacteria that grow in improperly canned food, prevents the release of a neurotransmitter called acetylcholine (ACh). Other drugs can act as agonists by stimulating the release of a neurotransmitter. Venom from the black widow spider, for example, causes massive ACh release.

Once the neurotransmitter is released into synapse, it must bind at receptor sites to produce an action. Some drugs act as agonists by binding with receptor sites and the activating them directly, mimicking neurotransmitters. Nicotine, for example, activates one of the acetylcholine receptor subtypes. Other drugs bind at receptor sites but do not activate them and thus prevent the neurotransmitter from any action. These drugs, called *receptor blockers*, and act as antagonists such as the anti-psychotic drugs.

Presynaptic membranes of some neurons have autoreceptors which help to regulate the amount of neurotransmitter that is released. Stimulation of these autoreceptors reduces the release of the neurotransmitter. There are drugs that selectively activate autoreceptors but do not activate the postsynaptic receptor sites and thus function as antagonists. One of the mechanisms of action of *LSD*, for example, is that it stimulates serotonin autoreceptors and thus, inhibits serotonin release.

As mentioned previously, enzymatic degradation essentially removes neurotransmitters from the synapse. Drugs that deactivate these enzymes will allow excess of neurotransmitters to remain in the synapse for a longer duration where they will continue to bind and stimulate receptor sites. For example, a drug called *phenelzine* blocks the enzyme that degrades the monoamine neurotransmitters and therefore is a monoamine agonist. Since enzyme degradation will reduce neurotransmitter activity, blocking the enzyme results in an increase in neurotransmitter activity and therefore the action would be considered an agonist.

The illustration on the next page shows how agonist and antagonist dynamics can occur. Whether induced artificially by drugs or not, neurotransmitter impact is also controlled by the sensitivity of the synapse as a whole. That is, there are some compensatory actions of the postsynaptic membrane receptor sites that take place in response to a particular level of neurotransmitter activity. The postsynaptic membrane has the capacity to either increase or decrease the number of receptor sites stimulated by the neurotransmitter, depending on the level and intensity of the neurotransmitter released.

In other words, the postsynaptic neuron can alter its sensitivity as a response to different levels of neurotransmitter release. It is as if the system as a whole, determined by it genetic DNA coding, inherently "knows" the optimal level of stimulation, so that when this level is not achieved, receptor sites attempt to compensate for the level of neurotransmitter release.

When the postsynaptic neuron decreases the number of receptors, usually in response to over-active stimulation of neurotransmitters, the temporary change is called postsynaptic subsensitivity or down regulation. Basically, this is the process in which postsynaptic neurons reduce their functioning by desensitizing receptor sites. This is actually what takes place during *cellular tolerance*. Since the number of receptor sites has been reduced, there are fewer "entry points" for substances to bind and stimulate. Therefore, more of the drug may be required to initiate an effect. The postsynaptic neuron also has the ability to increase the number of its receptors, usually in response to an underactive stimulation of neurotransmitters. When this occurs it is called postsynaptic supersensitivity, or up regulation.

How drugs might produce an agonist or antagonist action (aka, *drug mechanism of action*) is illustrated in the image below.

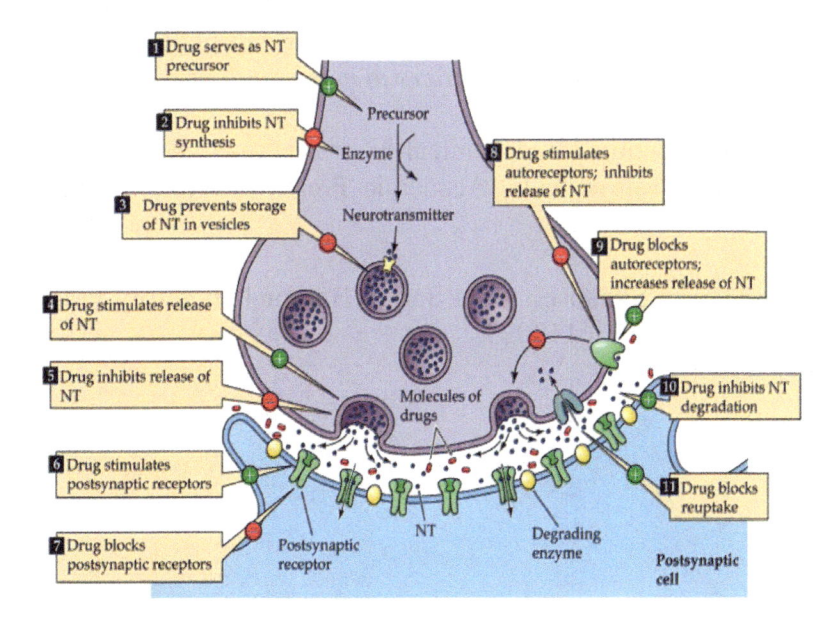

We have talked about several ways the synapse can regulate its level of activity — from the synaptic defenses to changes in postsynaptic receptors. This flexibility and resilience helps maintain synaptic activity at optimal levels (homeostasis). Balance in the nervous system largely determines how well a person will respond and overcome distress produced by drugs, neural damage or even defective genes.

## SUGGESTED READINGS ON THIS TOPIC

Cowan, WM. Synapses. The Johns Hopkins University Press. 2001. ISBN-10: 0801864984.

Julien, RM. Julien's Primer of Drug Action. Macmillan. 2023. ISBN: 9781319244866

Kandel, E. Principles of Neural Science. McGraw Hill. 2021. ISBN-10 : 1259642232.

Luengo-Sanchez, S., Bielza, C., Benavides-Piccione, R., Fernaud-Espinosa, I., DeFelipe, J., & Larrañaga, P. (2015). A univocal definition of the neuronal soma morphology using Gaussian mixture models. *Frontiers in neuroanatomy, 9*, 137.g

Moihni, J. Functional and Clinical Neuroanatomy: A Guide for Health Care Professionals. Academic Press; 1st edition. 2020. ISBN-10: 0128174242.

Sheng, M. The Synapse. Cold Spring Harbor Laboratory Press. 2012. ISBN-10: 1936113023.

# CHAPTER 6. THE CHEMISTRY OF BEHAVIOR: NEUROTRANSMITTERS

## Key Concepts

| | |
|---|---|
| Acetylcholine (Ach) | (ACh) is a white crystalline derivative of choline that is released at the ends of nerve fibers in the somatic and parasympathetic nervous systems and is involved in the transmission of nerve impulses in the body. ACh associated with the biochemistry of memory and movement. |
| Catecholamines | Dopamine, norepinephrine, and epinephrine are physiologically active molecules known as catecholamines. Catecholamines act both as neurotransmitters and hormones vital to the maintenance of homeostasis through the autonomic nervous system. |
| Dopamine(DA) | (DA) is a monoamine neurotransmitter formed in the brain by the decarboxylation of dopa and essential to the normal functioning of the central nervous system specific to the behaviors of mood, movement, motivation and pleasure. |
| Endocannabinoids | Endogenous cannabinoids, or endocannabinoids, are naturally occurring, lipid-based neurotransmitters. They are a part of the endocannabinoid system (ECS) in the brain which primarily influences neuronal synaptic communication, and affects eating, anxiety, learning and memory, reproduction, metabolism, growth and development and an array of actions throughout the nervous system. |
| Endorphins | Endogenous morphine, combining these two words into one - *endorphins*, are opioid neuropeptides that are naturally produced in |

the body that serve a primary function of blocking the perception of pain and present in sensations of pleasure. Created in the pituitary gland and hypothalamus, endorphins are a type of neurotransmitter. They attach to the brain's opioid receptors and carry signals across the nervous system. There are more than 20 types of endorphins in the body that are categorized into 3 groups: *alpha-endorphin, beta-endorphin, and gamma-endorphin.* Of the three endorphin types, beta-endorphins have been the most studied and prevalent, accounting for the majority of the functional properties of endorphin

| | |
|---|---|
| Gamma amino butyric acid (GABA) | (GABA) is the primary inhibitory neurotransmitter in the central nervous system. It plays an important role in regulating neuronal excitability. GABA is also directly responsible for the regulation of muscle tone. |
| Glutamate(Glu) | (Glu) is an amino acid, the salt (glutamate) of which functions as a neurotransmitter. Glu is secreted in many areas of the brain and by some neurons in the spinal cord where its effects are generally excitatory. |
| Histamine(H) | A biologically active amine that is formed by the decarboxylation of the amino acid histadine. It is widely distributed in nature and is found in tissues as well as in venoms. In humans, histamine is a mediator of inflammatory reactions, and it functions as a stimulant of hydrochloric acid secretion in the stomach. |
| Indolamines: | Indolamines are a family of neurotransmitters share a common molecular structure of indolamine. A common example of an indolamine is the neurotransmitter serotonin, which is involved in mood, sleep, appetite, and other behaviors. Another example of an indolamine is melatonin, which regulates the |

| | |
|---|---|
| | sleep-wake cycle (circadian rhythm) in humans. |
| Large molecule neurotransmitters | Neuroactive peptides weighing above 1000M, including the endorphins. |
| Leu-enkephalin | Leucine -enkephalin, critical to pain sensation and suppression (analgesia). |
| Met-enkephalin | Methionine-enkephalin, critical to pain sensation and suppression (analgesia). |
| Monoamines | The group of 3 neurotransmitters, norepinephrine, dopamine, and serotonin, made from a single amino precursor. |
| Monoamine oxidase | (MAO) is the enzyme that degrades any of the monoamine neurotransmitters. |
| Neurotransmitters | Neurotransmitters are endogenous(made from within) chemicals that allow neurons to communicate with each other throughout the body. They enable the brain to provide a variety of functions, through the process of synaptic transmission. These chemicals are integral in shaping everyday life and functions. |
| Norepinephrine (NE) | (NE) is both a hormone and neurotransmitter, secreted by the adrenal medulla and the nerve endings of the sympathetic nervous system to cause vasoconstriction and increases in heart rate, blood pressure, and the sugar level of the blood. Also called noradrenaline. Centrally, NE needed for mood, sleep, memory, attention and sensation. |
| Small molecule neurotransmitters | Individual amino acids, such as glutamate and GABA, as well as the transmitters acetylcholine, serotonin, and histamine, are much smaller than neuropeptides and have therefore come to be called small-molecule neurotransmitter. |

Serotonin(5-HT) — Also known as 5-hydroxytryptamine (5-HT), is a neurotransmitter derived from an indole-containing amino acid, tryptophan. 5-HT important in the behaviors of mood, sleep, appetite, and pain sensation.

# CHAPTER 6

## Functional Chemistry of Behavior: Neurotransmitters

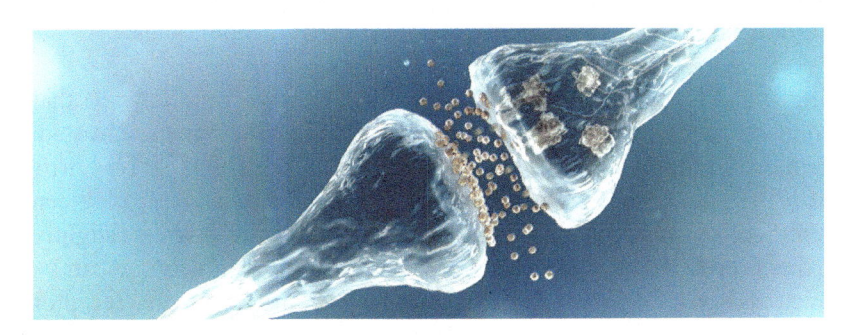

Chemical messengers that communicate neurological information from neuron to neuron are called *neurotransmitters.* That is, these chemical messengers transmit important neurological information throughout the body. While there are over 100 different types of neurotransmitters in the brain and body, only a few have been extensively studied with respect to their relationship in substance use and co-occurring disorders.

Neurotransmitters produce two general effects on the postsynaptic membrane — either excitation (depolarization) or inhibition (hyperpolarization). Since there are only two general effects, one might imagine that there only needs to be two types of neurotransmitters. However, the type of behavior that a neurotransmitter produces is not simply a matter of whether it excites or inhibits.

In fact, behavior is determined by the *locus of activity* (location in the nervous system where an event takes place) and the neurotransmitter involved. Thus, the same neurotransmitter in a different part of the nervous system might create different effects, and different neurotransmitters in the same area of the nervous system will produce different behaviors. For example, the neurotransmitter dopamine in the midbrain substantia nigras coordinates movement, whereas dopamine in the medial forebrain bundle has more to do with emotions and pleasure.

Further complicating the neurobiology of behavior is the fact that no single neuron releases all neurotransmitters. Each neuron stores and releases only one or two neurotransmitters, and neurons that release a particular neurotransmitter are clustered together to form neural pathways (i.e. the "dopamine pathway"). Postsynaptic neurons, on the other hand, receive a number of different neurotransmitters at various chemical synapse at receptor sites.

Finally, there are an abundance of *receptor subtypes* that produce a variance of different behavioral responses when activated. Some postsynaptic neurons have a large number of receptor subtypes, like the serotonin system which has at least eighteen identified receptor subtypes. Since these subtypes possess slightly different protein structures, drugs selective for a given subtype can be developed. Drugs with greater selectivity to target specific receptor subtypes can have significantly reduced unwanted side effects.

Many of the newer psychiatric medications, for example, have a much greater selectivity to specific receptor subtypes where the therapeutic effect is obtained with fewer side effects. Clozapine, for example, was the prototypical antipsychotic and has more selective actions at certain receptor sites than previous generations of these drugs. Today, there are even more selective medicines and the more selective they can target receptor sites, the more compliance is achieved with patients experiencing fewer side effects than the older medicines.

A drug's action relates to the neurotransmitters it affects. Behavioral pharmacology seeks to understand a particular drug's mechanism of action by identifying which neurotransmitter systems the drug targets, whether it is an agonist or antagonist, and what are the observed behavioral changes, some of which may be toxic. To qualify as a neurotransmitter, a chemical must meet four criteria as outlined in the box below

---

**NEUROTRANSMITTER CRITERIA**

1. It is synthesized within the neuron and present within the axon endings.
2. It is released in sufficient amounts that produce a defined action on the postsynaptic receptor sites
3. When administered from the outside (exogenously), such as a drug, it mimics the action of endogenously (from within) released neurotransmitters by activating the same ion channels or second-messenger systems in the postsynaptic neuron.
4. Specific mechanisms exist for the removal of the substance from its site of action (the synapse).

**Small and Large-Molecule Neurotransmitters**

Neurotransmitters are classified into two general groups, based on their molecular weights and chemical composition: small-molecule and large-molecule neurotransmitters. The ***small-molecule neurotransmitters*** are those normally associated with the term "neurotransmitter". The primary small-molecule neurotransmitters are dopamine, norepinephrine, serotonin, acetylcholine, glutamate, GABA (y-aminobutyric acid), and histamine (H). ***Large-molecule neurotransmitters*** (also called neuroactive peptides) are proteins that have molecular weights above 1000M, including endorphins, enkephalins, methionine, cholecystokinin, ACTH (adrenocortocotropic hormone), vasopressin and Substance P. The general effects on behavior of both the small and large-molecule neurotransmitters are shown in the charts below.

| Principal Small-Molecule Neurotransmitters |||
|---|---|---|
| Type | Receptor Sites | General Functions |
| Dopamine (DA) | Designated *D1* and *D2* | Mood, movement reward, pleasure, olfaction, concentration, attention |
| Norepinephrine (NE) | Alpha 1, Alpha 1a, Beta 1, Beta 2, and Beta 3 | Mood, sleep, learning, memory, attention, concentration, mental alertness, anxiety and sensory processing |
| Serotonin (5-HT) | 18 identified receptors designated into 8 families 5-HT1 through 5-HT 8 | Mood, sleep, pain processing, appetite, sex, and aggression. |
| Acetylcholine (ACh) | Muscarinic (M1 through M5) and Nicotinic (NN and NM) | Movement, motor coordination, memory, and sensory processing |
| Gamma-amino butyric acid (GABA) | GABA A and GABA B | Major inhibitory function within CNS |
| Glutamate (Glu) | NMDA, Quisqualate and Kainate | Memory, major excitatory function within the nervous system |
| Histamine (H) | H1 and H2 | Sleep, sedation, temperature |

| Principal Large-Molecule Neurotransmitters ||
|---|---|
| Type | General Functions |
| Endorphins | Suppression of pain, learning, memory and pleasure |
| Enkephalins Leucine | Suppression of pain, learning, memory and pleasure |
| Cholecystokinin | Regulation of food intake |
| Adrenocorticotropic hormone (ACTH) | Energy production, water intake, learning and memory |
| Vasopressin | Learning and memory, vasocontrcition, raises blood pressure, and reduces excretion of urine. |
| Substance P | Perception of pain. Transmission of pain impulses from peripheral receptors to the central nervous system. |

The following provides an overview of the small-molecule neurotransmitters and their general functions within the nervous system. Included also is an overview of the receptor sub-types for each of the neurotransmitters discussed.

**Dopamine**

Dopamine (DA) is made from the amino acid *tyrosine*. In the CNS, DA originates in two brain areas: the substantia nigras and the ventral tegmental area (VTA). It is then extended by three major pathways into other areas of the brain including the hypothalamus, the frontal lobes and the medial forebrain bundle (MFB). DA in the midbrain substantia nigras, the nigrostriatal pathway, is involved in the control of fine skeletal muscle movement (basal ganglia).

DA activity in the hypothalamus would suggest that it plays a role in autonomic functions. Degeneration of dopamine within the substantia nigras has been linked with Parkinson's disease, a movement disorder characterized by symptoms of tremors, muscle rigidity, compromised balance and difficulty in initiating movements. In the frontal lobes, DA is important in regulating thought and, via the nucleus accumbens within the MFB, is a principal substance that provides the chemical basis for the reward circuitry. DA has also been of great interest in its association with the thought disorder of schizophrenia.

Research studies from the 1960s discovered that antipsychotic drugs were effective in alleviating some of the symptoms of schizophrenia. There was evidence that antipsychotics were interfering with transmission of DA synapses. Studies have shown that the primary mechanism of action of antipsychotic drugs is binding and blocking a DA receptor sub-type called D2.

Interestingly, in contrast to the blocking actions of the antipsychotic drugs, DA agonist drugs such as cocaine or amphetamine, that mimic the actions of DA, can induce psychotic features. While it is tempting indeed to believe that schizophrenia is the result of a hyperactive DA system, studies have shown that DA, by itself, is not the single cause of the disorder. Nonetheless, DA is strongly associated with the condition of schizophrenia, although the disorder includes other systems and neurotransmitters.

It is generally agreed upon that the brain's reward circuitry is the main area where DA reinforces drug abuse, the DA-rich circuit that involves the mesolimbic pathway, the nucleus accumbens and the ventral tegmental area. Studies have demonstrated that drugs which have the potential for abuse demonstrate their agonist actions within the mesolimbic pathway involving the reward circuitry. DA's role in governing the brain's pleasure center is well documented, and the section on the neurobiology of reward will provide a detailed account of that information.

Most DA, when released into synapse, is eliminated through reuptake. However, there are two enzymes that are active in degrading excess DA. The first is called *monoamine oxidase* (MAO), found in both presynaptic and postsynaptic membranes. The second enzyme is called *catechol-O-methyltransferase* (COMT) located in the synaptic gap.

The five different dopamine receptors can subdivide into two categories. D1 and D5 receptors group together, and D2, D3, and D4 are together in a separate subgrouping. The overall basic function of each dopamine receptor:

- D1: memory, attention, impulse control, regulation of kidney function, movement

- D2: movement, attention, sleep, memory, learning

- D3: cognition, impulse control, attention, sleep

- D4: cognition, memory, fear, impulse control, attention, sleep

- D5: decision making, cognition, attention

**The Dopamine Pathways in the Brain**
Dopamine is transmitted via three major pathways. The first extends from the substantia nigra to the caudate nucleus-putamen (striatum) and is concerned with sensory stimuli and movement.

The second pathway projects from the ventral tegmentum to the mesolimbic forebrain and is associated with cognitive, reward and emotional behavior. The third pathway is concerned with neuronal control of the hypothalmic-pituatory endocrine system. The dopamine pathways in the brain are shown by the figure below.

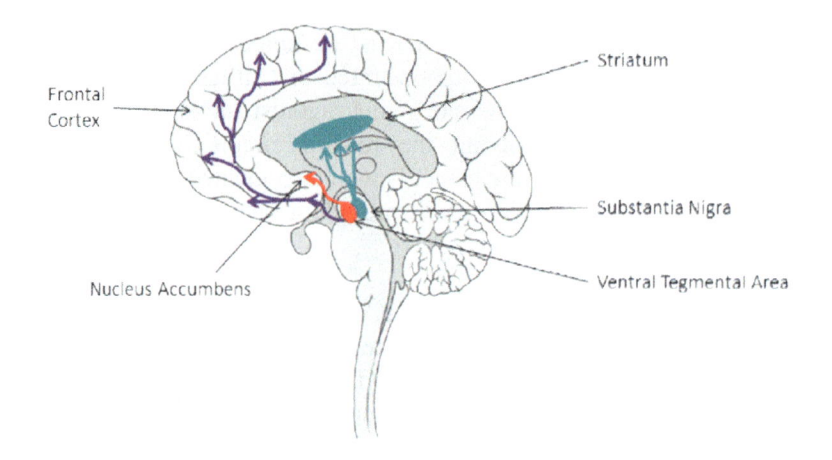

## Norepinephrine
Norepinephrine (NE) is found in both the peripheral and central nervous systems, and is synthesized from the amino acid *tyrosine,* as is dopamine. In fact, DA can be considered a precursor to norepinephrine because it is the second step of a three-step process in converting tyrosine to NE. In the autonomic nervous system, NE is the main neurotransmitter within the sympathetic nervous system, and is the primary substance where nerves innervate at target organs (involved in the fight-or-flight response). In the CNS, NE is involved in mood control, cortical arousal, pleasure, and cognitive behaviors of attenuation, concentration and focusing.

## The Noradrenaline Pathways in the Brain
Many regions of the brain are supplied by the noradrenergic systems. The principal centers for noradrenergic neurons are the locus coeruleus and the caudal raphe nuclei. The ascending nerves of the locus coeruleus project to the frontal cortex, thalamus, hypothalamus and limbic system. Noradrenaline is also transmitted from the locus coeruleus to the cerebellum. Nerves projecting from the caudal raphe nuclei ascend to the amygdala and descend to the midbrain.

Synapses that use NE are called *adrenergic* or *noradrenergic* synapses. With depolarization and Ca+ intake, the NE is released and acts on postsynaptic receptors, called -*alpha*-adrenergic receptors (α1). This primarily affects Ca+ channels mediated through second messengers. In addition, the released NE acts on presynaptic axon endings at receptors called α2-adrenergic receptors. It is known that α2-adrenergic receptors will control the activity at synapse. In norepinephrine systems, there is a second type of adrenergic receptor called the *beta* (β) receptor. This receptor differs from the alpha receptor mainly by being primarily postsynaptic and connected to the c-AMP second messenger system.

Stimulant drugs act as agonists within the NE system, but with a variety of different mechanisms. Cocaine will increase NE synaptic activity by increasing biosynthesis and release of newly formed NE molecules then blocking reuptake. Methamphetamine will do the same, but will also inhibit enzyme degradation. Contrasting this, noradrenergic antagonists, such as some antipsychotic drugs, will reduce NE activity, thus significantly reducing excitement and hypomania.

The alpha receptors, located in the PNS (peripheral nervous system) affect sympathetic responses including blood vessel constriction. As such, antagonist drugs specific to these receptors are useful in treating high blood pressure. Other adrenergic receptors within the PNS govern additional sympathetic responses. β receptors located on the heart muscle can be antagonized by "beta-blockers" to treat cardiac arrhythmia (irregular heart beat). NE activity is terminated by two mechanisms: reuptake (the primary method of terminating the NE), and enzymatic degradation by both MAO and COMT (the same enzymes that terminate DA).

Currently there are five NE receptor sub-types which are grouped into two categories: the *alpha-adrenergic* and *beta-adrenergic* receptors. Within the a-adrenergic system are the receptors Alpha 1 and Alpha 1a. Within the β-adrenergic systems are the receptors Beta 1, Beta 2, and Beta 3.

**Serotonin**

Approximately 98% of serotonin (5-HT, for *5- hydroxytryptamine)* is located outside of the CNS and in the gastrointestinal tracts. 5-HT is synthesized from the amino acid *tryptophan.* The storage, release and termination of serotonin is essentially the same as for DA and NE, with the exception that 5-HT is only metabolized by MAO enzymes. The reuptake process for 5-HT is also identical to the termination of DA and NE

The interest in the behavioral actions of 5-HT began in the 1950s with the realization that its molecular structure resembled *d-lysergic acid diethylamide* (LSD), and the discovery that LSD antagonized intestinal smooth muscles. 5-HT has been the focus of research in the 1980s and 1990s, with many new discoveries about its extensive role in behavior. The 5-HT system has the largest number of receptor subtypes, numbering eighteen to date, which are divided into eight families or categories.

**The Serotonin Pathways in the Brain**
The principal center for serotonergic neurons is the raphe nuclei. From the raphe nuclei axons ascend to the cerebral cortex, limbic regions and specifically to the basal ganglia. Serotonergic nuclei in the brain stem give rise to descending axons, some of which terminate in the medulla, while others descend the spinal cord.

## Serotonergic Pathways in the Brain

**Serotonin** (5-hydroxytryptamine, **5-HT**) cell bodies are mainly found in the **raphe nuclei,** and their **serotonergic** fibers project widely.

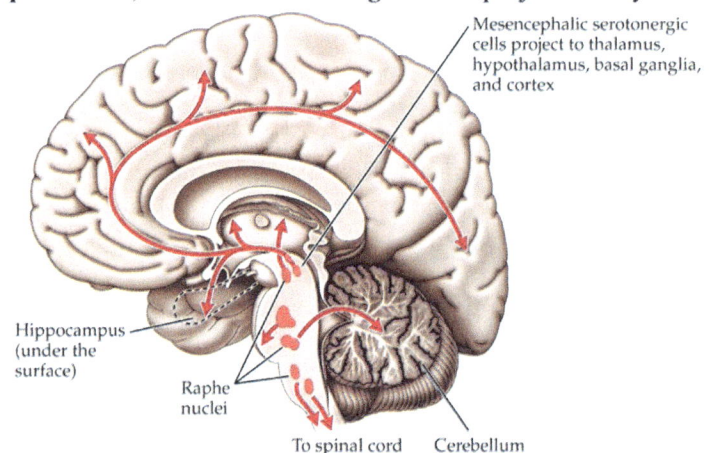

Mesencephalic serotonergic cells project to thalamus, hypothalamus, basal ganglia, and cortex

Hippocampus (under the surface)

Raphe nuclei

To spinal cord    Cerebellum

Serotonin is produced in presynaptic neurons by conversion of l-tryptophan. Serotonin is then incorporated into vesicles, where it resides until it is needed for neurotransmission. After axonal transmission, serotonin is released into the synaptic space, then binds to postsynaptic receptors to effect neurotransmission. A reuptake mechanism returns serotonin to the presynaptic neuron, where it is reintroduced into vesicles.

The following briefly summarizes the current understanding of the most widely studied serotonin (5-HT) receptors. Note that some 5-HT receptors affect other neurotransmitter systems. For example, when a particular 5-HT receptor site is stimulated, it may act as an antagonist to other neurotransmitter systems (i.e 5-HT3 receptors will cause a decrease in acetylcholine).

- **5-HT1 Receptors.** These receptors appear to be involved in the processes of smooth muscle relaxation, contraction of some cardiac and vascular smooth muscle, inhibition of neurotransmitter release, and effects in the CNS. Receptor subtypes have been identified.
- **5-HT1A.** This represents perhaps the most widely studied 5-HT receptor subtype. These receptors are located primarily in the CNS. This receptor has also been implicated in depression. When multiple 5-HT agonist drugs are used concurrently, such as the antidepressants Prozac, Zoloft and Paxil, the overactivity can result in the serotonin syndrome, marked by symptoms of confusion, hyperreflexia, ataxia and hypertension. Over activation of the 5-HT1A receptors is most likely the cause of this syndrome.
- **5-HT1B.** These may serve as autoreceptors; thus, their activation causes inhibition of neurotransmitter release. Agonists inhibit aggressive behavior and food intake in rodents. 5-HT1B receptors, which have been identified only in rodents and are apparently absent in humans, are therefore only of theoretical interest at present.
- **5-HT1c.** These receptors belong to the same receptor subfamily as the 5-HT2 receptor and have been recently renamed as 5-HT2c receptors. They are located in high density in the choroid plexus and may regulate cerebrospinal fluid production and cerebral circulation. This subtype is speculated to be involved in the regulation of analgesia, sleep and cardiovascular function.
- **5-HT1D.** Located primarily in the CNS, this subtype may play a role inhibiting neurotransmitter release by mediating a negative feedback effect. This subtype is the most abundant 5-HT1 receptor in the CNS but is also found in vascular smooth muscle mediating contraction.
- **5-HT2 Receptors.** Located primarily in vascular smooth muscles, platelets, lungs, CNS, and the GI tract, these appear to be involved in gastrointestinal and vascular smooth muscle contraction, blood platelet aggregation, hypertension, migraine, and neuronal depolarization. Antagonists have potential use as antipsychotic agents. Because these receptors belong to the same receptor subfamily as the former 5-HT1c receptors, they have been recently renamed as 5-HT2A receptors. The activation of the

5-HT2A receptors seems to increase the release of the neurotransmitters dopamine, acetylcholine, GABA and glutamate.
- 5-HT2A receptors are implicated in behavioral problems of hallucinations and depression, and may play a role in sleep as well. 5-HT2B receptors are located in the cortex, hypothalamus, and parts of the limbic system, and also found on postsynaptic membranes in these areas. These receptors are involved in anxiety states.

**Acetylcholine**

Acetylcholine (ACh) is perhaps the most widely distributed neurotransmitter in the nervous system. In the 1930's, scientists determined that the nerve impulse could not be an entirely electrical event, contrary to popular belief at that time. Scientists confirmed this notion with the discovery of the neurotransmitter acetylcholine (then identified as *vagus stuffe* since it was obtained from the vagus nerve). ACh is synthesized from *acetyl co-enzyme A (acetyl-CoA)* and choline, and is stored in vesicles much like other neurotransmitters. When released into synapse, ACh chemically binds at receptor sites and is terminated by the enzyme *acetylcholinesterase*.

The degradation of acetylcholine results in the liberation of choline, which is then taken back into the presynaptic axon ending and is re-synthesized into newly formed ACh. There are seven acetylcholinergic (also called *cholinergic*) receptor sub-types. These are divided into two families based on whether they are blocked by nicotine or muscarine. The two families are therefore called *muscarinic,* with receptors M1 through M5, and *nicotinic,* containing the receptors NN and NM. The nicotinic cholinergic receptors in the autonomic nervous system are significant in the coordination of movement, where ACh has an excitatory role in the control of skeletal muscles.

Direct binding of ACh at the nicotinic cholinergic receptors in the autonomic nervous system, along with the rapid degradation of the substance at synapse, facilitate quick action as needed for control of the skeletal muscles. In contrast to the nicotinic receptors, muscarinic receptors are typically found where the synapse actions are slower such as in the synapses of motor nerves onto the autonomic ganglia, glands, cardiac and smooth muscle.

**CHOLINERGIC PATHWAYS**

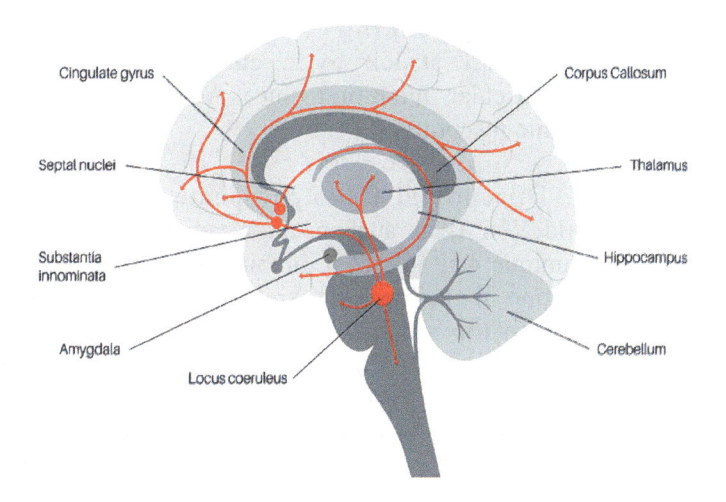

Remember that the key substance which chemically drives the autonomic nervous system is acetylcholine. In the CNS, ACh is found in several areas including the brain stem, midbrain regions, hypothalamus, cortical areas and the spinal cord. In the hindbrain, ACh is located within the reticular formation where it is involved in the control of the level of arousal. In the hypothalamus, ACh is involved in the release of *antidiuretic hormone* (ADH) and *adrenocorticotropic hormone* (ACTH) and plays a role in the regulation of body temperature.

The behavioral effects of ACh have been determined by using certain drugs, such as atropine, an antagonist to muscarinic receptors. Muscarinic receptors are largely found in the CNS. Atropine is a drug used medically by ophthamologists who administer it in eye drops to dilate the pupils. Large doses of atropine, however, where excessive muscarinic cholinergic receptor sites have been blocked, will produce an *atropine psychosis* characterized by symptoms of memory impairment, confusion, hallucinations, slurred speech and drowsiness.

Two other cholinergic drugs produce interesting behavioral effects: *curare, a* cholingeric antagonist, and *"nerve gas"* (di-isopropyl fluorophosphate, or *DFP),* a cholinergic agonist. Curare *(d-tubocurarine)* is the substance used by the Jivaro Indians of South America, where they place it on the tips of arrows to paralyze prey. The mechanism of action of curare is an antagonist at the nicotinic cholinergic receptor sites. Nicotinic receptors are largely found in the PNS, as mentioned previously. Curare occupies nicotinic receptors in skeletal muscles and therefore prohibits ACh from binding (an antagonist function). Therefore, the animal struck by a curare-soaked arrow is paralyzed from muscular inhibition since ACh cannot bind and stimulate the nicotinic receptors.

The other drug, Diisopropyl fluorophosphate (DFP), is a nerve gas used in World War II as a chemical weapon. This cholinergic agonist acts in a unique way in that it inhibits the synaptic defense of enzymatic degradation in cholinergic systems. As you recall, when ACh is released into the synapse it is rapidly removed by the enzyme acetylcholinesterase (AChE). DFP essentially disables AchE, resulting in a hyperactivity of ACh stimulation of postsynaptic neurons. The constant stimulation of receptors produces a flurry of action potentials in the nerves of skeletal muscles which become unable to relax. Constriction of muscles in this way leads to paralysis and eventually asphyxiation.

Some psychiatric medications can inadvertently decrease ACh activity and produce side effects called the anticholinergic syndrome. This syndrome is characterized by urinary retention, dry mouth, photosensitivity, delirium, motor incoordination and tachycardia (rapid heartbeat). Drugs such as the typical antipsychotics (i.e. the phenothiazines) and some anti-depressant drugs have greater liability for producing the anticholinergic syndrome. Marijuana produces anticholinergic *symptoms,* but not the syndrome as defined above.

**Gamma Aminobutyric Acid**
GABA (gamma aminobutyric acid*)* is considered the most important inhibitory neurotransmitter in the CNS. When binding at the postsynaptic receptor site, it hyperpolarizes the neuron by facilitating chloride (Cl-) ions through the channels which prevents the neuron from depolarization. GABA is terminated at synapse through reuptake into the presynaptic neuron and also in the glial cells. Because GABA is a powerful neural inhibitor, GABA agonists have been developed as sedatives, tranquilizers, antiseizure drugs and anesthetics. Two categories of GABA receptors have been identified: GABA$_A$ and GABA$_B$. Many subunits were found within GABAA receptors, categorized into three different groups *a (alpha), fi (beta)* and *y (gamma).* Each group

contains several different subunits, but the exact composition of most GABA$_A$ receptors is not known.

In addition, different subunits within each group also differ in pharmacological properties (sensitivity). As a result, the specific subunit composition of a GABA$_A$ receptor determines its overall characteristics. GABA$_A$ receptors in different parts of the brain also differ in their pharmacological properties. GABA$_A$ receptors are found in abundance throughout the brain. This wide distribution may be related to the spectrum of behaviors (i.e., sedation, relaxation or staggering gait) produced by various drugs that are GABA$_A$ agonists such as alcohol, benzodiazepines, the barbiturates. Alcohol significantly alters GABA neurotransmission, and provides some evidence that the GABA$_A$ receptors may play a critical role in the tolerance and dependence on alcohol while contributing to the predisposition to alcoholism. GABA$_B$ is the other receptor type of which not much is known.

**GABA Pathways in the Normal Brain**
GABA is the main inhibitory neurotransmitter in the central nervous system (CNS). GABAergic inhibition is seen at all levels of the CNS including the hypothalamus, hippocampus, cerebral cortex and cerebellar cortex. As well as the large well-established GABA pathways, GABA interneurons are abundant in the brain, with 50% of the inhibitory synapses in the brain being GABA mediated.

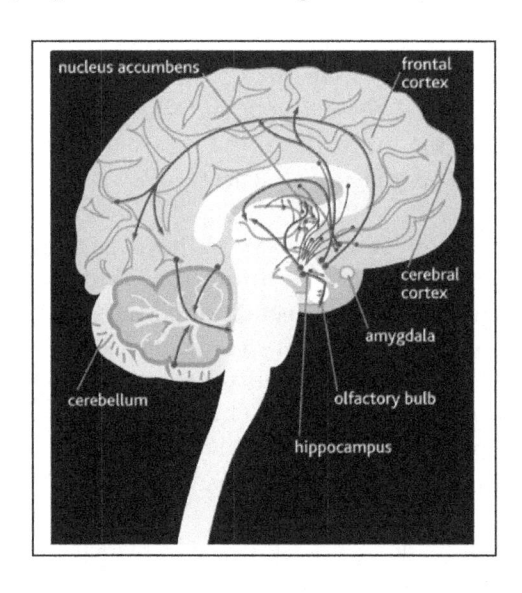

## Glutamate

Glutamate (Glu) is a potent neural excitatory substance. It has been known for some time that glutamic acid (Glu) is highly concentrated throughout the brain. Glu is synthesized from glutamine, stored in vesicles, and released depending on the presence of Ca+. Glu acts on postsynaptic receptors that are linked directly to those channels that depolarize the neuron's membrane and create action potentials. Glu is terminated from synapse by reuptake into both the presynaptic neuron and by glial cells as well.

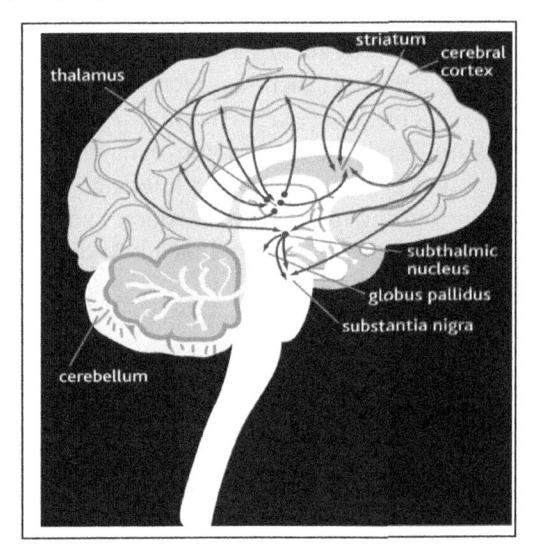

Glu has three receptor subtypes: NMDA (N-methyl-d-aspartate), AMPA (alpha-amino-3- hydroxy-5-methyl-4-isoxazole proprionic acid) and kainate. Of these receptors, NMDA plays a particularly important role in controlling the brain's ability to adapt to environmental and genetic influences.

Glu and its receptor subtype NMDA have been recently studied extensively for their role in addiction. Alcohol, for example, is a potent inhibitor of the function of NMDA receptor. Following chronic exposure of animals to alcohol, there is evidence for an up-regulation of NMDA receptors and a change in the NMDA receptor subunit composition. The time elapsed for this up-regulation parallels the cycle of alcohol withdrawal seizures, which can be attenuated by NMDA receptor antagonists.

Another recent study has provided evidence that the drug *dextromethorphan* – an uncompetitive NMDA antagonist, may facilitate detoxification from heroin and inhibit cravings. Also, after repeated exposure to amphetamine, dopamine neurons within the ventral tegmental area (VTA) are supersensitive to the excitatory effects of Glu and AMPA. Increases in excitatory drive may also reflect effects of amphetamine within the VTA, since studies demonstrate a delayed response in Glu eflux after local amphetamine.

The drug, *acamprosate (Campral) (calcium acetyl-homotaurinate)* is being used as an anti-craving medicine in the treatment of alcoholism. Acamprosate, a synthetic compound similar in structure to GABA, is thought to act via several mechanisms affecting multiple neurotransmitter systems including the inhibition of neural excitability by antagonism of NMDA activity and the reduction of Ca+ ion fluxes.

## Histamine (H)
Histamine (H) is found in high concentration in both the hypothalamus and reticular formation. Within these areas, H is made from *histadine* and increases cAMP levels by stimulation of adenyl cyclase. The effects of histamine at these sites is primarily inhibitory. There are currently two identified H receptor subtypes: Hi and H2. In the periphery, H is released as part of the body's reaction to allergens (producing common allergy symptoms including coughing and sneezing).

## Endocannabinoids
Endogenous cannabinoids, or endocannabinoids, are naturally occurring, lipid-based neurotransmitters. The endocannabinoid system (ECS) is an important *neuromodulatory* system and includes endogenous cannabinoid neurotransmitters (endocannabinoids), cannabinoid receptors, and enzymes responsible for the synthesis and degradation of endocannabinoids. There are two endocannabinoid neurotransmitters that have been discovered and studied: anandamide and 2-arachidonoyl glycerol (2-AG).

The effects of these endocannabinoids are primarily mediated by CB1 receptors, which are mostly found in the central nervous system and CB2 receptors, which are mostly found in the peripheral nervous system, especially immune cells. The ECS regulates and controls many of our most critical bodily functions such as the cognitive functions of learning and memory, emotional processing, mood, sleep, temperature control, pain control, inflammatory and immune responses, and eating. More on this during the talk on cannabinoid pharmacology.

**Nitric Oxide: A rather novel neurotransmitter**

Nitric oxide (NO), an endogenous substance, relaxes blood vessels, the lungs, the gut, and the genitourinary tract. It is also involved with immunologic defense, and appears to play a role in the function of neurotransmission, insulin secretion, and memory formation.

NO is a very small compound, not stored in vesicles, and diffuses from its formation directly to its site of action (since it is both water and lipid soluble, it diffuses freely within tissues). As discussed, neurotransmitters are large molecules stored in vesicles and released by specific properties, after which they move to a site of action and bind at a postsynaptic receptor.

In the CNS, NO is a neuronal mediator that may be involved in neurotransmitter release and even memory formation. NO formation in the CNS can be triggered by stimulation of the glutamate receptor. Glutamate, as you recall, is an excitatory neurotransmitter implicated in brain damage after *cerebral ischemia* and stroke. It now appears that stimulation of the glutamate receptor during ischemia causes a prolonged release of NO, with subsequent tissue damage. Thus, NO can be considered both beneficial (by protecting, enhancing, and mediating neural activity) as well as toxic, where under certain conditions, it indiscriminately destroys neurons.

In the peripheral nervous system, NO seems to function as a transmitter substance of sorts. It is located in nerves of the gastrointestinal (GI) and urogenital systems (so-called nitrogenic neurons) where it is involved in GI peristalsis and penile erection. NO may also cause insulin release, and excess NO may destroy 13 cells during the development of diabetes. More information on this rather unique and new transmitter substance is being discovered as the research continues.

**Neuropeptides and Endorphins**

A peptide is a small protein consisting of amino acid chains (many amino acids linked together in a specific sequence). Neuropeptides simply mean those peptides that are neuroactive (i.e. act in the nervous system). A variety of neuropeptides have been discovered and characterized as you noticed in the illustration of large-molecule neurotransmitters.

Endogenous morphine, coined by the combining of the two descriptive terms into *endorphins*, are opioid neuropeptides that are naturally produced in the body that serve a primary function as an agent blocking the perception of pain and, additionally, present in cases of pleasure. Created in the pituitary gland and hypothalamus, endorphins are a type of neurotransmitter. They attach to the brain's opioid receptors and carry signals across the nervous system.

There are more than 20 types of endorphins in the body that are categorized into 3 groups: *alpha-endorphin, beta-endorphin, and gamma-endorphin.* Of the three endorphin types, beta-endorphins have been the most studied and prevalent, accounting for the majority of the functional properties of endorphins as generalized and understood as a whole. Additionally, beta-endorphins have been found to be associated with states of pleasure, including such emotions brought upon by laughter, love, sex, and even appetizing food.

**SUGGESTED READINGS ON THIS TOPIC**

Blows, WT. The Biological Basis of Mental Health. Routledge; 4th edition. 2021. ISBN-10 : 0367563185

von Bohlen, O. Neurotransmitters and Neuromodulators. Wiley-Blackwell. 2006. ISBN-10: 3527313079.

Iversen, L. Amino Acid Neurotransmitters. Springer. 2013. ASIN: B00FAXEMFG.

Nowaczyk, A. Neurotransmitter: Related Molecular Modeling Studies. Mdpi AG. 2022. ISBN-10 : 3036542779.

Lembke, A. Dopamine Nation: Finding Balance in the Age of Indulgence. Dutton Pub. 2023. ISMN-10: 1524746746.

# CHAPTER 7. THE NEUROSCIENCE OF SUBSTANCE USE DISORDERS

## Key Concepts

| | |
|---|---|
| Abuse liability | A measure of the likelihood that repeated use of drug will result in continued use despite adverse consequences caused by or exacerbated by the drug. |
| Addiction | Not a term used much anymore but is equivalent to what is now called severe substance use disorder. |
| Cued reactivity | A learned conditioned response where both internal and external triggers are associated with the anticipation of drug reward. Explains the dynamics of relapse. |
| Drug discrimination | The perception of the specific effects of a drug, usually in relation to a placebo. |
| Genetic component | Multiple genes that control biological drug creating predisposition to use drugs. |
| MLP | The brain's pleasure or reward circuitry called the mesolimbic pathway or MLP. |
| Pharmacological equivalence | Drug products are considered equivalents if they have the same active ingredients, the same dosage form and are identical in strength, quality, purity, and identity as the brand-name product, but they may differ in characteristics such as shape, packaging, and excipients (e.g., colors, flavors, and preservatives). |
| Physical dependence | Through repeated drug use, the development of tolerance to the drug's effects and a withdrawal syndrome upon abrupt cessation. Physical dependence by itself is not a strong association for substance use disorder. |

| | |
|---|---|
| Residual neuroadaptation | Cellular adaptations to drugs with symptoms that last for months or years in abstinence. |
| Sensitization | When the drug effects increase after repeated use, the opposite of tolerance. |
| Substance Use Disorder (SUD) | Substance use disorder (SUD) is a treatable behavioral health disorder that affects a person's brain and behavior, leading to their inability to control their use of psychoactive substances of legal or illegal drugs. SUD is a spectrum disorder where symptoms can be mild, moderate or severe. |
| Tolerance | The body's adaptive process to repeated exposure of drugs and alcohol. As a result, there are reduced effects that require progressively larger doses to achieve desired effect. |
| Withdrawal syndrome | The body's de-adaptive process drug use is discontinued or reduced. Anxiety, insomnia, nausea, perspiration, body aches, and tremors are a few of the common symptoms. |

# CHAPTER 7

## The Neuroscience of Substance Use Disorders

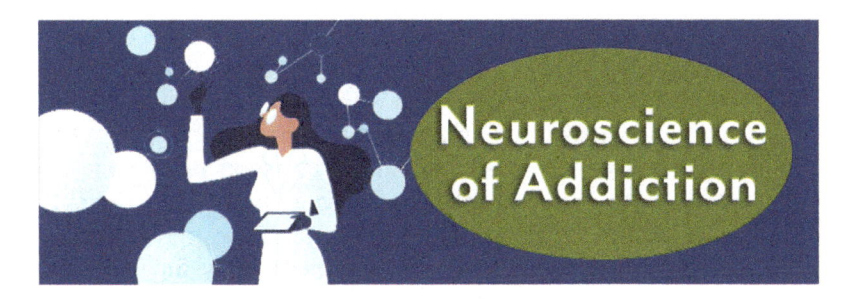

According to the American Society of Addiction Medicine (ASAM, 2019.), addiction is a treatable, chronic medical disease involving complex interactions among brain circuits, genetics, the environment, and an individual's life experiences. People with addiction use substances or engage in behaviors that become compulsive and often continue despite harmful consequences. Prevention efforts and treatment approaches for addiction are generally as successful as those for other chronic diseases.

At one time however, addiction was viewed as a failure of willpower or a flaw of moral character. It was not recognized as a disease of the brain, in the same way that mental illnesses previously were not viewed as such. Medical authorities have now accepted drug addiction as a chronic, relapsing condition that alters normal brain function, just as any other neurological or psychiatric illness. Its development and expression are influenced by genetic, biological, psychosocial, and environmental factors. Outwardly, addiction is often characterized by impaired control over continued drug use, compulsive use despite harmful consequences, and drug craving.

To understand substance use disorders today, adopting the largest possible perspective of the related science, the current research that shapes our perceptions, and the evidence-based approaches to treatment. At the Brookhaven National Laboratory in New York, for instance, Nora D. Volkow, MD, has found that even 100 days after a cocaine addict's last dose, there is significant disruption in the brain's frontal cortical area, which governs such attributes as impulse, motivation and drive. Dr. Volkow says that "the disruption of the dopamine pathways leads to a decrease in the reinforcing value of normal things, and this pushes the individual to take drugs to compensate." Other researchers have found the physiological basis for the craving, one of the diagnostic considerations for substance use disorders (SUD).

Herbert D. Kleber, MD, past medical director of the National Center on Addiction and Substance Abuse in New York, says that the brain-disease concept fits with his experience with thousands of addicts over the years. "No one wants to be an addict," he says. "All anyone wants to be able to do is knock back a few drinks with the guys on Friday or have a cigarette with coffee or take a toke on a crack pipe. But very few addicts can do this. When someone goes from being able to control their habit to mugging their grandmother to get money for their next fix, that convinces me that something has changed in their brain."

From the evidence of the newer science on substance use disorders (SUD), it seems that addiction (the severest form of SUD) is a brain disease expressed as compulsive behavior; both in its development and in the recovery from it depend on the individual's behavior. Substance use begins with an individual's conscious choice, but addiction is not simply using alcohol and drugs in excess. Research provides overwhelming evidence that not only do alcohol and other drugs interfere with normal brain functioning by creating powerful feelings of pleasure, but they also have long-term effects on brain metabolism and activity.

At some point, changes occur in the brain that produce conditioned urges to repeat drug use, while simultaneously reducing awareness, caution and judgment. It is clear that these are predictable, physiological consequences of substance use, and they explain why those with SUD suffer from a compulsive craving for, and use of, these substances and cannot quit by themselves. Treatment is generally necessary.

The word "treatment" may be a misleading as it implies a one-time strategy to eliminate the adverse effects of a physiological condition. Like other chronic illnesses such as heart disease, diabetes and hypertension, treatment of moderate to severe forms of SUD actually refers to an extended process of diagnosis, treatment of acute symptoms, identification and management of circumstances that initially may have promoted the substance use, and development of life-long strategies to minimize the likelihood of ongoing use and its attendant consequences.

There is gaining momentum in the SUD treatment arena that is shifting from long-standing pathology and intervention paradigms to a client-centered solution-focused recovery paradigm. The shift toward a recovery paradigm is evident in a number of quarters: the international growth of SUD recovery mutual aid societies, a new recovery advocacy movement, and calls to shift the design of SUD treatment from a model of acute biopsychosocial stabilization to a model of sustained recovery management.

From the scientific research, it is generally agreed that those drugs with abuse potential possess reinforcing properties due to actions within a common neural circuitry. While the mechanisms for all drugs of abuse are not completely described, many activate the mesolimbic pathway (MLP). Such drugs include cocaine, amphetamines, opiates, sedatives, and nicotine. For other drugs of abuse, the precise relationship, if any, to the brain reward system is unclear.

Repeated administration of all drugs with abuse potential is associated with neuro-adaptive responses. In general, tolerance develops to at least some of their effects, although the details of the biological mechanisms underlying these changes are not completely understood. A prominent aspect of SUD is tolerance to the reinforcing properties of drugs, where higher doses are needed to achieve the same result.

Withdrawal is associated with most cases of SUD though the severity varies. Alcohol, stimulants, opiates and benzodiazepines produce pronounced and sometimes severe withdrawal symptoms, while those for nicotine and caffeine are less intense. A withdrawal syndrome has also been established for cannabis use disorder, while there is no evidence of a withdrawal syndrome related to LSD. Certain aspects of withdrawal, such as changes in mood and motivation induced by the chronic drug state, are key factors to relapse and drug-seeking behavior.

Psychoactive drugs alter the brain's normal balance and level of biochemical activity by altering one or more of the brain's synaptic defenses. As you know, synaptic defenses are specific neurobiological mechanisms that work in concert to keep the chemistry stabilized at synapse in order to maintain behavioral homeostasis. Drugs of abuse interrupt this delicate process and compromise homeostasis.
Drugs alter the neuropharmacological activity in the brain and body through different mechanisms. They effect the production, release or reuptake of the neurotransmitters, they can mimic or block the

neurotransmitters at a receptor, or they can interfere with other cellular activity. Prolonged substance use potentially alters these processes, and the ultimate effect either excites or inhibits activity in various brain regions. Both the immediate and long-term effects of substance use will change normal brain behavior, and ultimately have very strong reinforcing effects that increase their use

*Reinforcement* is defined as the increased likelihood that the consequences of taking the drug will increase the behavior directed toward that drug. More simply stated, individuals who use drugs experience some effect, such as pleasure, detachment or relief from distress that initially establishes and then maintains drug use. Thus, taking the drug enhances the prospect that it will be relied upon for some real or perceived effect which creates a need state, hence engendering compulsive self-administration.

What separates substances with abuse potential from other psychoactive drugs is that these drugs act, at least in part, on those areas of the brain that mediate feelings of pleasure and reward. By stimulating the brain reward system, drugs of abuse create positive reinforcement that provoke and supports their continued use and abuse.

Beyond their immediate rewarding effects, several drugs used in a chronic, long-term basis can cause either permanent changes in the brain or alterations that may take hours, days, months, even years, to reverse after the drug use has stopped. These changes are adaptive responses that occur in the brain to counter the immediate effects of a drug. When drug taking is stopped, these changes often appear opposite to the initial pleasurable drug response. The continued administration of drugs to avoid aversive effects of drug cessation creates negative reinforcement which also contributes to an individual's addiction to a drug.

In addition to their reinforcing effects, drugs of abuse can have a variety of pharmacological actions in other areas of the brain and the body. The ultimate effect of a drug will also be shaped by other factors including the dose of the drug, the route of administration, the health status of the user, and the environmental context in which the drug is taken.

**The Brain Reward Circuitry**
Eating, drinking, sexual and maternal behaviors are essential for the survival of the individual and the species. To ensure these

behaviors occur, natural selection has ensured their powerful rewarding properties. Bioanthropologists also suggest that the brain reward circuitry apparently evolved to process these natural reinforcers.

Recent studies have shown that direct stimulation of certain areas of the brain produces extreme pleasure. Such stimulation activates neural pathways that carry natural rewarding stimuli. The fact that lab animals will forego food and drink or willingly experience pain to receive the reward attests to the power of these reinforcing characteristics. In the case of addiction, administration of most drugs of abuse reduces the amount of electrical stimulation needed to produce self-stimulation responding.

The reward system is made up of various brain structures. The central component is a neural pathway that interconnects structures in the middle part of the brain (hypothalamus and ventral tegmental area [VTA]) to structures in the front part of the brain (frontal cortex and limbic system). A key part of this drug reward pathway appears to be the mesolimbic pathway (MLP).

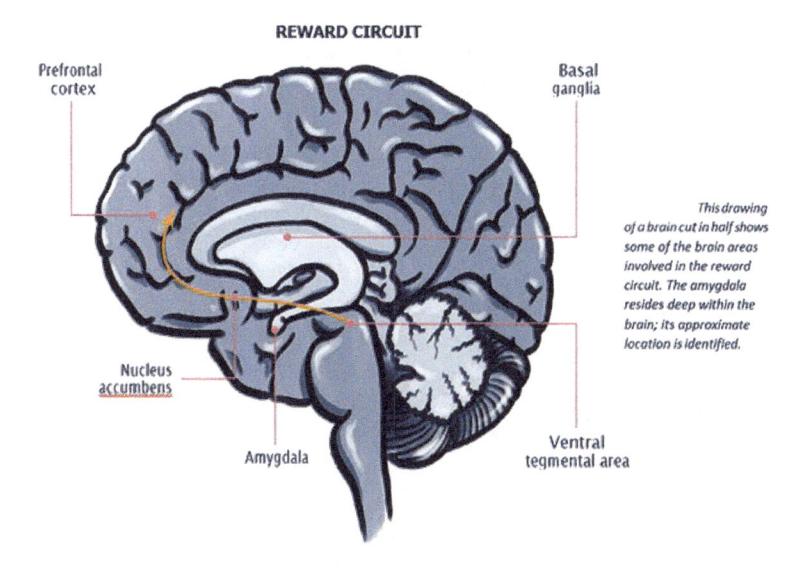

**REWARD CIRCUIT**

*This drawing of a brain cut in half shows some of the brain areas involved in the reward circuit. The amygdala resides deep within the brain; its approximate location is identified.*

Labels: Prefrontal cortex, Basal ganglia, Nucleus accumbens, Amygdala, Ventral tegmental area

The MLP is made up of the axons of neuronal cell bodies in the ventral tegmental area projecting to the nucleus accumbens, a nucleus in the limbic system. The limbic system is a network of brain structures that controls emotion, behavior and specifically perception, motivation, gratification, and memory. MLP also connects the ventral tegmental area with parts of the frontal cortex (medial prefrontal cortex).

The VTA consists of dopaminergic neurons which respond to glutamate. These cells respond when stimuli indicative of a reward are present. The VTA supports learning and sensitization development and releases dopamine into the forebrain. These neurons also project and release dopamine into the nucleus accubems through the MLP. Ventral tegmental neurons release dopamine to regulate activity of cells in the nucleus accumbens and the prefrontal cortex. Virtually all drugs causing substance use disorders increase the dopamine release in the MLP in addition to their specific effects.

The nucleus accumbens (NAcc), consisting of mainly of GABA neurons, is associated with acquiring and eliciting conditioned behaviors and involved in the increased sensitivity to drugs as addiction progresses. The prefrontal cortex, more specifically the anterior cingulate and orbital frontal cortices, is important for the integration of information which contributes to whether a behavior will be elicited. It appears to be the area in which motivation originates and the salience of stimuli are determined.

The basolateral amygdala projects into the NAcc and is important for motivation as well. More evidence is pointing towards the role of the hippocampus in drug addiction because of its importance in learning and memory. Much of this evidence stems from investigations manipulating cells in the hippocampus alters dopamine levels in NAcc and firing rates of VTA dopaminergic cells.

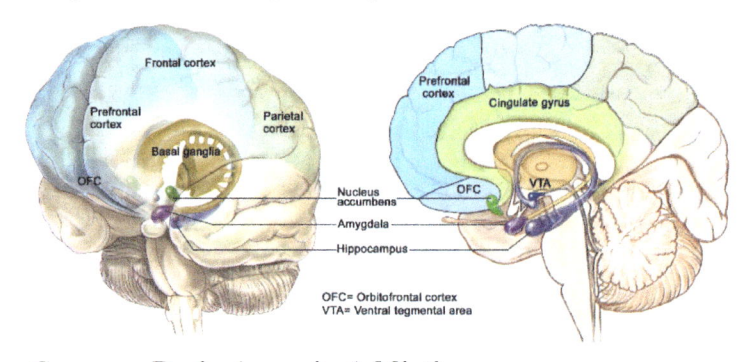

### Key Common Brain Areas in Addiction
- *Nucleus Accumbens Central Nucleus of the Amygdala* – Forebrain structures involved in the rewarding effects of drugs of abuse and drive the binge intoxication stage of

addiction. Contains key reward neurotransmitters: dopamine and opioid peptides.
- *Amygdala* – Composed of central nucleus of the amygdala, bed nucleus of the stria terminalis, and a transition zone on the medial part of the nucleus accumbens. Contains "brain stress" neurotransmitter, corticotropin-releasing-factor (CRF) that controls hormonal, sympathetic, and behavioral responses to stressors, and is involved in the anti-reward effects of drug addiction.
- *Prefrontal Cortex* – neurobiological substrate for "executive function" that is compromised in drug addiction and plays a key role in facilitating relapse. Contains major glutamatergic projection to nucleus accumbens and the amygdala.

These structures play a significant role in reinforcing drug use, although some precise mechanisms involved lack thorough description. The MLP is critical in reinforcing stimulant drugs as well, like cocaine and amphetamines. Also, both the ventral tegmental area and the nucleus accumbens appear to be important for opiate reward, while these same structures and their connections to other limbic areas, like the amygdala may play a role in the rewarding aspects of barbiturates and alcohol. PCP is also a strong reinforcer but its relationship, if any, to activity in MLP has not been well established.

Other drugs are either weak reinforcers or have not been shown to support self-administration in animal experiments at all. Nicotine activates dopamine neurons in the MLP system; however, when compared with cocaine or amphetamine, this effect is modest. Likewise, caffeine is a weak reinforcer, but the precise mechanisms of its reinforcement still remain unclear. Finally, while cannabis and lysergic acid diethylamide (LSD) produce positive effects that clearly support their use, there is currently little empirical evidence that they act as reinforcers in controlled experiments. Interestingly, a new study has shown that while dopaminergic pathways of the brain's reward circuitry do indeed play a major role in the reinforcing effects of many drugs, they are not the only mechanisms involved.

**Cycle of Addiction**
As addiction develops, neuroplastic brain reward systems eventually become transformed. This is what some refer to as the "dark side" of

drug addiction. That is, the decline in normal reward-related neural mechanisms and persistent recruitment of the brain's anti-reward systems that accompany drug use. Progressive worsening of the brain reward system perpetuates compulsive use of the drug.

Substance use disorders (SUD) have elements of both an impulse control disorder and a compulsive disorder that are mediated by separate but overlapping neural circuits. The individual with an impulse control disorder experiences an increasing sense of tension or arousal before committing the impulsive act such as drug-taking; pleasure, gratification or relief during the act; and in some cases, regret, self-reproach or guilt following the act. The individual with a compulsive disorder feels anxiety and stress before the compulsive, repetitive act, and relief from stress by performing the act. In the progression from an impulsive disorder to a compulsive disorder, the motivation for the behavior shifts from positive reinforcement to negative reinforcement, when removal of the aversive state increases the probability of the behavior. SUD follows this pattern in a cycle involving 3 stages (see illustration below):

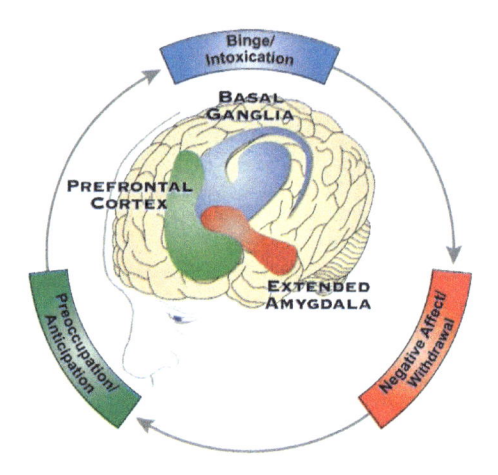

SUD involves a long-term persistent plasticity of the neural circuits that control two different reward systems: declining function of brain reward systems driven by natural rewards and stimulation of anti-reward systems that bring on aversive states. Studies on the acute reinforcing effects of drugs in the binge/intoxication stage have identified the neurobiological substrates involved in the reward response.

Drugs with the potential for abuse, such as the opioid analgesics, initially produce positive reinforcing effects from actions at the ventral tegmental area in the midbrain and the nucleus accumbens and amygdala of the basal forebrain. Activation of the MLP is the primary route of positive reinforcement in addiction for psychostimulant drugs, but the opioid peptides (endorphins), serotonin, and gamma-aminobutyric acid (GABA) have key roles for nonstimulant drugs. These so-called "reward neurotransmitters" induce hedonic effects of euphoria and a feeling of well-being.

| Reward Neurotransmitters Implicated in the Motivational Effects of Substance Use ||
| --- | --- |
| Positive Pleasurable Effects | Negative Unpleasant Effects of Withdrawal |
| Increased dopamine | Decreased dopamine (dysphoria) |
| Increased opioid peptides | Decreased opioid peptides (pain) |
| Increased serotonin | Decreased serotonin (dysphoria) |
| Increased GABA | Decreased GABA (anxiety, panic attacks) |

**Craving and Relapse**
The preoccupation/anticipation stage of the addiction cycle is mediated via afferent projections to the extended amygdala and nucleus accumbens. There are different stimuli for craving a drug of abuse, leading to relapse. It can be drug-induced, cue-induced, or stress-induced. Chronic relapse is a significant problem in substance use disorders (SUD), with about half of all addicts relapsing into drug taking. Persons with SUD often return to compulsive drug taking long after acute withdrawal exhibiting behavior that corresponds to the preoccupation/anticipation stage of addiction. Drug-related cues and stressors are a powerful inducement to return to drug use. Areas of the brain associated with drug and cue-induced reinstatement are the prefrontal cortex (orbitofrontal, medial prefrontal, prelimbic/cingulate), and the amygdala. See the pioneering work by Anna Rose Childress of the University of Pennsylvania cited in the Suggested Reading section at the end of this chapter. Amazing work!

The neurotransmitters involved in relapse include dopamine, opioid peptides, glutamate, and GABA. Relapse can also be precipitated by stress and the release of CRF, glucocorticoids and norepinephrine. Many different stressors can provoke drug craving and drug-seeking behavior

**Neurobiological Actions**
One thing is certain – changes will occur in the brain when it is exposed to drugs. Beyond the immediate reward, chronic and long-term drug abuse can cause alterations in brain function that can take years to reverse or improve, if at all. These changes are adaptive

responses to the pharmacological action of drugs in order to counter their disruptive effects. Remember, the biological system is genetically coded to always find and maintain healthy balance. Therefore, the adaptive responses to repeat drug exposure are biological expressions of the system attempting to regain its homeostasis.

One such adaptive response is *tolerance*, where the intensity of the drug's effects are reduced. Tolerance can contribute to drug-taking behavior by requiring that an individual take progressively larger doses of a drug to achieve a desired effect. While it is unclear from available data whether or not tolerance develops to cocaine's rewarding effects, the notion is supported by experiments and anecdotal reports that the drug's euphoric actions diminish with repeated use. This decrease of effects may be related to decreasing levels of available dopamine to work on.

*Dependence* is when cells adapt to prolonged use of a drug so that use is required to maintain comfortable body functioning. Upon abrupt cessation of the drug, neurons may behave abnormally, causing a *withdrawal syndrome*. Generally, the withdrawal syndrome is characterized by signs and symptoms that are *opposite* to those of the acute effects of the drug.

The figure below provides an example.

| Substance | Acute Effects | Withdrawal Effects |
|---|---|---|
| *Stimulants* (amphetamines, cocaine) | Euphoria, increased energy, insomnia, decreased appetite | dysphoria, depression, fatigue, increased appetite |
| *Sedatives* (alcohol, benzodiazepines) | Sedation, sleep inducing, anti-seizure, anti-anxiety | irritability, insomnia, anxiety, agitation, seizure |
| **Opiates** (morphine, heroin) | Euphoria, analgesia, constipation | dysphoria, depression, hypersensitivity to pain, diarrhea |

Understanding the basic acute symptoms of drugs will lend to understanding withdrawal symptoms because they are generally the opposite in nature. Withdrawal also creates a craving state where there is a strong desire for the drug. Drug craving behaviors play a strong role in patterns of relapse, and also in maintaining drug seeking behavior to forestall the withdrawal syndrome.

*Sensitization* occurs when the effects of a given dose of a drug will increase after repeated administration; sensitization is the opposite of tolerance. Sensitization to a drug's behavioral effects seem also to play a significant role in supporting drug-taking behavior. For example, while tolerance to some of the effects of cocaine and amphetamines develops, sensitization to other effects can also occur.

The *abuse liability* of a drug is a measure of the likelihood that its use will result in addiction. Many factors ultimately play a role in a person's drug usage. Nevertheless, abuse potential of a drug is due to its intrinsic rewarding properties and neuroadaptive responses that result from its prolonged use. Drugs can be screened for their abuse liability using animals as models. The criteria to classify a drug as addictive include: pharmacological equivalence to known drugs of abuse, demonstration of reinforcing effects, tolerance, and physical dependence. The reinforcing capacity is essential in determining abuse potential, whereas tolerance and physical dependence might occur, but are not absolutely required to make this determination.

The main feature of all drugs with abuse potential is that they are *self-administered.* In fact, self-administration to the point where behavior becomes obsessive. Indeed, a primary diagnostic considerations for SUD is the continued compulsive use despite adverse consequences caused by or exacerbated by the continued drug use (NIDA. 2011). Another contributing factor to abuse liability is the notion of craving and the tendency of individuals to relapse to drug use during withdrawal. Although craving is a difficult term to quantify, once a drug is voluntarily or involuntarily withdrawn, the desire to take the drug can create relapse to substance abuse.

Another measure in the assessment of abuse liability is *drug discrimination,* the perception of the specific effects of a drug. Specifically, animal or human subjects that can discriminate a drug from a *placebo* show a remarkable ability to distinguish that drug from other drugs with different properties. These procedures also permit the subject to consider the drug to be the equivalent of another drug. *Pharmacological equivalence* is when drugs of a particular class, such as stimulants or depressants, cause a series of similar effects on the body that collectively constitute their pharmacological profile.

**Residual Tolerance**
In general, expression of tolerance and dependence has been considered to be *rate-limited* in that adaptation to drugs gradually

dissipates with time as the brain readapts to the disappearance of the drug; withdrawal peaks within hours or days after discontinued use but then disappears. However, there is a significant amount of evidence indicating that there may be persistent or *residual neuroadaptation* that lasts for months or years. For example, craving and drug-seeking behavior have been reported to last for years with nicotine, alcohol and cocaine, suggesting some residual effect of drug use that may not dissipate with time. Moreover, there is a phenomenon that characterizes specific drug-dependent individuals.

Specifically, with repeated cycles of abstinence and reinitiation of drug use, the time required to elicit drug dependence grows shorter and shorter. Furthermore, there is evidence that naloxone (Narcan), a drug that blocks the actions of opiates (an antagonist), can elicit a withdrawal syndrome in individuals who have abstained from opiate use for an extensive time. These findings indicate that some residual neuroadaptive changes induced by drugs can persist for as yet undefined periods of time. Little information is available about the mechanisms involved in this effect, but it is clear that long-term residual changes do persist for some recovering patients, which may account for the striking relapses that occur after long-term abstinence.

**Learned Conditioned Responses**
Another significant factor in drug abuse is the *learning* that can occur during an individual's drug-taking activity. In addition to producing pleasant feelings, drugs of abuse produce changes in numerous organ systems such as the cardiovascular, digestive, and endocrine systems. The effects of a drug occur in the context of an individual's drug-seeking and drug-using environment. As a result, there are environmental cues present before and during a person's drug use that are consistently associated with behavioral and physiological effects. With repetition, these cues become *conditioned stimuli* that automatically change organ systems and cause severe craving even after long-term absence of the drug.

This is analogous to Pavlov's classical conditioning experiments in which dogs salivate on the cue of a bell, following repeated association of food with a ringing bell. Evidence for this effect is seen in numerous studies showing that animals seek out places associated with reinforcing drugs, and that the physiological effects of drugs can be classically conditioned in both animals and humans. Thus, exposure to environmental cues associated with drug use in the past can act as a stimulus for voluntary drug-seeking behavior. If the individual succeeds in finding and taking the drug, the chain of behaviors is further reinforced by the drug-induced reward and the effects of the drug on other organ systems. Drug conditioning can explain why many drug abusers often return to environments associated with drug use, even after being counseled not to. The effects of environmental stimuli are similar to the priming effects of a dose of the drug.

Also, it has long been known that conditioning may stimulate withdrawal effects of drugs. It was observed that opiate addicts who were drug free for months and thus should not have had any signs of opiate withdrawal developed withdrawal symptoms (e.g., yawning, sniffling, tearing of the eyes, etc.) when talking about drugs in group therapy sessions. This phenomenon, termed *conditioned withdrawal,* results from environmental ability to elicit signs and symptoms of pharmacological withdrawal.

Conditioned withdrawal can also play a role in relapse to drug use in abstinent individuals. The emergence of withdrawal symptoms resulting from conditioned exposure can motivate a person to seek out and use drugs. Relapse prevention protocols address this conditioning process to re-condition cellular response.

Studies have also demonstrated that conditioned associations are difficult to reverse. In theory, repeated presentation of the environmental cues, without the drug, should extinguish the conditioned association. Animal studies indicate that extinction is difficult to achieve and does not erase the original learning. As a result, once established, the extinction is easily reversed. Research has found that various aspects of extinguished responses can either be reinstated with a single pairing of the drug and environmental cue, a single dose of drug in the absence of the environmental cue, or can spontaneously recover.

The biological mechanisms underlying conditioned drug effects are just beginning to be understood. Recent evidence links the mesolimbic pathway (MLP) to these effects. Studies have found increased release of dopamine in the nucleus accumbens \associated with anticipated voluntary alcohol consumption. Other studies have presented evidence that destruction of the MLP blocks the conditioned reinforcing effects of opiates.

**A brief mention of the evidence-based treatment for SUD based on the science**

The Diagnostic and Statistical Manual of Mental Disorders, Fifth Edition, text revision, often called the DSM-5-TR, is the latest version of the American Psychiatric Association's gold-standard text on the names, symptoms, and diagnostic features of every recognized mental illness—including addictions. The DSM-5-TR criteria for Substance Use Disorders are based on decades of research and clinical knowledge. The DSM-5-TR was published in 2013, and in 2022, a text revision was published that included updated criteria for more than 70 disorders, including the requirements for stimulant-induced mild neurocognitive disorder.

**DSM-5-TR Substance Use Disorder Criteria**
Substance use disorders span a wide variety of problems arising from substance use, and cover 11 different criteria.

1. Taking the substance in larger amounts or for longer than you're meant to
2. Wanting to cut down or stop using the substance but not managing to
3. Spending a lot of time getting, using, or recovering from use of the substance
4. Cravings and urges to use the substance
5. Not managing to do what you should at work, home, or school because of substance use
6. Continuing to use, even when it causes problems in relationships
7. Giving up important social, occupational, or recreational activities because of substance use
8. Using substances again and again, even when it puts you in danger
9. Continuing to use, even when you know you have a physical or psychological problem that could have been caused or made worse by the substance
10. Needing more of the substance to get the effect you want (tolerance)
11. Development of withdrawal symptoms, which can be relieved by taking more of the substance

The 11 criteria outlined in the DSM-5-TR can be grouped into four primary categories: physical dependence, risky use, social problems, and impaired control.

**Substance Use Disorder As a Spectrum Disorder**
The DSM-5-TR allows clinicians to specify how severe or how much of a problem the substance use disorder is, depending on how many symptoms are identified.
- **Mild**: Two or three symptoms indicate a mild substance use disorder.[5]
- **Moderate**: Four or five symptoms indicate a moderate substance use disorder.
- **Severe**: Six or more symptoms indicate a severe substance use disorder.

**A Clinical Assessment prior to treatment planning**
A thorough substance use assessment includes a detailed inventory of the type, amount, frequency, and consequences of the patient's substance use, their perception of their use, and readiness to change. Additionally, we review past medical and psychiatric history and assess for co-occurring psychiatric disorders. Two of the best clinical assessment tools are:

- The ASAM Criteria's strength-based multidimensional assessment takes into account a patient's needs, obstacles and liabilities, as well as their strengths, assets, resources, and support structure. This information is used to determine the appropriate level of care across a continuum.
- The ASUS (Adult Substance Use Survey) is a 64-item self-report survey designed to assess an individual's perceived alcohol and other drug use.

**Difference between Screening and Assessment:**
The purpose of screening is to determine whether a person needs services in general. The purpose of an assessment, however, is to gather detailed information needed for a treatment plan that meets the individual needs of the person.
- *Screening* is a process for evaluating the possible presence of a particular problem. The outcome is a simple yes or no.
- *Assessment* is a process for defining the nature of that problem, determining a diagnosis, and developing specific treatment recommendations for addressing the problem or diagnosis.

**What is the treatment for substance use disorder?**
The three main forms of treatment include:
1. Withdrawal management
2. Cognitive and behavioral therapies
3. Medication-assisted treatment

There are also several different levels of care for treatment, depending on the client's clinical need, including:
- Outpatient
- Intensive outpatient
- Inpatient
- Long term therapeutic communities

**Withdrawal Management (WM)**
In WM, the client stops taking the substance(s), allowing them to leave the body. Depending on the severity of the SUD, the substance or an alternative may be tapered off to lessen the effects of withdrawal. It's the first major step of treatment for SUD. WM can take place in both inpatient and outpatient settings.

**Cognitive and behavioral therapies**
Counseling can help treat SUD and any other co-occurring mental health conditions. Therapy also teaches healthy coping mechanisms. Treatment providers may recommend cognitive and behavioral therapies alone or in combination with medications.

Some examples of evidence-based cognitive and behavioral therapies for SUDs include:
- **Cognitive behavioral therapy (CBT)**: CBT is a structured, goal-oriented type of psychotherapy. This approach helps the client look closely at their thoughts and emotions and how thoughts affect behavior.
- **Dialectical behavior therapy (DBT)**: DBT is especially effective for people who have difficulty managing and regulating their emotions. DBT has proven to be effective for treating and managing various mental health conditions, including SUD.
- **Motivational Interviewing (MI)**: MI is an effective counseling method that enhances motivation through the resolution of ambivalence. It draws on the phrase 'ready, willing and able' to outline three critical components of motivation which are: the importance of change for the patient

(willingness); the confidence to change (ability) and; whether change is an immediate priority (readiness).
- **Couples and Family Counseling:** The treatment field has adapted family systems approaches to address the unique circumstances of families in which SUDs occur. Clients and their family members learn about how to initiate and sustain recovery from SUDs through active involvement in treatment. When family members change their thinking about substance use and their behavioral responses to substance use, the entire family system changes.
- **Contingency Management (CM):** CM encourages healthy behaviors by offering rewards for desired behaviors. Most commonly, the treatment provides something of monetary value to people with SUD to incentivize them not to use substances. For instance, upon a negative drug test result, you earn a chance to receive a prize or gift card.

**Medication-Assisted Treatment (MAT):** The use of medications, in combination with counseling and behavioral therapies, to provide a "whole-patient" approach to the treatment of substance use disorders. Medications used are approved by the FDA and are clinically driven and tailored to meet each patient's needs. Research shows that a combination of medication and therapy can successfully treat substance use disorders for longer periods of symptoms-free living and sustained recovery. Medications are also used to prevent or reduce opioid overdose. Participating in self-help programs, like Narcotics Anonymous, can also play a significant role in a person's response to SUD treatment.

## SUGGESTED READINGS ON THIS TOPIC

American Psychiatric Association. Diagnostic and Statistical Manual of Mental Disorders, Text Revision DSM-5-tr 5th Edition. Amer Psychiatric Pub Inc; 5th edition. 2022. ISBN-10 : 0890425760.

American Society of Addiction Medicine (ASAM). https://www.asam.org/quality-care/definition-of-addiction

Brasler, P. The Clinician's Guide to Substance Use Disorders: Practical Tools for Assessment, Treatment & Recovery. PESI Publishing, Inc. 2022. ISBN-10 : 1683735676.

Chandler, TL. Co-occurring Mental Illness and Substance Use Disorders: Evidence-based Integrative Treatment and Multicultural Application. Routledge. 2022. ISBN-10 : 103211651X.

Childress, AM. Limbic Activation During Cue-Induced Cocaine Craving. Am J Psychiatry 1999; 156:11–18.

Filbey, FM. The Neuroscience of Addiction. Cambridge University Press. 2019. ISBN-10 : 1107567335.

Galanter M, Kleber H. Psychotherapy for the Treatment of Substance Abuse. American Psychiatric Publishing, Inc.; 1st edition. 2010. ISBN-10: 1585623903.

Grisel, J. Never Enough: The Neuroscience and Experience of Addiction. Anchor; Reprint edition. 2020. ISBN-10 : 0525434909.

NIDA. 2024, January 5. Drug Misuse and Addiction. Retrieved from https://nida.nih.gov/publications/drugs-brains-behavior-science-addiction/drug-misuse-addiction on 2024, March 4

O'Brien, C.P., Childress, A.R. and McLellan, A.T., et al. Classical Conditioning in Drug-Dependent Humans. P.W. Kalivas and H.H. Samson (editors), The Neurobiology of Drug and Alcohol Addiciton, Annals of the American Academy of Sciences, Volume 654: 400-415, 1992.

Volkow, N. Drug Addiction: The neurobiology of behaviour gone awry. Nature. Rev./Neurosci. 5: 963-970, 2004.

# CHAPTER 8. ALCOHOL AND OTHER SEDATIVES

## Key Concepts

| | |
|---|---|
| Acetaldehyde | Metabolite that alcohol oxidizes into and of which circulates through the system. |
| Aldehyde dehydrogenase | Enzyme that metabolizes acetaldehyde into acetic acid, where it can be excreted. |
| Antabuse | (disulfiram) A drug that inhibits alcohol's full metabolism resulting in a buildup of acetaldehyde causing extreme discomfort. |
| Anxiolytics | The benzodiazepine class of drugs introduced in the 1960s as anti-anxiety agents. |
| Blood Alcohol Concentration (BAC) | The concentration of alcohol in one's bloodstream, expressed as a percentage. The BAC is used to determine whether a person is legally intoxicated. |
| Cardiac Arrhythmias | (Irregular Heart Beat) One of the direct effects of alcohol on the heart muscle. |
| Cardiomyopathy | (Heart Swelling) One of the direct effects of alcohol on the heart muscle. |
| Delirium Tremens | (DTs) Severe, potentially fatal symptom of delirium of the alcohol withdrawal syndrome. |
| Hepatitis | Inflammation of the liver. There are several type of hepatitis HCA, HCB, HV, etc. with varying severity levels. |
| MEOS | (Mixed Enzyme Oxidizing System) Liver enzymes that converts alcohol into acetaldehyde. |
| Peripheral neuropathy | Thiamine deficiency in alcoholics, caused by demyelination of peripheral nerve fibers. |

# CHAPTER 8

## Alcohol and Other Sedatives

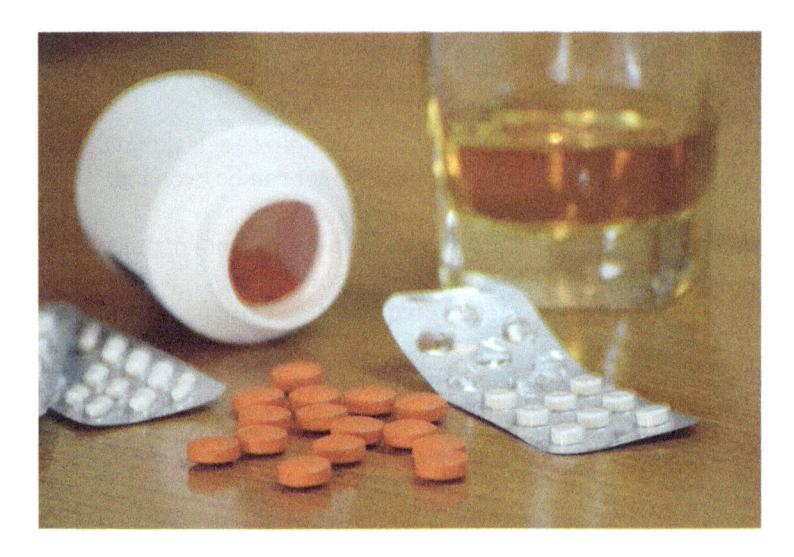

For this chapter about alcohol and alcohol use disorders, I want to begin by referencing the 2 premier federal agencies dedicated to the research and publications on substance use-related, addiction and co-occurring disorders. These are the National Institute on Alcohol Abuse and Alcoholism (NIAAA) and the National Institute of Drug Abuse (NIDA). Both are part of the National Institutes of Health (NIH).

According to the 2023 National Institute for Drug Abuse (NIDA), alcohol is among the most used drugs, plays a large role in many societies and cultures around the world, and greatly impacts public health. More people over age 12 in the United States have used alcohol in the past year than any other drug or tobacco product, and alcohol use disorder is the most common type of substance use disorder in the United States.

From the 2023 data set of the National Institute on Alcohol Abuse and Alcoholism (NIAAA)**,** the prevalence of Lifetime Drinking can be summarized as follows:

### *People Ages 12 and Older*
According to the 2022 National Survey on Drug Use and Health (NSDUH), 221.3 million people ages 12 and older (78.5% in this age

group) reported that they drank alcohol at some point in their lifetime. This includes:
- 110.2 million males ages 12 and older (79.7% in this age group)
- 111.1 million females ages 12 and older (77.3% in this age group)
- 976,000 American Indian or Alaska Native people ages 12 and older (66.7% in this age group)
- 10.1 million Asian people ages 12 and older (59.1% in this age group)
- 24.1 million Black or African American people ages 12 and older (69.8% in this age group)
- 144.1 million White people ages 12 and older (84.2% in this age group)
- 4.5 million people of two or more races ages 12 and older (76.0% in this age group)
- 36.8 million Hispanic or Latino people ages 12 and older (72.3% in this age group)
- Estimates for Native Hawaiian or other Pacific Islander people ages 12 and older were not presented because they were based on a relatively small number of respondents or had a large margin of error.

**Understanding Alcohol Use Disorder (AUD)**
Alcohol use disorder (AUD) is a medical condition characterized by an impaired ability to stop or control alcohol use despite adverse social, occupational, or health consequences. It encompasses the conditions that some people refer to as alcohol abuse, alcohol dependence, alcohol addiction, and the colloquial term, alcoholism.

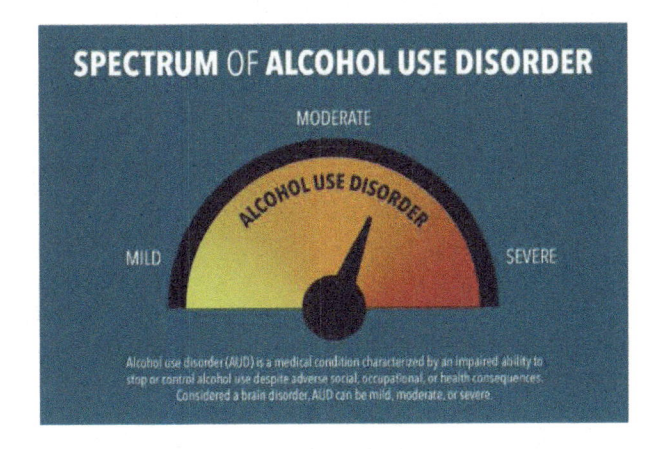

Considered a spectrum disorder, AUD can be mild, moderate, or severe. Lasting changes in the brain caused by alcohol misuse perpetuate AUD and make individuals vulnerable to relapse. The good news is that no matter how severe the problem may seem, evidence-based treatment with behavioral therapies, mutual-support groups, and/or medications can help people with AUD achieve and maintain recovery. According to the 2022 National Survey on Drug Use and Health, 28.8 million adults ages 18 and older (11.2% in this age group) had AUD in 2021. Among youth, an estimated 753,000 adolescents ages 12 to 17 (2.9% of this age group) had AUD during this time frame.

**What Increases the Risk for Alcohol Use Disorder?**
A person's risk for developing AUD depends in part on how much, how often, and how quickly they consume alcohol. Alcohol misuse, which includes binge drinking and heavy alcohol use, over time increases the risk of AUD. Other factors also increase the risk of AUD, such as:
- Drinking at an early age. A recent national survey found that among people ages 26 and older, those who began drinking before age 15 were more than three times as likely to report having AUD in the past year as those who waited until age 21 or later to begin drinking. The risk for females in this group is higher than that of males.
- Genetics and family history of alcohol problems. Genetics play a role, with hereditability accounting for approximately 60%; however, like other chronic health conditions, AUD risk is influenced by the interplay between a person's genes and their environment. Parents' drinking patterns may also influence the likelihood that a child will one day develop AUD.
- Mental health conditions and a history of trauma. A wide range of psychiatric conditions—including depression, post-traumatic stress disorder, and attention deficit hyperactivity disorder—are comorbid with AUD and are associated with an increased risk of AUD. People with a history of childhood trauma are also vulnerable to AUD.

**The Pharmacology**
Alcohol, barbiturates, and benzodiazepines are drugs that depress (slow down) CNS activity. Although all these drugs have different specific mechanisms of action in the brain, they all share the ability to enhance the activity of the inhibitory neurotransmitter, gamma amino butyric acid (GABA). In some cases, GABA

activation in turn alters other inhibitory pathways. Thus, the final outcome of inhibiting an inhibitory pathway is the net activation of a brain region. This mechanism of interfering with other inhibitory pathways is thought to play a role in the abuse of these drugs.

Alcohol (ethyl alcohol or ethanol) differs from most other drugs of abuse in that it has no known target receptor system in the brain. Ethanol affects a number of neurotransmitter systems through its action on membranes of neurons and the ion channels inside, particularly calcium (CA+) and chloride (CL-). In general, ethanol inhibits receptors for excitatory neurotransmitters and augments activity at inhibitory neurotransmitters. For example, ethanol enhances the activity of GABA by slowing ion channels associated with GABA$_A$ receptor subtype and the excitatory amino acid neurotransmitter glutamate, through inhibition of the NMDA receptor. The net effect of ethanol is to depress activity in the brain, producing paradoxical sedative and intoxicating effects. A similar spectrum of effects is seen with benzodiazepines and barbiturates.

**Dopamine and Alcohol**
Studies have found up to 30 percent lower levels of dopamine in the nucleus accumbens and the olfactory tubercle in alcohol-preferring rats. No other differences in dopamine content have been observed in other brain areas. This data suggest an abnormality in the dopamine system projecting from the ventral tegmental area to limbic regions (nucleus accumbens) of rats bred to prefer alcohol.

Since this system is thought to mediate various drugs of abuse, and ethanol is thought to increase dopamine levels in the system, it may indicate that abnormal functioning of mesolimbic pathway (MLP) where dopamine promotes AUD behaviors. That is, alcohol preference may be due, in part, to neuroadaptation to compensate for a reduction of GABA receptor sensitivity and an increase in glutamate balancing.

Differences in dopamine receptors within the AUD cohort population have been reported. Two genetically determined alcoholic lines of rats had fewer of one type of dopamine receptor (the D2 receptor) in their limbic system compared with the nonalcoholic rats. 20 percent fewer D2 receptors were also observed in the nucleus accumbens of these rats. These studies, along with genetic linkage studies, provide a foundation for relating the D2 receptor to alcohol preference.

**Serotonin and Ethanol**
Evidence suggests that the serotonin system is involved in regulating the activity of the dopamine system. Further examination has indicated a relationship between high alcohol preference and a deficiency in CNS serotonin. A number of studies have reported 10 to 30 percent lower levels of serotonin and its metabolites in the brains of alcohol-preferring rats. Only one study, using a strain of rats not used in any other tests, did not find lower brain serotonin levels. Areas of the brain found to have low serotonin include the cerebral cortex, frontal cortex, nucleus accumbens, anterior and corpus striatum, septal nuclei, hippocampus, olfactory tubercle, thalamus and hypothalamus.

Since several of these CNS regions may be mediate the rewards of drugs of abuse, these findings suggest a relationship between lower brain serotonin and high alcohol preference. Also, some of the areas found to have less serotonin (the hypothalamus and hippocampus) may be involved in mediating the aversive effects of ethanol. Since tolerance is a possible characteristic of alcoholic abuse, a deficiency in serotonin in these areas may be an innate factor promoting tolerance to the aversive effects of ethanol in alcohol-preferring lines of rodents.

Overall, the animal data shows an inverse relationship between the functioning of the CNS serotonin system and alcohol behavior. Thus, innate low functioning of the serotonin system may be associated with high alcohol preference. In support of this concept, some studies found lower serotonin metabolite concentrations in cerebrospinal fluid of alcoholics than in various control populations.

**GABA and Ethanol**
Research indicates that alcohol can exert some of its anti-anxiety and intoxicating effects by potentiating the actions of the neurotransmitter gamma amino butyric acid (GABA) receptor. GABA receptors seem to be involved in mediating alcohol drinking behavior of alcohol-preferring rats. A recent study examined the density of GABA fibers in the nucleus accumbens and other brain areas of both alcoholic and non-preferring rats. The results of this study indicated a higher density of GABA fibers in the nucleus accumbens of the alcohol-preferring rats. There was no difference between the respective lines in the other regions. These results suggest alcohol preference may involve an innate,

abnormal GABA system within the nucleus accumbens.

Alcohol, as with all depressants, induces a dose-response relationship leading to disinhibition, ataxia, impaired judgment, sedation, slurred speech, and eventually coma, respiratory depression and death.

**Blood Alcohol Concentrations (BAC)**

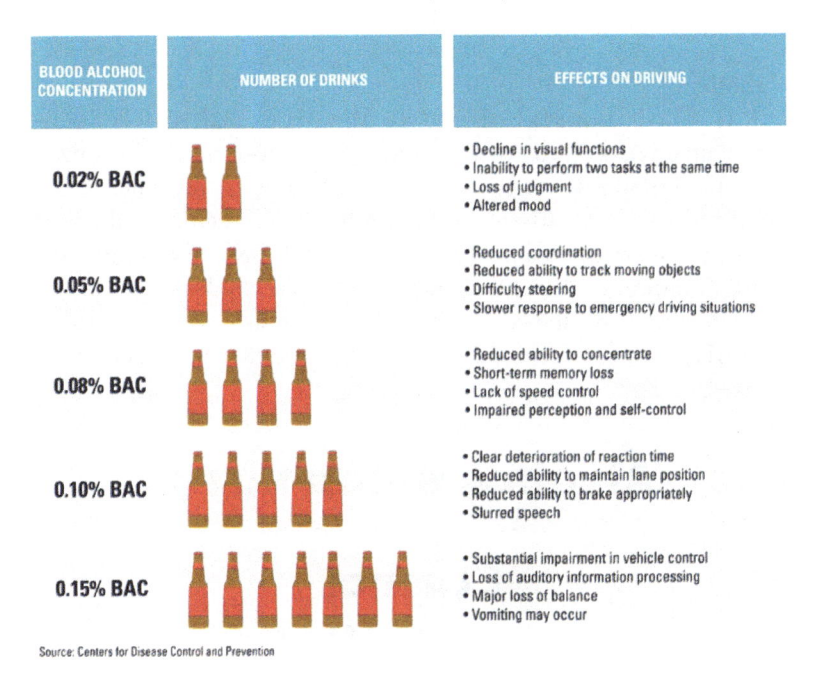

| BLOOD ALCOHOL CONCENTRATION | NUMBER OF DRINKS | EFFECTS ON DRIVING |
|---|---|---|
| 0.02% BAC | 2 | • Decline in visual functions<br>• Inability to perform two tasks at the same time<br>• Loss of judgment<br>• Altered mood |
| 0.05% BAC | 3 | • Reduced coordination<br>• Reduced ability to track moving objects<br>• Difficulty steering<br>• Slower response to emergency driving situations |
| 0.08% BAC | 4 | • Reduced ability to concentrate<br>• Short-term memory loss<br>• Lack of speed control<br>• Impaired perception and self-control |
| 0.10% BAC | 5 | • Clear deterioration of reaction time<br>• Reduced ability to maintain lane position<br>• Reduced ability to brake appropriately<br>• Slurred speech |
| 0.15% BAC | 7 | • Substantial impairment in vehicle control<br>• Loss of auditory information processing<br>• Major loss of balance<br>• Vomiting may occur |

Source: Centers for Disease Control and Prevention

The illustration above shows that effects of alcohol with the corresponding blood alcohol levels (BALs).

Once absorbed, alcohol is distributed rather uniformly through all tissues and fluids. Measuring the levels of alcohol in the body is accomplished by evaluating the amount of alcohol in the blood. Blood-levels of alcohol are measured in grams of alcohol present in 100 milliliters (mls) of blood. That is, .08 g percent is 80 mg of alcohol in 100 mls of blood. The dose-response relationship effects of alcohol are related to the blood alcohol level (BAL) which is the concentration of alcohol in the blood.

**Absorption**
After ingestion, alcohol is absorbed from the stomach and small intestine, and is then distributed uniformly throughout the body. Absorption of alcohol from the stomach will increase as gastric alcohol increases. As alcohol concentrations rise, the rate of absorption decreases as the astringent actions of alcohol will restrict the blood supply to the stomach. Carbohydrates may actually enhance alcohol absorption by the small intestines. The complete absorption of alcohol takes from 2 to 6 hours.

**Metabolism**
Most alcohol is metabolized in the liver. Alcohol is oxidized into acetaldehyde with the assistance of a zinc-containing enzyme called alcohol dehydrogenase. When alcohol is present in large concentrations, another liver-enzyme system, called the *microsomal ethanol oxidizing system* (MEOS), is induced to convert alcohol into the metabolite of acetaldehyde. *Aldehyde dehydrogenase* is the enzyme that assists in the further metabolization of acetaldehyde into acetic acid where it then becomes excreted.

## Alcohol Metabolism

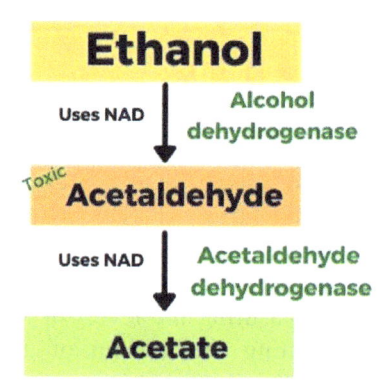

**Ethanol**
Uses NAD — Alcohol dehydrogenase
↓
Toxic **Acetaldehyde**
Uses NAD — Acetaldehyde dehydrogenase
↓
**Acetate**

**Alcohol Effects on the Brain**
Alcohol has two major actions on the brain: increasing neuronal inhibition mediated through the inhibitory gamma-aminobutyric acid (GABA), glycine, and adenosine—prolonged alcohol use down-regulates these receptors and decreases inhibitory neurotransmission; and inhibiting excitatory neurotransmission by inhibiting both N-

methyl-d-aspartate (NMDA) and non-NMDA (kainite and α-amino-3-hydroxy-5-methisoxizole-4-propionic acid [AMPA]) receptors. Up-regulation of these glutamate receptors compensates for alcohol's antagonistic effect after prolonged exposure and results in increased neuroexcitation. Cessation or reduction of alcohol use initiates an imbalance between the decreased neural inhibition and increased neural excitation. This causes the clinical manifestations of the alcohol withdrawal syndrome (AWS).

**Alcohol Withdrawal Syndrome (AWS)**
Alcohol withdrawal symptoms usually appear when an individual with alcohol use disorder (AUD) discontinues or reduces alcohol intake after a period of prolonged consumption. In most cases, mild symptoms may start to develop within hours of the last drink. An Alcohol Withdrawal Syndrome (AWS) occurs when patients stop drinking or significantly decrease their alcohol intake after long-term dependence. Withdrawal has a broad range of symptoms from mild tremors to a condition called delirium tremens, which results in seizures and could progress to death if not recognized and treated promptly. The reported mortality rate for patients who experience delirium tremens is anywhere from 1 to 5%. AWS represents a group of symptoms that usually arise 1–3 d after the last drink. Sometimes, the symptoms are already present when the alcohol blood level is above 0 (0.5‰ or even more). See chart below.

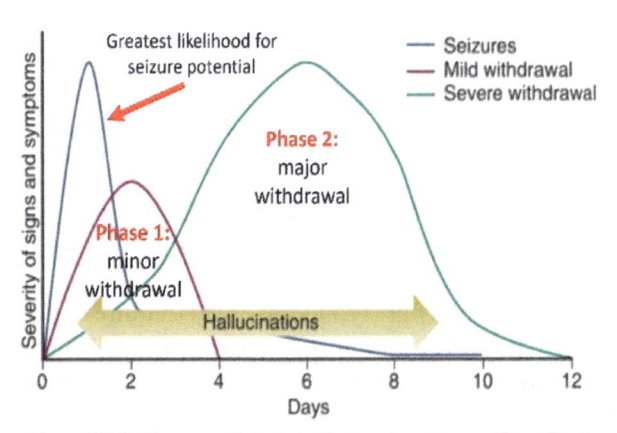

**Figure 26-5.** Progress of alcohol withdrawal syndrome. *(From Frank L, Pead J. New concepts in drug withdrawal: a resource handbook. Melbourne, 1995, University of Melbourne.)*

Stern TA, et al. Massachusetts General Hospital - Comprehensive Clinical Psychiatry, Second Edition. Elsevier 2016

The Diagnostic and Statistical Manual of Mental Disorders (DSM-5) outlines diagnostic criteria for AWS using two main components so that the AWS is diagnosed when the following two conditions are met:
1. A clear evidence of cessation or reduction in heavy and prolonged alcohol use.
2. The symptoms of withdrawal are not accounted for by a medical or another mental or behavioral disorder.

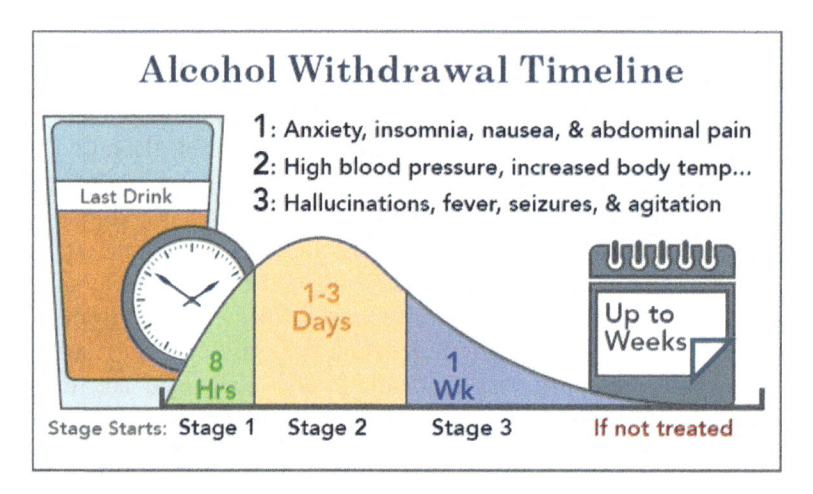

## Alcohol Withdrawal Timeline

1: Anxiety, insomnia, nausea, & abdominal pain
2: High blood pressure, increased body temp...
3: Hallucinations, fever, seizures, & agitation

Last Drink

Stage Starts: **Stage 1** (8 Hrs) **Stage 2** (1-3 Days) **Stage 3** (1 Wk) **If not treated** (Up to Weeks)

Managing the AWS requires a physical examination and investigations should be directed toward detecting common signs and symptoms of AWS. Patients should be kept calm in a controlled environment to try to reduce the risks of progression from mild symptoms to hallucinations. With mild to moderate symptoms, patients should receive supportive therapy.

The hallmark of management for severe symptoms is the administration of long-acting benzodiazepines. The most commonly used benzodiazepines are diazepam or lorazepam for management.

Patients with severe withdrawal symptoms may require escalating doses and intensive care level monitoring. Early consultation with a toxicologist is recommended to assist with aggressive management as these patients may require benzodiazepine doses at a level higher than the practitioner is comfortable with to manage their symptoms.

## The Alcohol Withdrawal Syndrome (AWS)

| Drug | Onset | Duration | Signs and Symptoms |
|---|---|---|---|
| ALCOHOL | 6-24 hours after last drink<br>• Onset may be delayed if benzodiazepines or other sedatives have been recently consumed.<br>• May also occur when blood alcohol is decreasing but not zero. | Usually 2-3 days, may continue up to 10 days if withdrawal is severe | **Autonomic overactivity**<br>• Sweating, tachycardia, tremor, fever<br>• Hypertension, insomnia.<br>**Gastrointestinal**<br>• Anorexia, nausea, vomiting, dyspepsia<br>**Cognitive and perceptual changes**<br>• Anxiety, vivid dreams, hallucinations, illusions<br>• Seizures occur in about 5% of people withdrawing from alcohol.<br>Note: seizures occur early (usually 7-24 hours after the last drink), are grand mal in type (i.e. not focal) and usually (though not always) occur as a single episode.<br>**Alcohol withdrawal delirium (AWD) is a medical emergency and may be a risk with some patients.** *Refer to section 7.4.4: Alcohol withdrawal delirium (previously known as delirium tremens) for further information.* |

In general, the Clinical Institute for Withdrawal Assessment for alcohol revised (CIWA-AR) assessment can be used to monitor AWS signs and symptoms severity over time to help in withdrawal management. The CIWA-AR protocol is the most common method of assessment, managing and treating the alcohol withdrawal syndrome.

The CIWA-AR is a tool used to assess the severity of alcohol withdrawal symptoms. The tool allows clinicians and counselors to monitor for the signs and symptoms of withdrawal and determine who needs medical therapy. The features that are used for the CIWA-Ar scale include the presence of:
- Nausea and vomiting
- Headache
- Auditory disturbances
- Agitation
- Paroxysmal sweating
- Visual disturbances
- Tremor
- Clouding of sensorium
- Anxiety

## Alcohol Withdrawal Assessment Scoring Guidelines (CIWA - Ar)

**Nausea/Vomiting** - Rate on scale 0 - 7
0 - None
1 - Mild nausea with no vomiting
2
3
4 - Intermittent nausea
5
6
7 - Constant nausea and frequent dry heaves and vomiting

**Tremors** - have patient extend arms & spread fingers. Rate on scale 0 - 7.
0 - No tremor
1 - Not visible, but can be felt fingertip to fingertip
2
3
4 - Moderate, with patient's arms extended
5
6
7 - severe, even w/ arms not extended

**Anxiety** - Rate on scale 0 - 7
0 - no anxiety, patient at ease
1 - mildly anxious
2
3
4 - moderately anxious or guarded, so anxiety is inferred
5
6
7 - equivalent to acute panic states seen in severe delirium or acute schizophrenic reactions.

**Agitation** - Rate on scale 0 - 7
0 - normal activity
1 - somewhat normal activity
2
3
4 - moderately fidgety and restless
5
6
7 - paces back and forth, or constantly thrashes about

**Paroxysmal Sweats** - Rate on Scale 0 - 7.
0 - no sweats
1 - barely perceptible sweating, palms moist
2
3
4 - beads of sweat obvious on forehead
5
6
7 - drenching sweats

**Orientation and clouding of sensorium** - Ask, "What day is this? Where are you? Who am I?" Rate scale 0 - 4
0 - Oriented
1 - cannot do serial additions or is uncertain about date
2 - disoriented to date by no more than 2 calendar days
3 - disoriented to date by more than 2 calendar days
4 - Disoriented to place and / or person

**Tactile disturbances** - Ask, "Have you experienced any itching, pins & needles sensation, burning or numbness, or a feeling of bugs crawling on or under your skin?"
0 - none
1 - very mild itching, pins & needles, burning, or numbness
2 - mild itching, pins & needles, burning, or numbness
3 - moderate itching, pins & needles, burning, or numbness
4 - moderate hallucinations
5 - severe hallucinations
6 - extremely severe hallucinations
7 - continuous hallucinations

**Auditory Disturbances** - Ask, "Are you more aware of sounds around you? Are they harsh? Do they startle you? Do you hear anything that disturbs you or that you know isn't there?"
0 - not present
1 - Very mild harshness or ability to startle
2 - mild harshness or ability to startle
3 - moderate harshness or ability to startle
4 - moderate hallucinations
5 - severe hallucinations
6 - extremely severe hallucinations
7 - continuous hallucinations

**Visual disturbances** - Ask, "Does the light appear to be too bright? Is its color different than normal? Does it hurt your eyes? Are you seeing anything that disturbs you or that you know isn't there?"
0 - not present
1 - very mild sensitivity
2 - mild sensitivity
3 - moderate sensitivity
4 - moderate hallucinations
5 - severe hallucinations
6 - extremely severe hallucinations
7 - continuous hallucinations

**Headache** - Ask, "Does your head feel different than usual? Does it feel like there is a band around your head?" Do not rate dizziness or lightheadedness.
0 - not present
1 - very mild
2 - mild
3 - moderate
4 - moderately severe
5 - severe
6 - very severe
7 - extremely severe

1. Assess and rate each of the 10 criteria of the CIWA-Ar scale. Each criterion is rated on a scale from 0 to 7, except for "Orientation and clouding of sensorium" which is rated on scale 0 to 4. Add up the scores for all ten criteria. This is the total CIWA-Ar score for the patient at that time. Prophylactic medication should be started for any patient with a total CIWA-Ar score of 9 or greater (ie. start on withdrawal medication). If started on scheduled or fixed dosage medication, additional one time medication should be given for a total CIWA-Ar score of 16 or greater.
2. Document vitals and CIWA-Ar assessment on the Withdrawal Assessment Sheet. Document administration of one time medications on the assessment sheet as well.
3. The CIWA-Ar scale is the most sensitive tool for assessment of the patient experiencing alcohol withdrawal. Nursing assessment is vitally important. Early intervention for CIWA-Ar score of 9 or greater provides the best means to prevent the progression of withdrawal.

## How Do You Score the CIWA-AR?

The CIWA-AR protocol items are scored on a scale of 0-7, with higher scores indicating more severe symptoms. The final item regarding orientation to time and place is rated from 0-4. The CIWA-AR score is based on the patient's self-reported symptoms

and observable signs. It takes two minutes to administer the assessment. Below are the total score ranges and their meaning:
- 7 or below: minimal to mild withdrawal
- 8-15: moderate withdrawal
- 16 or more: severe withdrawal (impending delirium tremens)

Scoring the CIWA protocol is simple and can be done by any healthcare professional who has been trained in its use.

Overview of Treatment of Alcohol Withdrawal, Based on CIWA-Ar score

| CIWA-Ar Score | Level of Withdrawal | Recommended Treatment |
|---|---|---|
| <10 | Mild | Supportive, non-pharmacologic therapy and close monitoring are indicated (unless patient has history of alcohol withdrawal seizures or co-morbid cardiovascular conditions). |
| 10–15 | Moderate | Medication (lorazepam) is indicated to reduce symptoms and the risk of major complications. |
| >15 | Severe | Strong consideration should be given to hospitalizing inmates who exhibit severe symptoms, as they are at increased risk for serious complications. |

Alcohol withdrawal is a classic example of *neuroadaptation,* often characterized by CNS hyperexcitability, resulting in anxiety, anorexia, insomnia, tremors and disorientation. In severe withdrawal a syndrome called *delirium tremens* may develop as well, marked by hallucinations, disorientation, and outbursts of irrational behavior. The syndrome peaks 24 to 48 hours after the drug is cleared. Potentially fatal convulsions and cardiovascular collapse can also occur after a week. Protracted abstinence syndrome generally follows and is often marked by depression and sleep disturbances.

The CNS hyperexcitability associated with alcohol withdrawal is thought to be related to alcohol-induced alterations in the sensitivity of GABA and glutamate receptors. Experimental evidence indicates that prolonged alcohol exposure decreases the sensitivity of GABA receptors and increases the sensitivity of glutamate receptors. With the cessation of alcohol intake, these changes are manifested throughout the brain as a decrease in the inhibitory neurotransmitter GABA and an increase in the excitatory amino acid neurotransmitter glutamate.

## Alcohol and Health

Alcohol is thought to enhance GABA activity in specific parts of the brain. GABA enhancement mirrors the reinforcing effects of alcohol, since drugs that block GABA activity also decrease alcohol intake, while drugs that increase GABA activity increase alcohol preference forestalling withdrawal. Part of alcohol's reinforcement is possibly due to increased GABA inhibition on other inhibitory neurons that decrease the activity of the dopamine neurons in the ventral tegmental area. This chain of action would have the ultimate effect of increasing the activity of the dopamine neurons. However, the experimental evidence supporting this idea is equivocal. While it is clear that both GABA and dopamine are involved in the reinforcing effects of alcohol, the relationship between these systems in this action is yet to be fully defined. The following medical conditions have been associated with chronic alcohol abuse.

Liver and organ effects are caused by enzyme depletion. Alcohol metabolism requires a coenzyme called *nicotinamide adenine dinucleotide (NAD)* which can get depleted in alcoholics. NAD depletion can result in the build-up of glutamate, maleate, and lactate which contribute to liver impairment and damage. This can lead to fatty liver (hyperlipemia), hepatitis and cirrhosis. Depletion of NAD can also lead to alcoholic hypoglycemia which contributes to alcohol's mental effects since the brain is an insulin-dependent organ. Alcohol also disrupts the gastrointestinal function by reducing the water-soluble vitamins, and increasing secretion of hydrochloric acid (HCL) and digestive juices that contribute to gastritis and pancreatitis.

Vitamin and mineral deficiencies can result from alcohol's "empty calories", which are of no nutritional value. The ingestion of large amounts of alcohol also results in limited or sporadic food consumption, resulting in vitamin deficiencies.

Secondary deficiencies may develop, due to impaired absorption and storage of vitamins. These alcohol-related defects involve the liver, which is the primary organ that stores and converts precursor forms of vitamins to their active metabolites. B vitamin deficiencies are common in chronic alcoholics. Vitamin B deficiency is associated with cardiovascular symptoms, alcohol neuritis, Korsakoff s psychosis and Wernicke's syndrome. *Peripheral neuropathy,* a thiamine deficiency, is actually demyelination of peripheral nerve fibers, also common in many alcoholics. This condition is associated with less sensory acuity, *paresthesias* and reduced conductance velocity.

Deficiencies in vitamins D, K and A are also common in chronic alcoholics. Alcoholics with liver damage such as hepatitis (fatty liver) have an 80% decrease in hepatic (liver) vitamin A levels. The combination of impaired vitamin D metabolism, chronic intake of antacids containing aluminum, and high corticosteroid levels may also result in osteoporosis in both alcoholic women and men. The metabolism of iron is impaired by alcohol, even when the person is well nourished and has no anemia. The loss of iron metabolism caused by chronic drinking is important in contributing to idiopathic hemochromatosis (iron overload).

High blood pressure and *cardiac irregularities* are observed in both acute and chronic alcohol ingestion due to the combined effects of more norepinephrine, depression of cardio regulatory centers *in* the brainstem, and the reflex response to peripheral vasodilation. The direct effects of alcohol on the heart muscle itself may eventually lead to *cardiomyopathy* (heart swelling) with associated *arrhythmias* (irregular beat). Peripheral neuropathies that accompany chronic use also contribute to cardiovascular impairment.

Alcohol-induced CNS depression produces a marked decrease in *antidiuretic hormone (ADH)* from the posterior pituitary. The sudden decrease in ADH, coupled with the increase in liquid volume consumption, can lead to a profound and dramatic diuresis.

**Alcohol and Body Temperature**
Contrary to what many believe, alcohol actually lowers body temperature. Even though the vasodilation from acute alcohol ingestion produces a warm sensation (due to increased vascular flow to the cutaneous vessels), the restricted blood flow to the periphery causes heat loss. Also, alcohol at high doses produces hypothalamic depression and will compromise the temperature-regulating systems of the body. These combined factors can be potentially fatal to the homeless alcoholic living on the street, because their systems cannot respond to changes in weather. There are also dangers when alcohol is used in combination with certain antipsychotic medications that further impair response to temperature changes. The dually diagnosed patient, for example, who is taking an anti-psychotic medication and is at risk for

alcohol relapse would require careful case management in this regard.

## Alcohol Use and Pregnancy

There is no known safe amount of alcohol use during pregnancy or while trying to get pregnant. There is also no safe time for alcohol use during pregnancy. All types of alcohol are equally harmful, including all wines and beer. Prenatal exposure to alcohol can produce a variety of problems for children. Fetal alcohol syndrome includes mental retardation, congenital heart defects, and abnormal morphological conditions including microencephaly, under-development and facial abnormalities.

Alcohol in the mother's blood passes to the baby through the umbilical cord. Alcohol use during pregnancy can cause miscarriage, stillbirth, and a range of lifelong physical, behavioral, and intellectual disabilities. These disabilities are known as fetal alcohol spectrum disorders (FASDs). Children with FASDs might have the following characteristics and behaviors:
- Abnormal facial features, such as a smooth ridge between the nose and upper lip (this ridge is called the philtrum)
- Small head size
- Shorter-than-average height
- Low body weight
- Poor coordination
- Hyperactive behavior
- Difficulty with attention
- Poor memory
- Difficulty in school (especially with math)
- Learning disabilities
- Speech and language delays
- Intellectual disability or low IQ
- Poor reasoning and judgment skills
- Sleep and sucking problems as a baby
- Vision or hearing problems
- Problems with the heart, kidney, or bones

Fetal Alcohol Spectrum Disorders (FASDs) are preventable if a baby is not exposed to alcohol before birth.

## High Risk Populations and Alcohol Use Disorder (AUD) - Vulnerability

Genetic influences on normal and pathological consumption of alcohol are shown in family studies, twin studies and adoption studies, as well as animal research. Animal studies have established that alcohol preference and the reinforcing actions of alcohol are influenced by genetic factors. While there have been fewer studies examining the genetic component of drug abuse, evidence from animal studies also supports a genetic influence on the use and abuse of drugs other than alcohol.

The study of nonalcoholic drug abuse in humans is more difficult because of substantially smaller populations that use these drugs and marked changes in exposure to these agents. Investigation in this area is further hampered by the complexity of subjects' drug use, since most drug abusers have used multiple agents. This has led researchers either to concentrate on one class of drug or to treat all illicit drug use as equivalent. The tendency to lump all illicit drugs into one category makes results difficult to interpret or compare. In the case of alcohol, studies indicate that low doses of alcohol are stimulating and produce a strong positive reward in animals susceptible to the alcohol addiction.

Another component of excessive alcohol consumption might be that alcoholics have a high threshold to the aversive effects of ethanol. This could be a result of an innate low sensitivity to medium and high doses of alcohol or acute tolerance to its aversive effects. Results from animal studies suggest an association between high alcohol preference and acute tolerance to high-dose effects of ethanol.

Neurobiological evidence points to common pathways mediating the positive reinforcing actions of alcohol and other drugs of abuse. Most evidence shows the involvement of the mesolimbic pathway(MLP) dopamine system in drug reinforcement. Other neural pathways that regulate MLP activity may also increase the rewarding effects of ethanol and other drugs of abuse. In the case of serotonin, innate genetic factors appear to reduce CNS activity of serotonin, and induce heavy drinking.

**Twin Studies**
Evidence from twin studies suggests genetic influences on drinking patterns and alcohol problems. Results from twin studies demonstrate genetic determination of alcohol consumption such as abstention, average alcohol intake or heavy alcohol use. Twin studies also indicate an inherited risk for smoking.

When evaluating how alcoholism develops, twin studies generally show mutual development of a disorder. One study found a higher concordance rate for alcohol abuse between identical twins (54 percent) versus fraternal twins (28 percent), while two subsequent studies found no such relationship. A 1991 study examined 50 male and 31 female identical twin pairs and 64 male and 24 female fraternal twin pairs, with 1 member of the pair meeting alcohol abuse or dependence criteria.

The study found that identical male twins differed from fraternal male twins in the frequencies of both alcohol abuse and dependence as well as other substance abuse and dependence. On the other hand, female identical and fraternal twins were equally likely to abuse alcohol and/or become dependent on other substances, but identical female twins were more likely to become alcohol dependent.

Another study of 356 twin pairs also found higher identical than fraternal rates of concordance for problems related to alcohol and drug use as well as conduct disorder. The same study also noted that among men, heritability was greater for early rather than late onset of alcohol problems, whereas no such effect was seen for women. Finally, a study of 1,030 female twin pairs found evidence for substantial heritability of liability to alcoholism, ranging from 50 to 60 percent.

Thus, twin studies provide general agreement that genetic factors influence certain aspects of drinking. Most twin studies also show genetic influence over pathological drinking, including the diagnosis of alcoholism, which appears (like many psychiatric disorders) to be moderately heritable. Whether genetic factors operate comparably in men and women, and whether severity of alcoholism influences twin concordance is less clear. How psychiatric comorbidity may affect heritability of alcoholism also remains to be studied.

**Adoption Studies**
Adoption studies have also supported the role of heritable factors in risk for alcoholism. The results from a series of studies conducted in Denmark during the 1970s are typical. Of 5,483 adoption cases from Copenhagen between 1924 and 1947, the researchers compared 20 adoptees with 30 nonadopted brothers.

They also studied 49 female adoptees, comparing them with 81 non-adopted daughters of alcoholics. Comparisons also were made with matched control adoptees.

The Copenhagen study revealed that adopted sons of alcoholic parents were *four times* as likely as sons of nonalcoholics to have developed alcoholism. Evidence also suggested that the alcoholism in these cases was more severe. The groups differed little on other variables, including prevalence of other psychiatric illness or heavy drinking. Being raised by an alcoholic biological parent did not further increase the likelihood of developing alcoholism. That is, rates of alcoholism did not differ between the adopted children and their nonadopted brothers.

In contrast, daughters of alcoholics were not at elevated risk of alcoholism. Among adoptees, 2 percent had alcoholism (another 2 percent had drinking problems), compared with 4 percent of alcoholism among the adopted controls and 3 percent among nonadopted daughters.

Another analysis examined factors promoting drug abuse as well. In this study, all classes of illicit drugs were collapsed into a single category of "drug abuse." Most of the 40 adopted drug abusers had coexisting anti-social personality disorder; the presence of ASPD correlated highly with drug abuse. For those without ASPD, family history of alcoholism accompanied drug abuse. Also, turmoil in the adoptive family (divorce or psychiatric disturbance) was also associated with increased drug abuse.

Finally, results from other adoption studies suggest two possible forms of alcohol abuse. The two forms have been classified as "milieu- limited" or *Type I alcohol abuse* in contrast to "male-limited" or *Type 2 alcohol abuse*. Type 1 alcohol abuse is generally mild, characterized by mild alcohol problems and minimal criminal behavior in the parents, but it can be occasionally severe, depending on a provocative environment. Type 2 is associated with severe alcohol abuse and criminality in biological fathers. In the adoptees, it was associated with recurrent problems and appeared to be unaffected by postnatal environment.

In summary, adoption studies of alcoholism clearly indicate the role of biological, presumably genetic, factors in the genesis of alcoholism. They do not exclude, however, a possible role for environmental factors as well. Moreover, evidence suggests several biological backgrounds are conducive to alcoholism. In particular, one pattern of inheritance suggests a relationship between parental antisocial behavior and alcoholism in the next generation. Thus, adoption studies, like other designs, suggest that even at the genetic level, alcoholism is not a homogeneous construct.

## BIOCHEMICAL ASSAYS

### Serotonin

Results over the last two decades from both human and animal studies have supported a relationship between low levels of serotonin in the central nervous system (CNS) and impulsive violent behavior. Since problematic drug use has long been associated with a wide range of violent behavior, scientists have examined the relationship between alcoholism and serotonergic abnormalities. While a consistent relationship is lacking between alcoholism and low CNS levels of serotonin and its metabolites, mounting evidence supports low serotonin in a subgroup of alcoholics with early-onset problems and a history of violence.

Because measures of serotonin activity are difficult to obtain, researchers have used pharmacological probes of serotonin function, such as hormonal response to drugs that affect serotonin. These indirect measures have also indicated a relationship between impulsivity, substance abuse, and abnormal serotonin function.

Given that early-onset alcoholism and ASPD overlap substantially, the specificity of the serotonin findings is unclear, especially as similar results have been found in substance abusers with ASPD. However, at least one report has indicated that, even after controlling for the presence of ASPD and illicit drug abuse, other neurochemical findings remained significantly associated with alcoholism. While research might delineate the relationship between decreased CNS serotonin levels and specific psychiatric syndromes, current evidence suggests relatively specific biological differences may exist between early- and late-onset alcoholics, raising the possibility of defining biologically homogeneous subgroups.

**Aldehyde and Alcohol Dehydrogenase**
Many Asians rapidly develop a prominent facial flush following ingestion of a small amount of alcohol. Continued drinking leads to nausea, dizziness, palpitations and faintness. This reaction is due to inactivity in the individuals' aldehyde dehydrogenase, an enzyme, as you will recall, that helps metabolize alcohol in the body. Ineffective enzyme activity results in a buildup of acetaldehyde in the blood following alcohol consumption which can be toxic. Interestingly, a mutant form of alcohol dehydrogenase also produces a transient increase in the acetaldehyde concentration after alcohol ingestion. This form of the enzyme also has been reported in Asian populations.

The two enzymes, aldehyde and alcohol dehydrogenase, interact in some individuals to amplify the adverse reaction to alcohol consumption. Since this reaction discourages heavy drinking and occurs in populations where alcoholism is relatively rare, this suggests that alcohol and aldehyde dehydrogenase mutations might be a major determinant of alcohol consumption, abuse, and dependence. This holds true in Taiwan and Japan where the reaction occurs in 30 to 50 percent of individuals.

The genetics of aldehyde and alcohol dehydrogenase are well described. Different forms of these enzymes are by variations of their normal genes. The presence of these gene variations in an individual accounts for variations in the metabolism of alcohol. Thus, these genes can also effect alcohol consumption. For example, the gene variation that code for the ineffective form of aldehyde dehydrogenase is not only rare in alcoholics, but is also rare in Japanese patients with alcoholic liver disease. Despite identification of such genes, the relationship between their inheritance and family transmission of alcoholism remains unstudied.

**Benzodiazepines**
Benzodiazepines, also known as the *anxiolytics* (reducing anxiousness), are a class of drugs introduced in the 1960s as anti-anxiety agents. They rapidly replaced barbiturates, which have significant abuse potential, to treat psychiatric conditions. Like barbiturates, they generally inhibit brain activity by enhancing GABA. However, unlike barbiturates, which create a nonspecific effect on chloride ion channels, benzodiazepines act by binding to a specific receptor (BDZ receptor) within the

GABA system. The presence of a BDZ receptor suggests a natural endogenous chemical that normally interacts with it.

The benzodiazepine receptor is coupled with the GABAA receptor. Stimulation of the BDZ receptor increases the frequency of chloride ion channel opening in response to GABA binding to the GABAA receptor. Also, benzodiazepines enhance GABA binding to its receptor, and the presence of GABA enhances benzodiazepine binding. The net effect of benzodiazepines augments activity at the GABAA receptor and enhances GABA action, creating sedative results.

**Acute Administration**
Most benzodiazepines support only modest levels of self-administration, much below the levels observed with barbiturates, when given intravenously in animal studies. When given orally, benzodiazepines do not induce self- administration in animal studies. Human studies, similar to those used for barbiturates, have demonstrated that benzodiazepines yield modest rankings of liking and that given a choice, subjects consistently prefer barbiturates over benzodiazepines. Since benzodiazepines act selectively on GABA activity, their mild reinforcing properties might be due to activating GABA mechanisms similar to those for alcohol. However, combining benzodiazepines with alcohol or other sedatives produces an additive effect that can be extremely toxic.

**Chronic Administration**
Prolonged exposure to benzodiazepines results in tolerance to their therapeutic effects. This may be due to a reduction in the functional activity of GABA as a result of a desensitization of the benzodiazepine receptor caused by prolonged exposure to the drug. As with alcohol and the barbiturates, a withdrawal syndrome can occur following benzodiazepine cessation. In general, the characteristics of benzodiazepine withdrawal are similar to barbiturate withdrawal but at therapeutic doses, the magnitude of the symptoms are less severe than with barbiturates. Nonetheless, since benzodiazepines are widely prescribed, their abuse potential physicians to use careful administration.

**Barbiturates**
Barbiturates are a class of drugs that depress CNS activity. First introduced in the early 1900s, barbiturates were widely prescribed as antianxiety agents and sleep aids, and treatment for

other psychiatric conditions. However, their lethal overdose potential and high abuse potential, coupled with the advent of the safer benzodiazepine compounds, curtailed their use starting in the 1960s.

The sedative effects of barbiturates result from their ability to increase GABA activity. Their mechanism of action is an augmentation of the activity of the GABAA receptor. This receptor is linked to a chloride ion channel. Stimulation of the receptor by GABA opens the channel and increases the flow of chloride into the neuron, which inhibits the cell's activity. Barbiturates increase the time the chloride channel stays open, thus increasing the inhibitory effects of GABA.

**Acute Administration**
The reinforcing properties of barbiturates have been clearly demonstrated in both animal and human studies. Animals readily self-administer barbiturates in a variety of different experimental paradigms. Human studies have demonstrated that drug-experienced subjects, blind to the identity of the drug, consistently give barbiturates high rankings when asked to rate a series of drugs. Human subjects will work to receive barbiturates and will do more work to receive the drug if the available dosage is increased. Since one of the major effects is to enhance GABA activity, barbiturates, like alcohol, may increase GABA inhibition of other inhibitory neurons, thus increasing the net activity of the dopamine neurons in the ventral tegmental area. Further studies are necessary to confirm this possibility.

**Chronic Administration**
With continued use, some tolerance develops to most effects of barbiturates. However, little tolerance develops to prevent a lethal dose. Unlike most other drugs of abuse, both metabolic and pharmacodynamic tolerance are important in the development of barbiturate tolerance. Barbiturate withdrawal is marked by a severe and sometimes life-threatening condition similar to alcohol withdrawal. Both anxiety and depression are common, and with prolonged use, the development of severe grand mal tonic epileptic seizures can occur.

The neurochemical changes responsible for the pharmacodynamic tolerance and withdrawal syndrome have yet to be clearly established, but may be related to rebounding NE systems. Some evidence suggests that tolerance is the result of the GABAA receptors becoming less sensitive to the effects of barbiturates. After cessation, the barbiturate stimulation of GABA activity ceases, and the desensitized receptors create an overall decrease in GABA activity causing withdrawal symptoms. The hyperexcitability that results is very similar to what occurs in the alcohol withdrawal. In fact, barbiturates are sometimes referred to as "solid alcohols" because of the similarity in mechanism of action.

## Types of Treatments for Alcohol Use Disorder

Several evidence-based treatment approaches are available for AUD. One size does not fit all and a treatment approach that may work for one person may not work for another. Treatment can be outpatient and/or inpatient and be provided by specialty programs, therapists, and health care providers.

### Behavioral Treatments

Behavioral treatments—including counseling therapy, and provided by licensed therapists—are aimed at changing drinking behavior. Examples of behavioral treatments are brief interventions and reinforcement approaches, treatments that build motivation and teach skills for coping and preventing a return to drinking, and mindfulness-based therapies.

### Mutual-Support Groups

Mutual-support groups provide peer support for stopping or reducing drinking. Group meetings are available in most communities at low or no cost, and at convenient times and locations—including an increasing presence online. This means they can be especially helpful to individuals at risk for relapse to drinking. Combined with medications and behavioral treatment provided by health care professionals, mutual-support groups can offer a valuable added layer of support.

**Note:** People with severe AUD often need medical help to avoid alcohol withdrawal if they decide to stop drinking. Alcohol withdrawal is a potentially life-threatening process that can occur when someone who has been drinking heavily for a prolonged period of time suddenly stops drinking. Doctors can prescribe medications to address these symptoms and make the process safer and less distressing.

**Medications**
Three medications are currently approved by the U.S. Food and Drug Administration to help people stop or reduce their drinking and prevent a return to drinking: naltrexone (oral and long-acting injectable), acamprosate, and disulfiram. All these medications are nonaddictive, and they may be used alone or combined with behavioral treatments or mutual-support groups.

**Disulfiram (Antabuse)**
Disulfiram (Antabuse) was the first medicine approved for the treatment of alcohol abuse and alcohol dependence by the U.S. Food and Drug Administration. Antabuse is prescribed to help people who want to quit drinking by causing a negative reaction if the person drinks while they are taking Antabuse.

As you have read, alcohol is metabolized by the liver into acetaldehyde, a very toxic substance that causes many hangover symptoms heavy drinker's experience. Usually, the body continues to oxidize acetaldehyde into acetic acid, which is harmless. Antabuse interferes with this metabolic process, stops the process with the production of acetaldehyde and prevents the oxidation of acetaldehyde into acetic acid. Because of this, Antabuse will cause a buildup of acetaldehyde five or ten times greater than normally occurs when someone drinks alcohol.

The high concentration of acetaldehyde that occurs when someone drinks while taking Antabuse can cause reactions that range in severity. Some of the principal symptoms that can occur with acetaldehyde buildup include flushing, nausea, vomiting, sweating, throbbing headache, breathing difficulty, chest pains, heart palpitations, tachycardia, hypotension, and blurred vision.

Antabuse serves merely as an aversive treatment for someone trying to stop drinking. It does not reduce the person's craving for alcohol, nor does it treat any of the alcohol withdrawal syndrome. Remember, some things seem to work more or less for some people some of the time. All treatment has a role in certain situations. And, like all other forms for behavioral healthcare, medications alone is not a best practice. Rather, medications combined with counseling is a standard of care.

**Vivitrol** (naltrexone)
The FDA has approved naltrexone extended-release injectable suspension (*Vivitrol*) for the treatment of alcohol dependence in patients who are able to abstain from drinking in an outpatient setting and who are not actively drinking on therapy initiation. It must be administered by a healthcare professional and used in combination with psychosocial support, such as counseling or group therapy.

Naltrexone is a medication that blocks the effects of drugs known as opioids. It competes with these drugs for opioid receptors in the brain. Originally used to treat dependence on opioid drugs, naltrexone is also approved by the FDA as treatment for alcoholism (Vivitrol). In clinical trials evaluating the effectiveness of naltrexone, patients who received naltrexone were twice as successful in remaining abstinent and in avoiding relapse as patients who received placebo-an inactive pill. Vivitrol must be administered by a healthcare professional. It is administered once a month or every 4 weeks as a gluteal IM injection. Vivitrol is contraindicated in patients receiving or dependent on opioids, in acute opioid withdrawal, and in those who have failed the naloxone challenge test or have a positive urine screen for opioids; and in those with previous hypersensitivity to naltrexone, PLG or any other components of the diluent.

**Acamprosate** (Campral)
Acamprosate has in vitro affinity for GABA type A and GABA type B receptors, so it's been assumed that the therapeutic effects of acamprosate are due to actions on GABA receptors. However, acamprosate does not share most of the other effects of GABA receptor modifying drugs, such as antianxiety, hypnotic, or muscle relaxant activity. It's therefore possible, perhaps likely, that the effects are mediated some other way. Acamprosate is structurally related to l-glutamic acid (l-glutamate), which is an excitatory neurotransmitter. It's been proposed that acamprosate decreases the effects of the naturally-occurring excitatory neurotransmitter glutamate in the body.

Since chronic alcohol consumption disrupts this system, and the changes last many months after alcohol ingestion is stopped, it's possible that acamprosate somehow restores the glutamate system towards normal. It's thought, no matter how it acts, that Campral decreases the pleasant "high" associated with alcohol consumption, and thus decrease the frequency of relapse during abstinence.

**Vitamins**
    a. Common nutritional deficiencies of alcoholic patients: e.g., magnesium, zinc, various vitamins.
    b. Administration of supplemental thiamine to all patients with a history of chronic alcoholism and in the treatment of Wernicke's encephalopathy, alcoholic amblyopia (a decrease of vision).
    c. Multiple mega-B therapy recommended for amblyopia.

(NOTE: Thiamine, 100 mg daily and a multivitamin supplement, provided patient shows no significant neurologic or hematologic problems secondary to chronic excessive alcohol intake is a rather standard vitamin regime for this population.)

**What is considered "normal" drinking"**
Low risk drinking (normal consumption) has been identified by the National Institute on Alcohol Abuse and Alcoholism (NIAAA) as no more than 4 drinks per day and no more than 14 drinks per week for men. For women, NIAAA defines low risk drinking as no more than 3 drinks per day AND no more than 7 drinks per week.

**Safe limits to avoid health consequences?**
The risks and harms associated with drinking alcohol have been systematically evaluated over the years and are well documented. The World Health Organization has now published a statement in January 2023 issue of The Lancet Public Health stating, *when it comes to alcohol consumption, there is no safe amount that does not affect health.*

The risk of developing cancer increases substantially the more alcohol is consumed. However, latest available data indicate that half of all alcohol-attributable cancers in the WHO European Region are caused by "light" and "moderate" alcohol consumption – less than 1.5 liters of wine or less than 3.5 liters of beer or less than 450 milliliters of spirits per week. This drinking pattern is responsible for the majority of alcohol-attributable breast cancers in women, with the highest burden observed in countries of the European Union (EU). In the EU, cancer is the leading cause of death – with a steadily increasing incidence rate – and the majority of all alcohol-attributable deaths are due to different types of cancers.

To identify a "safe" level of alcohol consumption, valid scientific evidence would need to demonstrate that at and below a certain level, there is no risk of illness or injury associated with alcohol consumption. The new WHO statement clarifies: currently available evidence cannot indicate the existence of a threshold at which the carcinogenic effects of alcohol "switch on" and start to manifest in the human body.

Moreover, there are no studies that would demonstrate that the potential beneficial effects of light and moderate drinking on cardiovascular diseases and type 2 diabetes outweigh the cancer risk associated with these same levels of alcohol consumption for individual consumers.

"We cannot talk about a so-called safe level of alcohol use. It doesn't matter how much you drink – the risk to the drinker's health starts from the first drop of any alcoholic beverage. The only thing that we can say for sure is that the more you drink, the more harmful it is – or, in other words, the less you drink, the safer it is," explains Dr Carina Ferreira-Borges, acting Unit Lead for Noncommunicable Disease Management and Regional Advisor for Alcohol and Illicit Drugs in the WHO Regional Office for Europe.

Despite this, the question of beneficial effects of alcohol has been a contentious issue in research for years.

Disadvantaged and vulnerable populations have higher rates of alcohol-related death and hospitalization, as harms from a given amount and pattern of drinking are higher for poorer drinkers and their families than for richer drinkers in any given society.
So, when we talk about possible so-called safer levels of alcohol consumption or about its protective effects, we are ignoring the bigger picture of alcohol harm in and the world.

Although it is well established that alcohol can cause cancer, this fact is still not widely known to the public in most countries. We need cancer-related health information messages on labels of alcoholic beverages, following the example of tobacco products; we need empowered and trained health professionals who would feel comfortable to inform their patients about alcohol and cancer risk; and we need overall wide awareness of this topic in countries and communities (The World Health Organization, (2023, January 23).

## SUGGESTED READINGS ON THIS TOPIC

Agarwal, DP. Alcohol Metabolism, Alcohol Intolerance, and Alcoholism: Biochemical and Pharmacogenetic Approaches. Springer. 2012.
ASIN : B00HWVOOIY.

ASAM Clinical Practice Guideline on Alcohol Withdrawal Management.\
https://www.asam.org/docs/default-source/quality-science/the_asam_clinical_practice_guideline_on_alcohol-1.pdf?sfvrsn=ba255c2_2

Grant, KA. The Neuropharmacology of Alcohol. Springer. 2019.
ISBN-10 : 3319965220.

Preedy, VR. Neuroscience of Alcohol: Mechanisms and Treatment. Academic Press. 2019. ISBN-10 : 012813125X.

Rose, ME. Alcohol: Its History, Pharmacology and Treatment. Hazelden. 2011. ISBN-10 : 1616491477.

Spineanu, E. Sedative and Hypnotic-Induced Mental Health Disorders: Understanding Behavioral Impacts. Independently published . ASIN : B0CQJV7JXZ.

World Health Organization, (2023, January 23). No level of alcohol consumption is safe for our health. January 2023.
https://www.who.int/europe/news/item/04-01-2023-no-level-of-alcohol-consumption-is-safe-for-our-health

# CHAPTER 9. STIMULANT DRUGS
## Key Concepts

| | |
|---|---|
| Cathinones | A monoamine alkaloid found in the Khat plant and is chemically similar to ephedrine, cathine, methcathinone and other amphetamines. |
| Cocaethylene | Reaction of the combined use of both cocaine and alcohol in the body that potentiates the toxic effects on the heart. |
| Ephedrine | Naturally occurring chemical from the ephedra plant that forms the foundation for amphetamines. |
| MDMA | (methylenedioxymethamphetamine) an analog of methamphetamine that is chemically related to mescaline and amphetamine. |
| Methylxanthines | A class of CNS stimulant compounds, to which caffeine belongs. |
| Monoamine Oxidase | (MAO) The enzyme that degrades the monoamine neurotransmitters but is inhibited by amphetamines, so that NE, DA and 5-HT activity is increased. |
| Stimulant | A class of drug that increases activity in the body's central nervous system. |
| Prescription Stimulants | Medications that are generally used to treat ADHD and narcolepsy. I.e. Adderall, Ritalin, pseudoephedrine, |
| Sympathomimetic | Drugs that activate the sympathetic nervous system increasing mental alertness, and increasing blood flow to muscles. Adverse effects of high doses include raised blood pressure, increased heart rate, and increased anxiety. |

# CHAPTER 9

## Stimulant Drugs

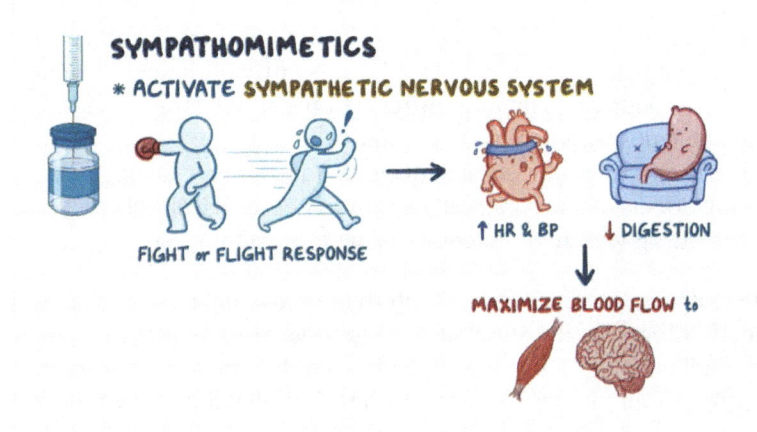

In this chapter we discuss the psychostimulants including methamphetamine and cocaine. To begin with, let's first review the data on this topic from the National Institute of Drug Abuse (NIDA), a division of the National Institutes of Health.

Psychostimulants (stimulants), is a category of prescription medications and illicit substances that increase energy and attention and decrease appetite. Stimulants such as methamphetamine and cocaine are potent substances with high potential for psychological or physical dependence. They produce increased feelings of energy, euphoria, and suppressed appetite and need for sleep. After continued use for several days, the body must crash with exhaustion, depression, and craving for more drug.

Methamphetamine—a potent and highly addictive stimulant—remains an extremely serious problem in the United States. In some areas of the country, it poses an even greater threat than opioids, and it is the drug that most contributes to violent crime. According to data from the 2022 National Survey on Drug Use and Health (NSDUH), more than 16.8 million people aged 12 or older (6.0% of the population) used methamphetamine at least once during their lifetime (2021 DT 1.1). In 2021, an estimated 2.5 million people reported using methamphetamine in the past 12 months (2021 DT 1.42A), and it remains one of the most commonly misused stimulant drugs in the world.

Developed early in the 20th century from its parent drug, amphetamine, methamphetamine was used originally in nasal decongestants and bronchial inhalers. Like amphetamine, methamphetamine causes increased activity and talkativeness, decreased appetite, and a pleasurable sense of well-being or euphoria. However, methamphetamine differs from amphetamine in that, at comparable doses, much greater amounts of the drug get into the brain, making it a more potent stimulant. It also has longer-lasting and more harmful effects on the central nervous system. These characteristics make it a drug with high potential for widespread misuse.

Methamphetamine, commonly referred to as meth or crystal meth, typically comes in the form of a white crystal-like 'rock' or powder. Methamphetamine is most commonly used by smoking, snorting, and injection. Common street names for methamphetamine include crank, crystal, ice, and speed. The methamphetamine molecule is structurally similar to amphetamine and to the neurotransmitter dopamine, a brain chemical that plays an important role in the reinforcement of rewarding behaviors, but it is quite different from cocaine. Although these stimulants have similar behavioral and physiological effects, there are some major differences in the basic mechanisms of how they work.

In contrast to cocaine, which is quickly removed from and almost completely metabolized in the body, methamphetamine has a much longer duration of action, and a larger percentage of the drug remains unchanged in the body. Methamphetamine therefore remains in the brain longer, which ultimately leads to prolonged stimulant effects.

Although both methamphetamine and cocaine increase levels of dopamine, administration of methamphetamine in animal studies leads to much higher levels of dopamine, because nerve cells respond differently to the two drugs. Cocaine prolongs dopamine actions in the brain by blocking the reuptake of the neurotransmitter by signaling nerve cells. At low doses, methamphetamine also blocks the re-uptake of dopamine, but it also increases the release of dopamine, leading to much higher concentrations in the synapse (the gap between neurons), which can be toxic to nerve terminals.

Some of the neurobiological effects of long-term methamphetamine use appear to be, at least, partially reversible. Abstinence from methamphetamine resulted in less excess microglial activation over time, and users who had remained methamphetamine-free for 2 years exhibited microglial activation levels similar to the study's control subjects. In addition to the neurological and behavioral consequences of methamphetamine misuse, long-term users also suffer physical effects, including weight loss, severe tooth decay and tooth loss, and skin sores.

Cocaine is another powerful stimulant drug. People abuse two chemical forms of cocaine: the water-soluble hydrochloride salt and the water-insoluble cocaine base (or freebase). Users inject or snort the hydrochloride salt, which is a powder. The base form of cocaine is created by processing the drug with ammonia or sodium bicarbonate (baking soda) and water, then heating it to remove the hydrochloride to produce a smokable substance.

The brain's *mesolimbic pathway* (MLP), its dopamine reward pathway, is stimulated by all types of reinforcing stimuli, such as food, sex, and many drugs of abuse, including cocaine. This pathway originates in a region of the midbrain called the ventral tegmental area and extends to the nucleus accumbens, one of the brain's key reward areas. Besides reward, this circuit also regulates emotions and motivation.

In the normal communication process, dopamine is released by a neuron into the synapse where it binds to specialized *dopamine receptors* on neighboring neurons. By this process, dopamine acts as a chemical messenger, carrying a signal from neuron to neuron. Another specialized protein called a *transporter* removes dopamine from the synapse to be recycled for further use.

As is the case with methamphetamine, repeated exposure to cocaine causes the brain to adapt so that the reward pathway becomes less sensitive to natural reinforcers. At the same time, circuits involved in stress become increasingly sensitive, leading to increased displeasure and negative moods when not taking the drug, which are signs of withdrawal. These combined effects make the user more likely to focus a priority on seeking the drug instead of relationships, food, or other natural rewards.

Persons in recovery from stimulus use disorder are at high risk for relapse, even following long periods of abstinence. Research indicates that during periods of abstinence, the memory of the cocaine experience or exposure to cues associated with drug use can trigger strong cravings, which can lead to relapse. (See the work on *cued reactivity* by Anna Rose Childress mentioned in the previous chapter).

**Pharmacology**

As the name implies, stimulant drugs have an energizing effect that promotes an increase in psychological and/or motor activity. Stimulants such as cocaine and the amphetamines have their most pronounced effect on the monoamine neurotransmitters like norepinephrine (NE), epinephrine (E), dopamine (DA) and serotonin (5-HT). This results from their combined actions as reuptake inhibitors, neurotransmitter releasers and monoamine oxidase inhibitors (MAOIs). The arousing and euphoric effects associated with these drugs are caused by these various actions. Stimulants also affect mechanisms triggered in stress situations (the fight-or-flight response) via activation of the sympathetic nervous system (sympathomimetic effects), including increases in heart rate (tachycardia), blood pressure (hypertension) and the release of various hormones.

## AMPHETAMINES

*Amphetamine* is a generic term that applies to a group of synthetic compounds derived from naturally occurring ephedrine found in the ephedra plant indigenous to Eastern Africa. Amphetamines are all classified as indirect-acting agonists at NE, DA and 5-HT synapses. Amphetamine users describe the euphoric effects of the drug in the same terms used by cocaine users, and in the laboratory, subjects cannot distinguish between the effects of cocaine and amphetamines. This is not to suggest that cocaine and amphetamines have the same mechanisms of action. They do not. For example, cocaine effects are relatively brief after intravenous injection, whereas those of methamphetamine may last for hours. Oral ingestion is a common route of amphetamine administration, but like cocaine, intravenous injection, smoking, and snorting are also common.

**Methamphetamines**
First synthesized in 1887 Germany, amphetamine was for a long time, a drug in search of a disease. Nothing was done with the drug, from its discovery (synthesis) until the late 1920's, when it was investigated as a cure or treatment against nearly everything from depression to decongestion. In the 1930's, amphetamine was marketed as Benzedrine, an over-the-counter inhaler to treat nasal congestion (for

asthmatics, hay fever sufferers, and people with colds). By 1937 amphetamine was available by prescription in tablet form.

**Adverse Effects**

Not surprisingly, the actions of amphetamines are similar to cocaine, but not the same. The reinforcing properties of these drugs result from their ability to enhance dopamine action in mesolimbic pathway (MLP). While amphetamines also block dopamine reuptake, their most significant action is to directly stimulate the release of dopamine from neurons (see Figure below). Thus, unlike cocaine, which blocks dopamine reuptake following normal release of the transmitter from the terminal, amphetamines increase dopamine activity independent from neuronal activity. As a result of this difference, amphetamines are more potent than cocaine in increasing the levels of dopamine in the synapse. Contributing to this as well, there is evidence that amphetamines, unlike cocaine, inhibits the enzyme monoamine oxidase, so newly released neurotransmitters remain in synapse longer where binding to and stimulating postsynaptic receptors occurs at a heightened frequency.

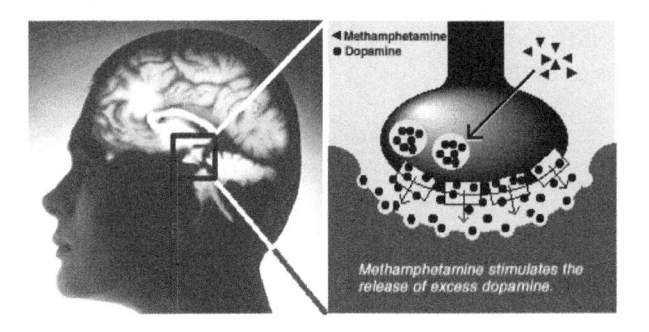

Amphetamines also directly stimulate the release of norepinephrine, epinephrine, and serotonin from neurons. Among the amphetamines, the balance between their actions on these different neurotransmitter systems varies. For example, methylenedioxymethamphetamine (MDMA, aka XTC) has a particularly potent effect on the serotonin system, which provides this drug with a psychedelic effect.

The central nervous system (CNS) actions that result from taking even small amounts of methamphetamine include increased wakefulness, increased physical activity, decreased appetite, increased respiration, hyperthermia, and euphoria. Other CNS effects include irritability, insomnia, confusion, tremors, convulsions, anxiety, paranoia, and aggressiveness. Hyperthermia and convulsions can result in death. Cardiovascular side effects, which include chest pain and hypertension, also can result in cardiovascular collapse and death. In addition, methamphetamine causes increased heart rate and blood pressure and can cause irreversible damage to blood vessels in the brain, producing strokes. Other effects of methamphetamine include respiratory problems, irregular heartbeat, and extreme anorexia.

Like cocaine, acute amphetamine administration results in mood elevation and increased energy. In addition, the user may experience feelings of markedly enhanced physical strength and mental capacity. Amphetamines also stimulate the sympathetic nervous system and produce the physiological effects associated with sympathetic activation. High doses of amphetamine produce a toxic syndrome that is characterized by visual, auditory, and sometimes tactile hallucinations. There is paranoia and disruption of normal thought processes. The toxic reaction to amphetamines can often be indistinguishable from an episode of schizophrenia.

The chart below shows the drug-induced neurotransmitter systems commonly affected by methamphetamine use and the behavioral toxic reactions as a result.

| Methamphetamine-Induced Behavioral Toxicity |||
| --- | --- | --- |
| Symptom | Complication | Neurotransmitter |
| paranoia | psychotic episode | increased DA |
| hypertension | cerebral hemorrhage | increased NE |
| tachycardia | cardiac arrhythmia | increased NE |
| increased physical energy | hyperexcitability | increased NE |
| anorexia | malnutrition | increased NE |
| hyperthermia | heat stroke | increased NE |
| insomnia | exacerbates paranoia | increased NE |
| euphoria | dysphoria | increased DA, then after repeated use, decreased DA |
| hypersexuality and increased susceptibility to STDs | hyposexuality and depression | increased DA, then after repeated use, decreased DA |

## Chronic Effects

As with cocaine, both sensitization and tolerance to different effects of amphetamines occur. Animal studies have shown that intermittent administration of amphetamines results in sensitization to the motor stimulating effects. This sensitization is thought to be due to an augmentation of dopamine release after intermittent, repeated drug administration.

Tolerance to the euphoric effects of amphetamine develops after prolonged, continuous use. Such tolerance is believed to be caused by depletion of stored neurotransmitters, especially dopamine, in the presynaptic terminals as a result of the continued stimulation of release from the stores by the drug. Drug craving is increased with continued amphetamine use.

Withdrawal from high doses produces prolonged sleep, dysphoria, severe depression, lassitude, increased appetite, and craving for the drug. Chronic abuse produces a psychosis resembling the primary symptoms of schizophrenia and is characterized by paranoia, and auditory and visual hallucinations. The most dangerous stage of the binge cycle is known as *tweaking*. Typically, during this stage, the abuser has not slept in three to fifteen days and is extremely irritable and paranoid. The "tweaker" has an intense craving for more methamphetamine; however, no dosage will help recreate the euphoric high. This causes frustration and can lead to unpredictability and a potential for violence.

Treatment enables people to counteract methamphetamine's disruptive effects on their brain and behavior and regain control of their lives - but it takes time.

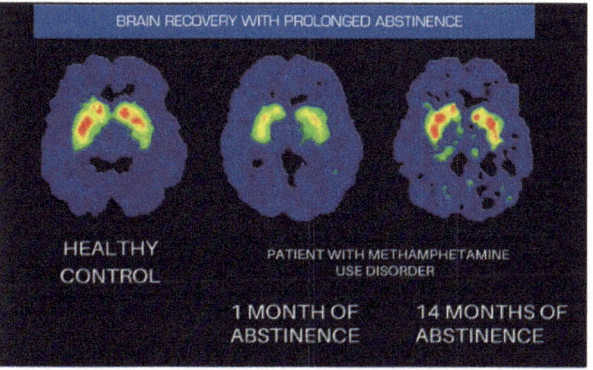

The images in the figure above showing the density of dopamine transporters in the brain illustrate the brain's remarkable ability to recover, at least in part, after a long abstinence from drugs—in this case, methamphetamine. Compare far left-slide to middle and far right-side images.

**Methamphetamine Analogs**
Several dozen analogs of amphetamine and methamphetamine are hallucinogenic; many have been scheduled under the

Controlled Substances Act (CSA). The methamphetamine analog most commonly used is MDMA (3,4- methylenedioxy-methamphetamine), also known as *Ecstasy or XTC*.

MDMA is structurally similar to both methamphetamine and mescaline, and stimulates hallucinations. MDMA was first synthesized in the early 1950s as an appetite suppressant, although it was never used as such. It was first made illegally in 1972, but was not widely abused until the 1980s. Beliefs about MDMA are reminiscent of similar claims made about LSD in the 1950s and 1960s, which proved to be untrue. According to its proponents, MDMA can make people trust each other and break down barriers between therapists and patients, lovers, and family members. In fact, various claims have been made by a few psychiatrists for the use of MDMA to enhance psychotherapy. However, no evidence has been presented to document these few anecdotal reports.

Many of the problems that users encounter with MDMA are similar to those found with the use of amphetamines and cocaine. These psychological difficulties include confusion, depression, sleep problems, drug craving, severe anxiety, and paranoia which sometimes occur weeks after taking MDMA along with psychotic episodes.

Physical symptoms include muscle tension, teeth-clenching, nausea, blurred vision, rapid eye movements, faintness, and chills. Increased heart rate and blood pressure pose a special risk for people with circulatory or heart disease.

**Cocaine**
Cocaine is found in the leaves of the *Erythroxylon coca* plant, a large shrub indigenous to South America. The compound is extracted from the leaves and processed into either rudimentary paste, powder or free-base form. Adding hydrochloric acid to the paste makes cocaine powder (cocaine hydrochloride). The only clinical application of cocaine is as a local anesthetic (in preparation to pass a tube in the nose or throat).

**Adverse Effects**
Physical effects of cocaine use include constricted peripheral blood vessels, dilated pupils, and increased body temperature, heart rate, and

blood pressure. The duration of cocaine's immediate euphoric effects, which include hyperstimulation, reduced fatigue, and mental clarity, depends on the route of administration. The faster the absorption, the more intense the high. On the other hand, the faster the absorption, the shorter the duration of action. The high from snorting may last 15 to 30 minutes, while that from smoking may last 5 to 10 minutes. Increased use can reduce the period of stimulation.

Some cocaine users report feelings of restlessness, irritability and anxiety. An appreciable tolerance to the high may develop, and many addicts report that they seek but fail to achieve as much pleasure as they did from their first exposure. Scientific evidence suggests that the powerful reinforcing property of cocaine is responsible for an individual's continued use, despite harmful physical and social consequences. In rare instances, sudden death can occur on the first use of cocaine or unexpectedly thereafter. However, there is no way to determine who is prone to sudden death.

High doses of cocaine and/or prolonged use can trigger paranoia. Smoking crack cocaine can produce a particularly aggressive paranoid behavior in users. When addicted individuals stop using cocaine, they often become depressed. This also may lead to further cocaine use to alleviate the depression. Prolonged cocaine snorting can result in ulceration of the mucous membrane of the nose and can damage the nasal septum enough to cause it to collapse.

Cocaine-related deaths are often a result of cardiac arrest or seizures followed by respiratory arrest. Other toxic effects of high doses of cocaine include delirium, seizures, stupor, cardiac arrhythmias, and coma. Seizures can sometimes result in sustained convulsions where multiple seizure episodes one right after the other (called, status epilepticus).

The most prominent pharmacological effect of cocaine is blocking dopamine reuptake back into the presynaptic terminal once it has been released from a neuron terminal, resulting in increased levels of dopamine at its synapses in the brain. The specific uptake site for dopamine has been identified and cocaine's actions on the mechanism that transports dopamine back into the neuron is an active area of research. Within the brain mesolimbic pathway (MLP), levels of dopamine increase in the synapses between the terminals of the neurons projecting from the ventral tegmental area and the neurons in the nucleus accumbens and medial prefrontal cortex. In addition to blocking dopamine reuptake, cocaine also blocks the reuptake of norepinephrine and serotonin.

The acute behavioral effects of cocaine are the result of these neurochemical actions. The acute reinforcing properties of cocaine are due to its capacity to enhance the activity of dopamine in MLP. The reinforcing properties of cocaine are mediated via dopamine activation of at least two receptor subtypes, the D1 and D2 dopamine receptor subtypes, and more recently there is evidence for an action at D3 receptors as well.

The increase in dopamine activity via D2 and DI receptors is also important in the other behavioral effects of cocaine. When combining cocaine and alcohol consumption, research shows that the human liver combines both drugs and makes a third substance, cocaethylene, that intensifies cocaine's euphoric effects, while potentially increasing the risk of sudden death.

**Chronic Effects**
Chronic administration of cocaine activates a number of brain neurochemical compensatory mechanisms. Both short and long-term changes in the dynamics of neurotransmission following repeated cocaine administration have been well documented. Animal studies indicate that continued administration results in a sustained increase in dopamine levels within the synapses of the nucleus accumbens. This is believed to be due to a decreased sensitivity of dopamine autoreceptors, which regulate the release of dopamine from the presynaptic terminal. In their normal state, these autoreceptors decrease the amount of dopamine released into the synapse. Changes also seem to occur in the number of postsynaptic receptors for dopamine, but the exact nature of these changes has yet to be characterized. Both increases and decreases in receptor numbers have been reported.

A number of changes occur in the intracellular mechanisms, including second messenger systems, involved in dopamine neurons in the ventral tegmental area and nucleus accumbens have been described following chronic cocaine administration. The changes are thought to be due to alterations in the expression of the genes that regulate and control the intracellular mechanisms. The net effect of these changes is to reduce the capacity of ventral tegmental neurons to transmit dopamine signals to the neurons in the nucleus accumbens. These represent a mechanism by which tolerance to the rewarding properties of cocaine would develop and could contribute to overall cocaine craving. Importantly, these changes are lacking in other dopamine pathways not involved in drug reward. Similar changes were observed following chronic morphine administration. These findings suggest a common physiological response to chronic administration of these drugs of abuse. Finally, repeated administration of cocaine changes the levels of other neurotransmitters, most notably the neuropeptides. These changes may result from alterations in dopamine transmission that affects other areas of the brain. These secondary responses indicate that the neurochemical adaptive response to repetitive cocaine administration involves a complex interaction between multiple neuronal pathways and neurotransmitter systems. Studies suggest that how the drug is administered affects whether sensitization or tolerance occurs.

A withdrawal syndrome occurs with the abrupt cessation of cocaine after repeated use. This syndrome is marked by prolonged sleep, depression, lassitude, increased appetite, and craving for the drug. In animal studies, cocaine withdrawal results in an increase in the level of electrical stimulation necessary to induce a rat to self-stimulate the brain reward system. It is suspected that the pharmacological mechanism underlying cocaine withdrawal is related to the hypoactivity in dopamine functioning within the brain reward system. Avoidance of the withdrawal reaction is another important determinant factor in continued cocaine use (negative reinforcement).

**Comparing PK differences between cocaine and methamphetamine**

| PK Differences Between Methamphetamine and Cocaine ||
|---|---|
| Methamphetamine | Cocaine |
| Stimulant | Stimulant and local anesthetic |
| Synthetic (human-made in a lab) | Plant-derived (botanical) |
| Inhaled, injected, snorted, oral | Same |
| Long acting (8 to 24 hours). 50% of the drug is removed from the body in 12 hours. Uses CYP2D6 pathway for metabolism. | Short acting (20 to 30 minutes). 50% of the drug is removed from the body in 1 hour. Uses CYP3A4 pathway for metabolism. |
| Reuptake blockade of dopamine, norepinephrine, and serotonin. Has MAOI-like activity inhibiting enzyme degradation | Reuptake blockade of dopamine and serotonin. Also alters mu opioid receptors. |
| Neurotoxic effects associated with damage to central monoamine systems, particularly dopamine signaling. Also involves oxidative stress, excitotoxicity, and neuroinflammation | Neurotoxic effects of combinations of cocaine with other drugs are also discussed. In summary, cocaine neurotoxicity may underlie brain dysfunction in cocaine and polydrug abusers and may predispose the brain to neurodegeneration |

## Synthetic Cathinones ("Bath Salts")

Synthetic cathinones are a class of lab-made stimulants chemically related to substances found in the khat plant. Khat is a shrub grown in East Africa and southern Arabia that some people consume for its stimulant effects. Illicit synthetic cathinones are more commonly known as "bath salts." People may ingest illicit synthetic cathinones intentionally—sometimes as cheaper or more accessible alternatives to other drugs—or unintentionally, as contaminants in other drugs. Research shows illicit synthetic cathinone use can be life-threatening and cause other serious health and safety problems. People who use synthetic cathinones regularly may develop stimulant use disorder.

## Caffeine

Caffeine is the most widely used psychoactive substance in the world. Surveys indicate that 92 percent of adults in North America regularly consume caffeine, mostly in coffee or tea. Caffeine belongs to a class of compounds called *methylxanthines,* CNS stimulants.

Caffeine blocks both the A1 and A2 receptors for inhibitory neurotransmitter adenosine, causing neural stimulation. Adenosine inhibits the release of various neurotransmitters, in particular the excitatory amino acid glutamate. Therefore, caffeine block of adenosine receptors results in increased glutamate activity.

Caffeine also increases the levels of norepinephrine and serotonin, which contributes to the drug's CNS stimulating effects. Caffeine's effects on dopamine are unclear in that increases, decreases, or no change in the release of dopamine have been observed following caffeine administration in various experiments.

In humans, caffeine has a general alerting affect, and it has been shown to increase locomotor activity in laboratory animals. However, evidence shows great individual variability in caffeine's effects, linked to differences in rates of caffeine absorption from the gastrointestinal system and metabolism in the body. Age also seems to affect the response to caffeine, in that older people show an increased sensitivity to caffeine's stimulating effects. This is particularly true of caffeine's disruptive effects on sleep.

Caffeine exhibits weak reinforcing effects in animal self-administration experiments. The level of responding induced by caffeine is much less than that seen with other stimulants such as amphetamine and cocaine. Caffeine's reinforcing actions are also minimal and dose-dependent. Low doses are mildly reinforcing with subjects reporting positive effects, while higher doses produce adverse effects. The results from human studies show that reinforcement occurs only under certain conditions and certain individuals.

The mechanism of caffeine's reinforcing actions is unknown. Tolerance may develop to many of the physical manifestations of caffeine's actions such as increased heart rate and higher blood pressure. There is, evidence that tolerance develops to its behavioral consequences including alertness and wakefulness. In animals, tolerance develops to some of caffeine's behavioral effects such as the stimulation of locomotor activity.\

A withdrawal syndrome has clearly and repeatedly been demonstrated after the cessation of chronic caffeine consumption. Changes in mood and behavior can occur with lethargy and headache being the two most common symptoms of caffeine withdrawal. These changes may be the result of a compensation increase in adenosine receptors resulting from the chronic blockade by caffeine. However, more studies are needed to confirm this possibility.

**Nicotine**
It is generally accepted that while people smoke tobacco for many social or cultural reasons, the majority of people smoke in order to experience the psychoactive properties of nicotine. Furthermore, a significant proportion of habitual smokers become dependent on nicotine and tobacco smoking has all the attributes of drug use considered to be addicting. Nicotine activates one of the receptor subtypes for the neurotransmitter acetylcholine. As a result, this receptor is called the nicotine receptor. The psychological effects of nicotine are fairly subtle and include mood changes, stress reduction, and some performance enhancement.

When tobacco is smoked, nicotine is readily absorbed by the lungs. Studies of smoking patterns have shown that habitual smokers tend to smoke more efficiently, because they inhale longer, have shorter intervals between puffs, and take a greater number of puffs per cigarette thus increasing the dose of nicotine they receive. Smokeless tobacco involves either chewing tobacco leaves or placing tobacco between the cheek and gums. The blood nicotine level achieved using smokeless tobacco can be as high as that achieved from smoking cigarettes. Because of the route of administration, however, blood nicotine levels remain higher longer.

Evidence indicates that the diseases related to the use of tobacco may be caused by different constituents of tobacco or tobacco smoke. For example, cardiovascular effects are related to carbon monoxide in the smoke, and the effects on the heart and various cancers are probably due to carcinogens in the tobacco.

Nicotine stimulates the release of dopamine from dopamine neurons in the MLP. Activation of nicotine receptors stimulates activity in dopamine neurons in the ventral tegmental area. However, when compared to the effects of cocaine or amphetamine, the nicotine increase in dopamine release is modest, and as a result, nicotine is a comparatively weak reinforcer in animal experiments. Nonetheless, nicotine reinforcing properties are thought to be the result of this action. Animal study results indicate that activation of nicotine receptors also stimulates the release of noradrenaline from neurons in the locus coeruleus and may reduce serotonin activity in the hippocampus. However, the exact nature of these changes and the role they may play in the behavioral effects of nicotine is unclear.

Tolerance develops to many of the effects of nicotine, and a withdrawal syndrome is marked by irritability, anxiety, restlessness, and difficulty concentrating. In addition, a craving for tobacco occurs but may subside in a few days although the mechanisms underlying these changes are unknown. Animal studies suggest that chronic administration of nicotine increases the number of nicotine receptors, yet the action that mediates this increase and its possible involvement in nicotine tolerance and withdrawal remains to be clarified. Within 12 hours after a smoker has his last cigarette, the levels of carbon monoxide and nicotine in the system declines rapidly, and the individual's heart and lungs begin to repair the damage caused by cigarette smoke. Within a few days, the individual probably will begin to notice some remarkable physical changes. The sense of smell and taste may improve. As a person's body begins to repair itself from the damages of smoking, the individual may feel worse for a while, before feeling better. Immediately after quitting, many ex-smokers experience "symptoms of recovery" such as temporary weight gain caused by fluid retention, irregularity, and dry, sore gums or tongue. They may feel edgy, hungry, tired, and short-tempered, with trouble sleeping and frequent coughing. These symptoms are the result of the body clearing itself of nicotine, and most of the nicotine is eliminated in 2 to 3 days.

**Treatment: Nicotine Replacement Therapy**
Nicotine gum and lozenges release nicotine slowly into the mouth. Nicotine patches applied to the skin and slowly release nicotine through the pores of the skin into the bloodstream. The nicotine inhaler has a holder that contains nicotine. The inhaler delivers a puff of nicotine vapor into the mouth and throat.

Nicotine replacement therapy (NRT) helps reduce nicotine withdrawal and craving by supplying the body with nicotine. It contains about one-third to one-half the amount of nicotine found in most cigarettes. Tars, carbon monoxide, and other toxic chemicals in tobacco cause harmful effects, not the nicotine. When tobacco smoke is inhaled, the nicotine in the smoke moves quickly from the lungs into the bloodstream. The nicotine in replacement products takes much longer to get into the system. This is why nicotine replacement medications are much less likely to cause dependence on nicotine than are cigarettes and other tobacco products. Nicotine by itself is not nearly as harmful as smoking which includes the inhalation of a variety of harmful and toxic substances.

**Chantix** (varenicline)
Chantix works by blocking the effect that nicotine has on the brain. As with other smoking cessation medications, Chantix also stimulates the release of low levels of dopamine in the brain to help reduce the symptoms of nicotine craving and withdrawal. In addition, Chantix blocks nicotinic receptors in the brain. The idea of blocking is that if the person relapses, the cigarette will not stimulate the brain's receptors with much intensity. Cigarettes, ideally, become markedly less pleasurable, and the desire to return to regular smoking is reduced.

**Zyban** (bupropion hydrochloride)
Zyban is a non-nicotine aid to smoking cessation. Zyban is chemically unrelated to nicotine or other agents currently used in the treatment of nicotine addiction. Initially developed and marketed as the antidepressant Wellbutrin. It works by increasing levels of brain dopamine and norepinephrine that is associated with the decrease in withdrawal intensity from nicotine.

**Prescription Stimulants**
According to the Substance Abuse and Mental Health Services

Association (SAMHSA), prescription stimulants belong to a larger class of drugs that includes both legal and illegal substances. Stimulants may temporarily increase alertness, attention, and energy, effects caused by the increased level of activity that occurs in the central nervous system as a result of stimulant use. Although all stimulants have similar behavioral and physiological effects, they differ in their mechanism of action or the ways in which they produce an effect.

Prescription stimulants such as amphetamine (Adderall) and methylphenidate (Ritalin) address the symptoms of attention-deficit hyperactivity disorder (ADHD). When taken as prescribed, prescription stimulants can increase a person living with ADHD's ability to pay attention and focus on tasks. When misused, for example by taking doses higher or more frequently than prescribed, prescription stimulants have the potential to lead to substance use disorder. Most prescription stimulants are amphetamine-type stimulants and primarily consist of medications used to treat ADHD and narcolepsy.

They also include diet aids, although most stimulant diet aids are no longer available in the United States. Prescription stimulants have several medical benefits for those who need them, including increased alertness, concentration, and attention. These effects make prescription stimulants a first line treatment for ADHD, which is characterized by inattention, distraction, and/or hyperactivity and impulsivity that can cause substantial functional impairment.

Of interest is the recent 2024 study from the University of Michigan, School of Nursing showing that the use of stimulant therapy by adolescents with ADHD was not associated with later prescription drug misuse (McCabe, et al. 2024.).

The study concluded that there were no significant differences between adolescents with or without lifetime stimulants in later incidence or prevalence of past-year prescription drug misuse during young adulthood.

The most robust predictor of prescription stimulant misuse during young adulthood was prescription stimulant misuse during adolescence; similarly, the most robust predictors of prescription opioid and prescription benzodiazepine misuse during young adulthood were prescription opioid and prescription benzodiazepine misuse (respectively) during adolescence. Prescription Stimulants are shown in the chart below:

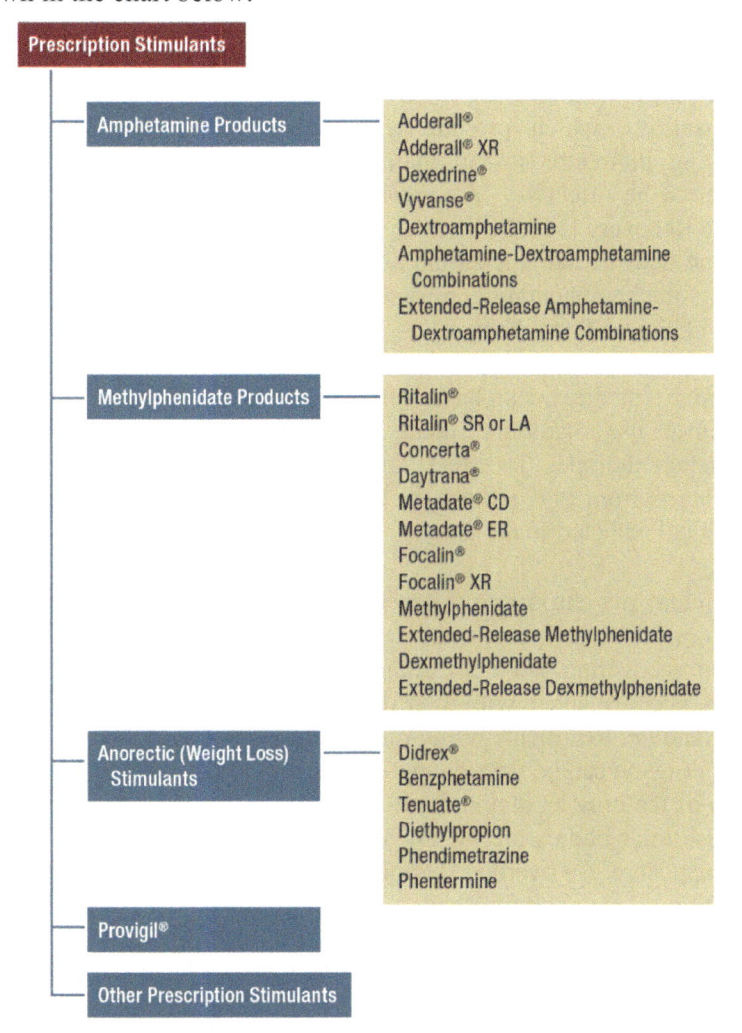

**Prescription Stimulants**

- **Amphetamine Products**
  - Adderall®
  - Adderall® XR
  - Dexedrine®
  - Vyvanse®
  - Dextroamphetamine
  - Amphetamine-Dextroamphetamine Combinations
  - Extended-Release Amphetamine-Dextroamphetamine Combinations

- **Methylphenidate Products**
  - Ritalin®
  - Ritalin® SR or LA
  - Concerta®
  - Daytrana®
  - Metadate® CD
  - Metadate® ER
  - Focalin®
  - Focalin® XR
  - Methylphenidate
  - Extended-Release Methylphenidate
  - Dexmethylphenidate
  - Extended-Release Dexmethylphenidate

- **Anorectic (Weight Loss) Stimulants**
  - Didrex®
  - Benzphetamine
  - Tenuate®
  - Diethylpropion
  - Phendimetrazine
  - Phentermine

- **Provigil®**

- **Other Prescription Stimulants**

**Treatment for Stimulant Use Disorder**

As NIDA states, "Like treatment for other chronic diseases such as heart disease or asthma, addiction treatment is not a cure, but a way of managing the condition. Treatment enables people to counteract addiction's disruptive effects on their brain and behavior and regain control of their lives. The chronic nature of addiction means that for some people *relapse,* or a return to drug use after an attempt to stop, can be part of the process, but newer treatments are designed to help with relapse prevention. Relapse rates for drug use are similar to rates for other chronic medical illnesses. If people stop following their medical treatment plan, they are likely to relapse."

The most effective treatments for methamphetamine addiction at this point are behavioral therapies, such as cognitive-behavioral and contingency management interventions. Contingency management interventions, which provide tangible incentives in exchange for engaging in treatment and maintaining abstinence, have also been shown to be effective. Motivational Incentives for Enhancing Drug Abuse Recovery (MIEDAR), an incentive-based method for promoting cocaine and methamphetamine abstinence, has demonstrated efficacy among methamphetamine misusers through NIDA's National Drug Abuse Clinical Trials Network.

Although medications have proven effective in treating some substance use disorders, there are currently no medications that counteract the specific effects of methamphetamine or that prolong abstinence from and reduce the misuse of methamphetamine by an individual addicted to the drug.

Treatment of chronic diseases involves changing deeply rooted behaviors, and relapse doesn't mean treatment has failed. When a person recovering from an addiction relapses, it indicates that the person needs to speak with their doctor to resume treatment, modify it, or try another treatment  While relapse is a normal part of recovery, for some drugs, it can be very dangerous—even deadly. If a person uses as much of the drug as they did before quitting, they can easily overdose because their bodies are no longer adapted to their previous level of drug exposure. An overdose happens when the person uses enough of a drug to produce uncomfortable feelings, life-threatening symptoms, or death.

A further note about treatment outcomes for persons recovering from stimulant use disorder.  A 2024 study was funded by the National Institute on Drug Abuse and the National Institute of Health and published in the January 10, 2024 Journal of Addiction, in patients with stimulant use disorder (SUD), even slight reductions in drug use can lessen depression and reduce cravings, this new analysis showed.

**Total abstinence not the only treatment goal in Stimulant Use Disorder**

Abstinence has long been the overall goal of SUD treatment, the investigators noted. The findings from this pooled analysis of randomized clinical trials support what investigators noted was a growing recognition that reducing stimulant use can lead to better outcomes. "This study provides evidence that reducing the overall use of drugs is important and clinically meaningful," study author Mehdi Farokhnia, MD, MPH, of the National Institute on Drug Abuse, North Bethesda, Maryland, wrote in a press release. "This shift may open opportunities for medication development that can help individuals achieve these improved outcomes, even if complete abstinence is not immediately achievable or wanted."

**Not the only indicator of success**
To compare clinical indicators of improvement among those with SUDs who achieved abstinence or reduced their use, investigators pooled data from 13 randomized clinical trials with more than 2000 patients seeking treatment for cocaine or methamphetamine use disorders at centers in the United States from 2001 to 2017. The trials used similar study protocols, including similar eligibility criteria, recruitment methods, and outcome measures. Participants were 18 or older and met criteria for methamphetamine or cocaine dependence at the beginning of each trial.

Among the participants, 1196 sought treatment for cocaine use disorder and 866 for methamphetamine use disorder. Of those, just 1487 had outcomes available by the end of the trial. Most participants had no change in the level of use or increased their use through the trial (68%) or transitioned from low (1-4 days a month) to high (5 or more days a month) frequency use. Nearly one third of participants (32%) stopped or reduced drug use, including 18% who cut down on stimulant use and 14% who abstained altogether.

Participants using methamphetamine were more likely to be in the abstinence vs reduced use category (21.3% vs 13.9%, respectively), whereas participants using cocaine were less likely to be in the abstinence vs reduced use category (9.1% vs 20.9%). Those who reached abstinence showed better clinical improvement than those who reduced use on most clinical measures ($P < .009$). However, there were no significant differences between groups on the Addiction Severity Index (ASI) psychiatric problems subscale and cravings for secondary drugs.

The findings from the study suggest that reduced frequency of stimulant use is also associated with improved psychosocial functioning. These findings suggest the need to re-evaluate the traditional approach of exclusively relying on total abstinence as the only indicator of successful treatment, a goal that may not be achievable for all patients, especially after one treatment episode.

Those who reduced drug intake showed a significant association with nearly all clinical indicators of improvement ($P < .010$) compared with those who didn't, except for the ASI psychiatric problems subscale and family/social relationship domains of the Problem Free Functioning scale, and HIV risk behavior.

## SUGGESTED READINGS ON THIS TOPIC

ASAM Management of Stimulant Use Disorder
https://downloads.asam.org/sitefinity-production-blobs/docs/default-source/quality-science/stud_guideline_document_final.pdf?sfvrsn=71094b38_1

Farokhnia M, et al. Reduced drug use as an alternative valid outcome in individuals with stimulant use disorders: Findings from 13 multisite randomized clinical trials. Society for the Study of Addiction. https://doi.org/10.1111/add.16409. January 10, 2024.

McCabe SE. Stimulants for ADHD Not Linked to Prescription Drug Misuse. University of Michigan School of Nursing. February 7, 2024. *Psychiatric Sciences*.

Moore, EA. The Amphetamine Debate. McFarland. 2010. ISBN-10 : 9780786458738.

National Institute on Drug Abuse. (2018). Prescription Stimulants DrugFacts. from
https://www.drugabuse.gov/publications/drugfacts/prescription-stimulants

National Institute on Drug Abuse. (2021). How is methamphetamine different from other stimulants, such as cocaine? from
https://www.drugabuse.gov/publications/research-reports/methamphetamine/how-methamphetamine-different-other-stimulants-such-cocaine

Substance Abuse and Mental Health Services Administration. (2020). 2019 National Survey of Drug Use and Health. from
https://www.samhsa.gov/data/release/2019-national-survey-drug-use-and-health-nsduh-releases

Taba, P. The Neuropsychiatric Complications of Stimulant Abuse. Academic Press. 2015. ISBN-10 : 0128029781.

Vosburg, S. K. et al. (2021) Characterizing pathways of non-oral prescriptions stimulant non-medical use among adults recruited from Reddit. Frontiers in Psychiatry, 11.

# CHAPTER 10. OPIOID DRUGS

## **Key Concepts**

| | |
|---|---|
| Analgesia | A reduction or absence of the sense of pain without loss of consciousness. |
| Bradycardia | Slowness of the heart rate, usually fewer than 60 beats per minute in an adult human. |
| Buprenorphine | Brand names, Buprenex®, Suboxone®, Subutex®, it is a semi-synthetic opiate with partial agonist and antagonist actions used in pain and addiction medicine. |
| COWS | The Clinical Opiate Withdrawal Scale (COWS) is a clinician-administered, pen and paper instrument that rates eleven common opiate withdrawal signs or symptoms. The COWS score was developed to assist clinicians in quantifying the degree of opiate withdrawal during their patient assessments. |
| Delta Opioid Receptor | Receptor subtype within the endogenous opioid system. Delta1 is responsible for analgesia and euphoria, delta2 only causes analgesia. |
| Fentanyl | A powerful synthetic opioid that is similar to morphine but is 50 to 100 times more potent. Used in virtually all other drugs as an adulterant, fentanyl is the most common drug involved fatal overdoses due to its extreme potency. |
| Kappa Opioid Receptor | Receptor subtype within the endogenous opioid system largely responsible for sedation and analgesia. |
| Methadone | Long-lasting synthetic opioid used in pain and addiction medicine. |

| | |
|---|---|
| Mu Opioid Receptor | Receptor subtype within the endogenous opioid system responsible for euphoria, sedation, analgesia and, if over stimulated, respiratory depression. |
| Nociception | The physiological system by which one feels the sensation of pain. |
| Nociceptors | A sensory receptor that responds selectively to potentially damaging stimuli. Its stimulation results in pain sensation. |
| Naloxone | Also called Narcan, it is a life-saving medication used to reverse an opioid overdose, including heroin, fentanyl and prescription opioid medications. |
| Naltrexone | A modified version of naloxone but with a longer half-life. Naltrexone is a medication that blocks the effects of opioids. It competes with these drugs for opioid receptors in the brain and disallows activation. Thus, it is used in the treatment of opioid addiction. Naltrexone is also used as an anti-craving medicine in the treatment of alcoholism. |
| Opioids | Opioids are a class of drugs naturally found in the opium poppy plant. Some opioids are made from the plant directly, and others, like fentanyl, are made in labs using the same chemical structure (semi-synthetic or synthetic). |
| Opioid Withdrawal Syndrome | Abrupt cessation or reduction of opioid use produces signs and symptoms of a withdrawal with symptoms of rhinorrhea, myalgia, diarrhea, nausea/vomiting, insomnia, autonomic hyperactivity (tachypnea, hyperreflexia, tachycardia, sweating, hypertension, hyperthermia). |

# CHAPTER 10

## Opioid Drugs

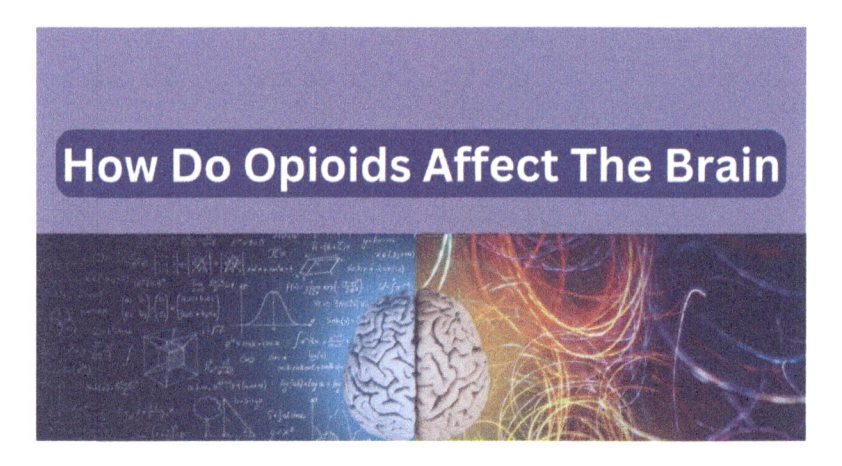

In this chapter, I'll review the opioids, their mechanisms of action for the endorphins and opioid receptors sites, and then discuss opioid use disorders and medication assisted treatment (MAT).

To start the discussion, opioids are a class of drugs that include the illegal drug heroin, synthetic opioids such as fentanyl, and pain relievers available legally by prescription, such as oxycodone (OxyContin®), hydrocodone (Vicodin®), codeine, morphine, and many others including fentanyl. All opioids have a similar mechanism of action (how they work). They activate an area of nerve cells in the brain and body called opioid receptors that block pain signals between the brain and the body.

Morphine is considered to be the archetypal opioid analgesic and the agent to which all other painkillers are compared. There is evidence to suggest that as long ago as 3000 BC the opium poppy, *Papaver somniferum*, was cultivated for its active opioid ingredient, opium.

The human body produces its own natural endogenous opioids, called endorphins, that when released, activate opioid receptors in the brain as part of the response to pain or other stress stimuli. Exogenous (coming from outside the body) opioid drugs activate this same system, and over time can change how the body responds to pain and pleasure.

Endorphins are proteins that are primarily the chemical response to physiologic stressors such as pain. They function through various mechanisms in both the central and peripheral nervous system to relieve pain when bound to their mu-opioid receptors. Opioid drugs function by mimicking the natural endorphins, competing for receptor site binding. In the acute setting, opioid drugs inhibit the production of endogenous opiates while in the chronic setting, opioid drugs inhibit the production of both endogenous opiates and mu-opioid receptors. Risks associated with chronic opiate use include opioid induced hyperalgesia, tolerance and opioid use disorder.

**Opioid Receptor Sites**
Several opioid receptor subtypes have been described and characterized. Analgesics are primarily used for their ability to reduce the perception of pain impulses by the Central Nervous System (CNS). Analgesic activity is mediated by opiate receptors in the CNS.

To date, five types of opioid receptors have been discovered which are: mu opioid receptor (MOR); kappa opioid receptor (KOR); delta opioid receptor (DOR); nociception opioid receptor (NOR) and; zeta opioid receptor (ZOR). Within these different types are a subset of subtypes, mu1, mu2, mu3, kappa1, kappa2, kappa3, delta1, and delta2. Opioids mediate their effects *via* opioid receptors: mu, delta, and kappa.

MOR: Classic opioids like morphine bind here preferentially. Also, the endogenous opioids Beta-Endorphin and Leu-Enkephalin, exerts some of its effects here. They are believed to be responsible for most of analgesic properties of opiates, as well as for euphoria, sedation, constipation, respiratory depression and dependence.

KOR Receptors: The endogenous opioid Dynorphin exerts some of its effects here. These specifically respond to pain from non-thermal stimuli.

DOR Receptors: These appear to be the preferential binding site for the
endogenous Met-Enkephalin, as well as several synthetic peptides. They are probably more important in the periphery and contribute to analgesic effects.

**Pure Agonists, Partial Agonists and Antagonists**
An opioid agonist is a substance that binds to any of the several subtypes of opioid receptor and produces some action. An opioid

antagonist is a substance that binds to receptor subtypes and inhibits an action. Opiates with an affinity for μ-receptors can be classified into **four** groups:

- Pure Agonists: These have high affinity for μ - receptors as well as strong intrinsic activity at said receptors. (e.g., heroin, morphine, and methadone)

- Partial Agonists: These drugs bind to the receptor but exert only a partial or even minimal action. Some of these have both agonist and antagonist activity at the μ - receptors (e.g., buprenorphine)
- Pure Antagonists: These bind to the opiate receptors but to do not exert any activity. All they do is to block the effects of agonists at μ - receptor sites by preventing any agonists from binding to the receptor. In dependent individuals, they precipitate withdrawal symptoms (e.g., naloxone, naltrexone)

- Mixed Agonist-Antagonists: These drugs act as agonists at one receptor whilst behaving as an antagonist at other receptors. (e.g., pentazocine, butorphanol, nalbuphine)

**Opioid Use Disorder (OUD)**
According to the DSM-5 TR, In order to confirm a diagnosis of OUD, at least two of the following should be observed within a 12-month period:
1. Opioids are often taken in larger amounts or over a longer period than was intended.
2. There is a persistent desire or unsuccessful efforts to cut down or control opioid use.
3. A great deal of time is spent in activities necessary to obtain the opioid, use the opioid, or recover from its effects.
4. Craving, or a strong desire or urge to use opioids.
5. Recurrent opioid use resulting in a failure to fulfill major role obligations at work, school, or home.
6. Continued opioid use despite having persistent or recurrent social or interpersonal problems caused or exacerbated by the effects of opioids.
7. Important social, occupational, or recreational activities are given up or reduced because of opioid use.
8. Recurrent opioid use in situations in which it is physically hazardous.

9. Continued opioid use despite knowledge of having a persistent or recurrent physical or psychological problem that is likely to have been caused or exacerbated by the substance.
10. Exhibits tolerance
11. Exhibits withdrawal

As you may recall from previous chapters, substance use disorders, including OUD, are spectrum disorders with varying levels of severity and number of manifesting symptoms. Determining the severity levels helps to define a best treatment level of care placement. The DSM-5 TR suggested this metric:   Mild: 2-3 symptoms. Moderate: 4-5 symptoms. Severe: 6 or more symptoms from the diagnostic criteria above.

**Note:** Tolerance is defined as either: 1) a need for markedly increased amounts of opioids to achieve intoxication or desired effect, or 2) a markedly diminished effect with continued use of the same amount of an opioid.

Withdrawal management (WM), (we no longer use the outdated and highly inaccurate term "detox"), refers to the medical and psychological care of patients who are experiencing withdrawal symptoms as a result of ceasing or reducing use of their drug of dependence. And, It is very common for people who complete withdrawal management to relapse to drug use. It is unrealistic to think that withdrawal management will lead to sustained abstinence. Rather, withdrawal management is an important first step before a patient commences treatment.  As stated by the American College of Emergency Physicians, opioid withdrawal manifests as 2 distinct yet reinforcing subsyndromes, psychological and physiologic. The physiologic findings include restlessness, nausea, vomiting, diarrhea, piloerection, diaphoresis, yawning, mydriasis, and mild autonomic hyperactivity. The psychological effects, including pain, anxiety, stress intolerance, irritability, and drug craving, coincide with the physiologic signs but may persist for weeks to months after physiologic normalization. Abstinence-related opioid withdrawal results from the discontinuation of opioid use in a patient with opioid dependent and is generally not life threatening.

Generally, to assess the severity of symptoms of the opioid withdrawal syndrome, the use of the ***Clinical Opiate Withdrawal Scale*** (COWS) is useful.  It can provide important information about treatment decisions during the patient's withdrawal occurrence. The COWS is an easy-to-use 11-item scale designed to be administered by a clinician. This tool can be used in both inpatient and outpatient settings to reproducibly rate common signs and symptoms of opiate withdrawal and monitor these symptoms over time. The summed score for the complete scale can be used to help clinicians determine the stage or severity of opiate withdrawal and assess the level of physical dependence on opioids.

Clients of opioid use disorder treatment programs often say in so many words, that using opioids calms their nerves, satisfies their cravings and helps them relax. Neuroscientists believe they now know why that might be. Namely, that ingesting opioids produces major changes in the flow of "feel good" chemicals in the brain (i.e. dopamine). Heroin is a semisynthetic opioid derived from dried sap of the opium poppy. Also derived from poppy, though not synthesized, are morphine and codeine.

Wesson & Ling, J Psychoactive Drugs. 2003 Apr-Jun;35(2):253-9.

## COWS Clinical Opiate Withdrawal Scale

| Resting Pulse Rate: ____ beats/minute Measured after patient is sitting or lying for one minute | | GI Upset: over last 1/2 hour | |
|---|---|---|---|
| 0 | Pulse rate 80 or below | 0 | No GI symptoms |
| 1 | Pulse rate 81-100 | 1 | Stomach cramps |
| 2 | Pulse rate 101-120 | 2 | Nausea or loose stool |
| 4 | Pulse rate greater than 120 | 3 | Vomiting or diarrhea |
| | | 5 | Multiple episodes of diarrhea or vomiting |

| Sweating: over past 1/2 hour not accounted for by room temperature or patient activity: | | Tremor observation of outstretched hands | |
|---|---|---|---|
| 0 | No report of chills or flushing | 0 | No tremor |
| 1 | Subjective report of chills or flushing | 1 | Tremor can be felt, but not observed |
| 2 | Flushed or observable moistness on face | 2 | Slight tremor observable |
| 3 | Beads of sweat on brow or face | 4 | Gross tremor or muscle twitching |
| 4 | Sweat streaming off face | | |

| Restlessness Observation during assessment | | Yawning Observation during assessment | |
|---|---|---|---|
| 0 | Able to sit still | 0 | No yawning |
| 1 | Reports difficulty sitting still, but is able to do so | 1 | Yawning once or twice during assessment |
| 3 | Frequent shifting or extraneous movements of legs/arms | 2 | Yawning three or more times during assessment |
| 5 | Unable to sit still for more than a few seconds | 4 | Yawning several times/minute |

| Pupil size | | Anxiety or irritability | |
|---|---|---|---|
| 0 | Pupils pinned or normal size for room light | 0 | None |
| 1 | Pupils possibly larger than normal for room light | 1 | Patient reports increasing irritability or anxiousness |
| 2 | Pupils moderately dilated | 2 | Patient obviously irritable anxious |
| 5 | Pupils so dilated that only the rim of the iris is visible | 4 | Patient so irritable or anxious that participation in the assessment is difficult |

| Bone or joint aches If patient was having pain previously, only the additional component attributed to opiates withdrawal is scored | | Gooseflesh skin | |
|---|---|---|---|
| 0 | Not present | 0 | Skin is smooth |
| 1 | Mild diffuse discomfort | 3 | Piloerrection of skin can be felt or hairs standing up on arms |
| 2 | Patient reports severe diffuse aching of joints/muscles | 5 | Prominent piloerrection |
| 4 | Patient is rubbing joints or muscles and is unable to sit still because of discomfort | | |

| Runny nose or tearing Not accounted for by cold symptoms or allergies | | | |
|---|---|---|---|
| 0 | Not present | | Total Score ____ |
| 1 | Nasal stuffiness or unusually moist eyes | | The total score is the sum of all 11 items |
| 2 | Nose running or tearing | | Initials of person completing Assessment:____ |
| 4 | Nose constantly running or tears streaming down cheeks | | |

Score: 5-12 mild; 13-24 moderate; 25-36 moderately severe; more than 36 = severe withdrawal

Obtain a copy of the COWS by going to:
https://www.asam.org/docs/default-source/education-docs/cows_induction_flow_sheet.pdf?sfvrsn=b577fc2_2

## The Pharmacology of Heroin and Medication-Assisted Treatment of Opioid Use Disorders

Heroin can be injected, smoked, swallowed or snorted. Intravenous injection produces the greatest intensity and most rapid onset of euphoria. Effects are felt within seconds. Even though effects for sniffing or smoking develop more slowly, beginning in 10 to 15 minutes, sniffing or smoking heroin has increased in popularity because of the availability of high-purity heroin and the fear of sharing needles. Also, users tend to mistakenly believe that taking heroin in ways other than IV use will not lead to addiction.

After ingestion, heroin rapidly crosses the blood-brain barrier. The blood-brain barrier is basically a layer of tightly packed cells that make up the walls of brain capillaries and prevent substances (i.e. toxins) in the blood from entering into the brain. These cells selectively filter out the molecules that are allowed to enter the brain, creating a more stable, nearly toxin-free environment. However, all psychoactive drugs freely pass the blood brain barrier and enter the brain.

While in the brain, heroin is converted to morphine, which rapidly binds to opioid receptors. Users tend to report feeling a "rush" or a surge of pleasurable sensations. The feeling varies in intensity depending on how much of the drug was ingested and how rapidly the drug enters the brain and binds to the natural opioid receptors. The rush is usually accompanied by a warm flushing of the skin, dry mouth, and a heavy feeling in the user's arms and legs. Following the initial effects, the user will be drowsy for several hours with clouded mental functioning and slow cardiac function. Breathing is slowed, and can possibly slow to the point of death.

Repeated use of heroin produces physical dependency, which means the development of tolerance to the drug's effects that necessitates ever larger amounts of the drug to achieve the same effect. A characteristic withdrawal syndrome upon abrupt cessation of use also develops. Withdrawal symptoms can begin within a few hours of last use and can include restlessness, body ache, muscle pain, insomnia, diarrhea, nausea, stomach cramps, vomiting, and hot/cold flashes. These symptoms peak between 24 and 48 hours after the last dose and subside after about a week, but may persist for up to a month. Heroin withdrawal is generally not fatal in an otherwise healthy adult, but can cause death to the fetus of a pregnant addict.

When purchased on the street, heroin is often adulterated with substances such as sugar, starch, powdered milk, strychnine and other poisons. These additives may not dissolve when injected in a user's system and can clog the blood vessels that lead to the lungs, liver, kidneys, or brain, infecting or even killing patches of cells in vital organs. In addition, many users do not know the heroin's actual strength or its true contents and are at risk of exposure to a tainted or contaminated quantity of heroin causing neurotoxic damage, drug overdose or even death.

Chronic heroin use can lead to medical consequences such as scarred and/or collapsed veins, bacterial infections of the blood vessels and heart valves, abscesses and other soft-tissue infections, and liver or kidney disease. Poor health conditions and depressed respiration from heroin use can cause lung complications, including various types of pneumonia and tuberculosis. Other long-term effects of heroin use can include arthritis and other rheumatologic problems and infection of blood borne pathogens such as HIV/AIDS and hepatitis B and C (which are contracted by sharing and reusing syringes and other injection paraphernalia). It is estimated that injection drug use has been a factor in one third of all HIV and more than half of all hepatitis C cases in the United States. Heroin use by a pregnant woman can result in a miscarriage or premature delivery. Heroin exposure *in utero* can increase a newborns' risk of SIDS (sudden infant death syndrome).

**Methadone Treatment**
Research from the National Institute of Drug Abuse (NIDA) has shown that opioid dependent individuals will compulsively continue to use despite adverse physical, emotional and life altering consequences because of at least two motivational factors: 1) the desire to self-manage the pain of withdrawal, and 2) to mitigate the force of drug craving that drives continued compulsive use. So, when behavioral therapies alone are underserving the severity of the client's addiction, medications are an important treatment option. Methadone is still considered the gold standard for heroin addiction and is especially useful for the treatment of heroin addiction with co-occurring mental health disorders.

The primary goals of methadone treatment are to stabilize clients on a sufficient dose of methadone to both treat the symptoms of withdrawal and to block the behaviors of drug craving – two precipitating dynamics for relapse behaviors. Once stabilized, clients can then begin the process of recovery by gaining new skills from counseling that will enable them to regain symptoms-free lifestyle and sustained recovery.

As used in maintenance treatment, methadone is not a heroin substitute. It is important to understand that methadone does not actually "replace" or "substitute" for other opioids. That's why the terms replacement and/or substitution therapy are inaccurate and misleading. Instead, these medications are able to suspend withdrawal symptoms, decrease drug craving behaviors and block the actions from other opioid drugs such as heroin.

The pharmacological effects of methadone are markedly different from those of heroin. Injected, snorted, or smoked, heroin causes an almost immediate "rush" or brief period of euphoria that wears off quickly, terminating in a "crash."

The cycle of euphoria, crash, and craving repeated several times a day leads to a cycle of addiction and severe behavioral disruption. These characteristics of heroin use result from the drug's rapid onset of action and its short duration of action in the brain. An individual who uses heroin multiple times per day subjects the brain and body to marked, rapid fluctuations as the opiate effects come and go (figure 1).

The individual also will experience an intense craving for more heroin to stop the cycle, fend off withdrawal and to reinstate the euphoria. Ultimately however, when tolerance to the drug has been established, the addicted person continues to use to avoid the pain of drug withdrawal and to feel relatively normal.

Methadone has a very gradual and slow onset of action compared with heroin. Because of this, patients stabilized on methadone do not experience the euphoric "rush" (figure 2).

Methadone is metabolized more slowly than heroin and thereby allows the brain and body to avoid the stressful ups and downs caused by heroin. When on a stabilized dose during maintenance treatment, there is also a marked reduction of the desire and craving for heroin.

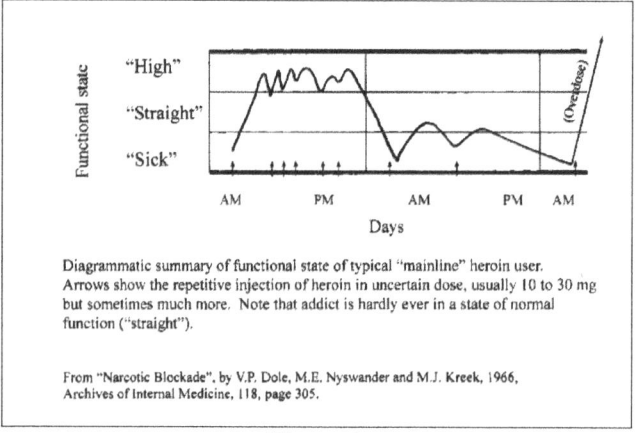

Figure 1

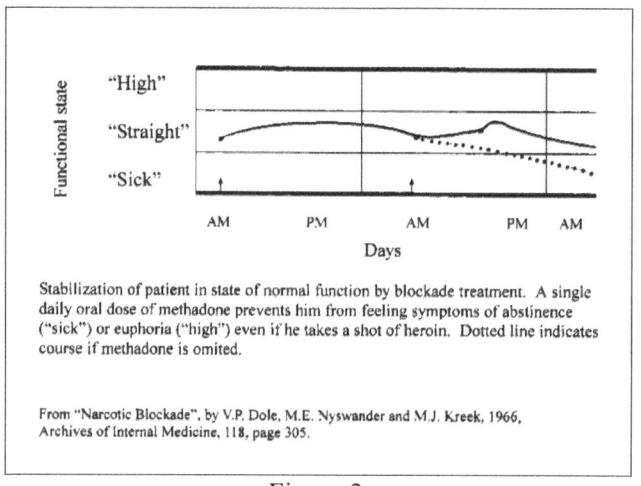

Diagrammatic summary of functional state of typical "mainline" heroin user. Arrows show the repetitive injection of heroin in uncertain dose, usually 10 to 30 mg but sometimes much more. Note that addict is hardly ever in a state of normal function ("straight").

From "Narcotic Blockade", by V.P. Dole, M.E. Nyswander and M.J. Kreek, 1966, Archives of Internal Medicine, 118, page 305.

Figure 2

Stabilization of patient in state of normal function by blockade treatment. A single daily oral dose of methadone prevents him from feeling symptoms of abstinence ("sick") or euphoria ("high") even if he takes a shot of heroin. Dotted line indicates course if methadone is omited.

From "Narcotic Blockade", by V.P. Dole, M.E. Nyswander and M.J. Kreek, 1966, Archives of Internal Medicine, 118, page 305.

Essentially all physiological systems are affected by opioid addiction. A characteristic syndrome occurs when an opiate addict goes through withdrawal. This syndrome includes perspiration, tremor, gooseflesh, restlessness, myalgia, anorexia, nausea, vomiting, abdominal cramps, diarrhea, fever, hyperpnea, and hypertension. Persistent symptoms such as sleep disturbances, irritability, restlessness, and poor concentration can continue for months or longer after the drug use has stopped. On one level, opioid dependency is an adaptation of the body to opiates. With repeated use, dependence develops when the body's various systems have adapted to the opioid where they require the drug to regulate a physiological balance.

Methadone, as used in the treatment of opioid addiction, has an affinity for *mu* opioid receptors in the brain where it blocks the withdrawal syndrome and diminishes craving behaviors which otherwise can lead to continued illicit drug use. Of importance is the fact that at *mu* receptor sites, methadone will also block the effects of other opioid drugs including heroin. This means that even if a patient on methadone ingests heroin, the blocking effect will disallow any heroin action and the patient is prevented from what might have otherwise been a long and torturous relapse.

**An Optimal Dose for Methadone Maintenance**
There have been many research studies comparing various doses of methadone for maintenance treatment. Reports have consistently shown that patients receiving higher doses of methadone compared to those receiving lower doses have much better outcomes – where outcomes are defined in terms of abstinence from illicit opioid use, length of treatment stay, and overall improvement in the quality of life.

Essentially, all of the research on dosing has concluded that there is no evidence of lower doses being adequate for the vast majority of patients. Vincent Dole, one of the co-discoverers of methadone for the treatment of opioid addiction, stated, "There is no compelling reason for prescribing doses that are only marginally adequate. As with antibiotics, the prudent policy is to give enough medication to ensure success.

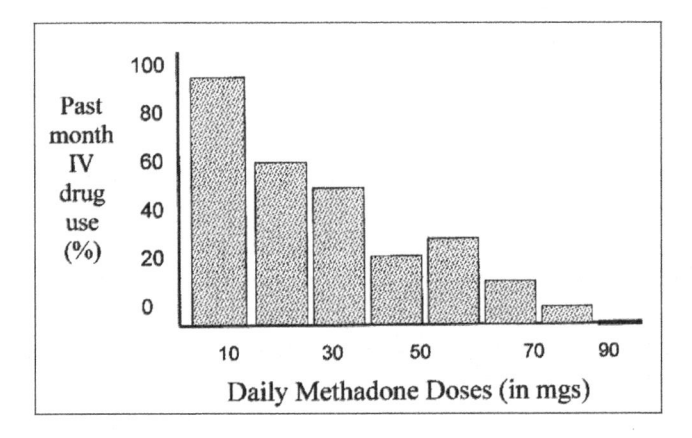

In terms of safety, a meta-analysis of methadone dosing studies found that patients having access to "high-dose maintenance" were actually at a greater reduced risk of fatal heroin overdose during treatment compared with those at lower doses. Remember, the goal of methadone is to stabilize the opioid addicted person so that withdrawal pain and drug craving behaviors are suspended. The optimal dose amount to initiate and maintain stabilization depends on individual patient needs.

**Buprenorphine**
In 2002, the U.S. Food and Drug Administration approved buprenorphine for the treatment of opioid addiction. Buprenorphine is intended for the treatment of pain (Buprenex®) and opioid addiction (Suboxone® and Subutex®). Buprenorphine has a unique pharmacological profile. It produces the effects typical of both pure mu agonists (like morphine) and partial agonists (like pentazocine) depending on dose, pattern of use and population taking the drug. It is about 20-30 times more potent than morphine as an analgesic and, like morphine it produces dose-related euphoria, drug liking, pupillary constriction, respiratory depression and sedation.

However, acute, high doses of buprenorphine have been shown to have a blunting effect on both physiological and psychological effects due to its partial opioid activity. The addition of naloxone in the Suboxone® product is intended to block the euphoric high resulting from the injection of this drug by non-buprenorphine maintained narcotic abusers.

Buprenorphine has a high affinity for opioid receptors. It is a partial mu-receptor agonist as well as a kappa-receptor antagonist. Mu opioid receptors mediate the common opioid effects such as analgesia, sedation, euphoria and respiratory depression. As a partial mu receptor agonist, buprenorphine results in less sedation than full mu-opioid agonists such as methadone and morphine, while still decreasing cravings for other opioids and preventing opioid withdrawal.

The clinical implication of the antagonist kappa receptor effect is not well understood, but it may result in buprenorphine having some mild antidepressant properties. As a partial agonist, buprenorphine has a "ceiling effect" (see figure below): there is a plateau to its opioid agonist effects at higher doses.

**Curve of Morphine and Buprenorphine**

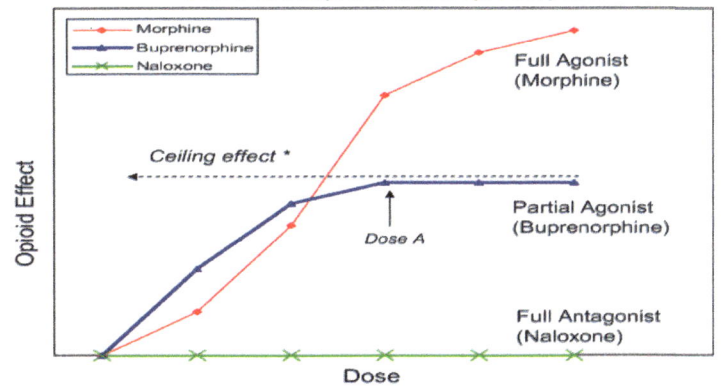

*The effects of morphine (analgesia, respiratory depression) increase with increasing doses. The effects of buprenorphine increase until "Dose A" is reached. No further effect is seen with an increase in dose beyond "Dose A."

Buprenorphine has a higher affinity for and lower intrinsic activity at opioid receptors than full μ-opioid agonists such as methadone, oxycodone and heroin. Hence, buprenorphine displaces agonists from opioid receptors and may precipitate withdrawal in patients physically dependent on opioids. The effect of buprenorphine peaks at 1–4 hours after the initial dose. Buprenorphine is metabolized mainly by cytochrome P4503A4 and its half-life is 24–60 hours.

Compared with methadone, buprenorphine has a relatively lower risk of abuse, dependence, and side effects, and it has a longer duration of action. Because buprenorphine is a partial opioid agonist, its opioid effects, such as euphoria and respiratory depression, as well as its side effects reach a ceiling of maximum effect, unlike with methadone or heroin.

Adverse effects are similar to those of other opioids and include nausea, vomiting and constipation. It is important to note that buprenorphine may precipitate opioid withdrawal symptoms if it is administered before other opioid agonist effects have subsided. Respiratory depression (and death) have been reported in the context of intravenous polysubstance, usually benzodiazepine, abuse.

| Buprenorphine vs. Methadone ||
|---|---|
| **Buprenorphine** | **Methadone** |
| Partial agonist and produces only a low level of euphoria. | Full agonist and can produce significant intoxication. |
| Has low dependence potential compared with full opioid agonists. | Potential to produce significant dependence. As tolerance increases, dose increases over |

|  | time are required. |
|---|---|
| Abstinence leads to mild withdrawal symptoms. | Abstinence leads to marked withdrawal symptoms. |
| At high doses, there is a ceiling effect. The risk of fatal respiratory depression by overdose of buprenorphine by itself is minimal. But when combined with benzodiazepines (diazepam), alcohol and other CNS depressants, respiratory depression has been reported. | Risk of fatal overdose by respiratory depression. |
| Sublingual tablets are effectively absorbed. It is not orally active. Sublingual tablets can be crushed, easily dissolved and injected. | Orally active. |

Buprenorphine will not replace methadone therapy. Rather, it is an important addition to the medications needed for the various types of opioid addicts. Methadone is still the "gold standard" in the treatment of many opioid addictions, particularly heroin. However, buprenorphine gives the addiction medicine physician an additional option in treating opioid use disorder, particularly in the treatment of addiction to long-acting prescription pain medications including Oxycontin or methadone.

Opioids are often used as medicines because they relax the body and can relieve pain. Prescription opioids are largely for moderate to severe pain, though some opioids (at different doses) can be used to treat coughing and diarrhea. According to NIDA, prescription opioids and heroin are chemically similar and can produce a similar high.

In some places, heroin is cheaper and easier to get than prescription opioids, so some people switch to using heroin instead. Data has shown that about 80 percent of people who used heroin first misused prescription opioids More recent data suggest that heroin is frequently the first opioid people use.

This suggests that prescription opioid misuse is just one factor leading to heroin use. In addition to medication assisted treatments I have talked about previously, behavioral therapies are very essential in helping the client with opioid use disorder find and sustain recovery through a newly developed symptoms-free lifestyle. If MAT is used for the treatment of OUD, behavioral therapies must also be used concurrently. This is a clinical bet practice standard of care.

## Prescription Pain Relievers

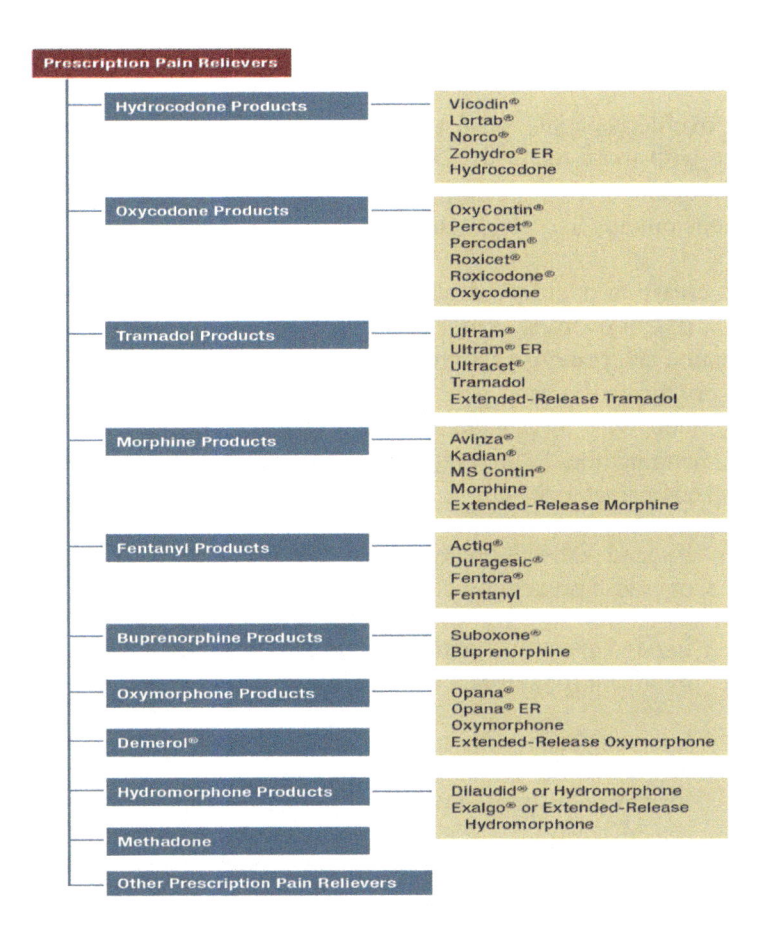

- **Hydrocodone Products**: Vicodin®, Lortab®, Norco®, Zohydro® ER, Hydrocodone
- **Oxycodone Products**: OxyContin®, Percocet®, Percodan®, Roxicet®, Roxicodone®, Oxycodone
- **Tramadol Products**: Ultram®, Ultram® ER, Ultracet®, Tramadol, Extended-Release Tramadol
- **Morphine Products**: Avinza®, Kadian®, MS Contin®, Morphine, Extended-Release Morphine
- **Fentanyl Products**: Actiq®, Duragesic®, Fentora®, Fentanyl
- **Buprenorphine Products**: Suboxone®, Buprenorphine
- **Oxymorphone Products**: Opana®, Opana® ER, Oxymorphone, Extended-Release Oxymorphone
- **Demerol®**
- **Hydromorphone Products**: Dilaudid® or Hydromorphone, Exalgo® or Extended-Release Hydromorphone
- **Methadone**
- **Other Prescription Pain Relievers**

For behavioral therapies in the treatment of OUD, research by NIDA and SAMHSA, have found that approaches such as contingency management and cognitive-behavioral therapy are effective in the treatment of heroin use disorder, especially when applied in concert with medications. Contingency management uses a voucher-based system in which patients earn "points" based on negative drug tests, which they can exchange for items that encourage healthy living.

Cognitive-behavioral therapy (CBT) is designed to help modify the patient's expectations and behaviors related to drug use and to increase skills in coping with various life stressors. An important task is to match the best treatment approach to meet the particular needs of the patient.

# OPIOID OVERDOSE PREVENTION – NALOXONE (NARCAN)

Drug overdose persists as a major public health issue in the United States, with more than 101,750 reported fatal overdoses occurring in the 12-month period ending in October 2022, primarily driven by synthetic opioids like illicit fentanyl.

The increase in overdose deaths highlights the need to ensure people most at risk of overdose can access care, as well as the need to expand prevention and response activities. CDC issued a <u>Health Alert Network Advisory</u> to medical and public health professionals, first responders, harm reduction organizations, and other community partners recommending the following actions as appropriate based on local needs and characteristics:

- Expand distribution and use of Narcan (naloxone) and overdose prevention education

- Expand awareness about and access to and availability of treatment for substance use disorders

- Intervene early with individuals at highest risk for overdose

- Improve detection of overdose outbreaks to facilitate more effective response

Narcan is a medicine that rapidly reverses an opioid overdose. It is an opioid antagonist. This means that it attaches to opioid receptors and reverses and blocks the effects of other opioids. Narcan can quickly restore normal breathing to a person if their breathing has slowed or stopped because of an opioid overdose. But, Narcan has no effect on someone who does not have opioids in their system, and it is not a treatment for opioid use disorder. Examples of opioids include heroin, fentanyl, oxycodone (OxyContin®), hydrocodone (Vicodin®), codeine, and morphine.

Administered when a patient is showing signs of opioid overdose Narcan is a temporary treatment and its effects do not last long. Therefore, it is critical to obtain medical intervention as soon as possible after administering/receiving Narcan.

**Opioid withdrawal symptoms include:**
- Feeling nervous, restless, or irritable

- Body aches
- Dizziness or weakness
- Diarrhea, stomach pain, or nausea
- Fever, chills, or goose bumps
- Sneezing or runny nose in the absence of a cold

**Features of the Opioid Withdrawal Syndrome (OWS)**

| Opioids | | | |
|---|---|---|---|
| | Short acting opioid (e.g. heroin), 6 – 24 hours after last dose. | 7-10 days | **Signs**<br>• Restlessness, yawning, sweating<br>• Rhinorrhea, dilated pupils, piloerection<br>• Muscle twitching, restless legs<br>• Vomiting, diarrhea |
| | Long-acting opioids, (e.g. methadone). 36 to 48 hours after last dose. | 3 – 4 weeks | **Symptoms**<br>• Anorexia, nausea, abdominal pain<br>• Hot and cold flushes<br>• Bone, joint and muscle pain, cramps<br>• Insomnia, disturbed and broken sleep<br>• Intense opioid craving |
| | Buprenorphine 3 to 5 days after last dose. | Several weeks | |

**Signs of opioid overdose:**
- unconsciousness
- very small pupils
- slow or shallow breathing
- vomiting
- an inability to speak
- faint heartbeat
- limp arms and legs
- pale skin
- bluesish or purple lips and fingernails

Narcan should be given to any person who shows signs of an opioid overdose or when an overdose is suspected. Naloxone can be obtained over-the-counter now as a nasal spray.

A concise, accurate and informative YouTube video on how to administer Narcan can be found at:
https://www.youtube.com/watch?v=B9Sv64FJPhg

**A NOTE ABOUT FENTANYL**
According to the Center for Disease Control (CDC), fentanyl is a synthetic opioid that is up to 50 times stronger than heroin and 100 times stronger than morphine. It is a major contributor to fatal and nonfatal overdoses in the U.S. There are two types of fentanyl:

pharmaceutical fentanyl and illegally made fentanyl. Both are considered synthetic opioids. Pharmaceutical fentanyl is prescribed by doctors to treat severe pain, especially after surgery and for advanced-stage cancer. However, most recent cases of fentanyl-related overdose are linked to illegally made fentanyl, which is distributed through illegal drug markets for its heroin-like effect. It is often added to other drugs because of its extreme potency, which makes drugs cheaper, more powerful, more addictive, and more dangerous.

As reported by the National Institute of Drug Abuse (NIDA), fentanyl is a powerful synthetic (human-made) opioid that is approved to treat severe and complex pain. Rather recently, fentanyl that is made and distributed illegally, as well as other illegally made synthetic opioids, are being seen in the drug supply.

During this time, fentanyl and related substances have contributed to a dramatic rise in drug overdose deaths in the United States. Illegally made fentanyl is available on the drug market in different forms, including liquid and powder. Powdered fentanyl looks just like many other drugs. It is commonly mixed with drugs like heroin, cocaine, and methamphetamine and made into pills that are made to resemble other prescription opioids. Fentanyl-laced drugs are extremely dangerous, and many people may be unaware that their drugs are laced with fentanyl.

In its liquid form, illegally made fentanyl can be found in nasal sprays, eye drops, and dropped onto paper or small candies

Fentanyl and other synthetic opioids are the most common drugs involved in overdose deaths. Even in small doses, it can be deadly. Over 150 people die every day from overdoses related to synthetic opioids like fentanyl. Drugs may contain deadly levels of fentanyl, and people wouldn't be able to see it, taste it, or smell it. It is nearly impossible to tell if drugs have been laced with fentanyl.

People both knowingly consume fentanyl and others will unknowingly consume it when it is combined with or sold as other drugs, such as heroin, cocaine, or counterfeit pills (i.e. Xanax, etc.). Because fentanyl is about 50 to 100 times more potent than morphine, using a drug that has been adulterated with or replaced by fentanyl can greatly increase one's risk of a fatal overdose.

*Fentanyl is the single deadliest drug threat our nation has ever encountered. Fentanyl is everywhere. From large metropolitan areas to rural America, no community is safe from this poison. We must take every opportunity to spread the word to prevent fentanyl-related overdose death and poisonings from claiming scores of American lives every day."*  - DEA Administrator Anne Milgram

**Potent sedative drugs showing up in other drugs including counterfeit pills.**

An animal tranquilizer called *xylazine* is increasingly being found in the US illicit drug supply and linked to overdose deaths. Xylazine can be life-threatening and is especially dangerous when combined with opioids like fentanyl. Xylazine, not an opioid, is a tranquilizer used in veterinary medicine for non-human animals only. It has recently been associated with an increased number of fatal overdoses nationwide in the evolving drug overdose crisis because more and more, xylazine is being added to illicit opioids, including fentanyl.

Sometimes referred to on the street as "tranq," xylazine is a central nervous system depressant that can cause drowsiness and amnesia and slow breathing, heart rate, and blood pressure to dangerously low levels. Taking opioids in combination with xylazine and other central nervous system depressants (alcohol or benzodiazepines) increases the risk of a fatal overdose. In the event of a suspected xylazine overdose, it is recommend giving the opioid overdose reversal medication Narcan because xylazine is frequently combined with opioids. However, because xylazine is not an opioid, naloxone does not address the impact of xylazine on breathing.

Also, as reported in May 2024, public health officials and the Center for Disease Control (CDC) find that Mexican cartels and gangs inside the U.S. are putting a dangerous sedative called *medetomidine* into fentanyl and other drugs sold illicitly on the street. Medetomidine is a drug used by veterinarians as an animal tranquilizer has been linked to recent increase in overdose outbreaks in Chicago and Pittsburgh. The CDC says, as with counterfeit fentanyl and xylazine, medetomidine, when mixed into counterfeit pills and powders sold on the street, slows the human heart rate to dangerous levels with potential lethality. And, it's impossible for users to detect. Xylazine and medetomidine don't respond to naloxone, the medication used to reverse most fentanyl overdoses. There's currently no way for users to know if their drugs are laced with this chemical or not.

Moving forward, physicians and other clinicians in emergency departments, urgent care centers, primary care settings, and substance use treatment facilities will need to be increasingly aware of the role of toxic adulterants in how patients who take street drugs present. They will also need to be increasingly mindful that toxic adulterants can cause unusual drug interactions, complications, and medical conditions, all of which may increase the risk of opioid-related overdose and death. Also, because health care providers and patients are best served by having a complete list of the drugs present in a patient's system, more complete toxicology panels, including those that test for a variety of adulterants, need to be available and used. Failure to recognize and identify toxic adulterants is likely to hinder timely and appropriate treatment, including life-saving measures.

In addition, public health professionals can work to build awareness and knowledge about the presence and dangers of toxic adulterants, particularly in populations most at risk for seeking illicit drugs. They can also continue to advocate for more comprehensive analyses of street drugs and their compositions, including toxic adulterants. Data from these analyses will provide a better understanding of the various factors that play a role in overdose deaths and will help identify emerging trends in the role of adulterants in the opioid epidemic.

Greater awareness and understanding of the developing role of toxic adulterants in the US opioid crisis is needed. Improved recognition of and knowledge about toxic adulterants could help clinicians take a more well-informed approach with their patients and guide public health professionals in formulating additional policies and programs to address the crisis.

**Clinicians and Providers Often Use Stigmatizing Language for Patients With Opioid Use Disorder**

About 85% of patients with opioid use disorder (OUD) are described in clinical notes as being abusers, addicts, junkies, or with other stigmatizing terms, preliminary results of a new study suggest.

Female healthcare providers and social workers used stigmatizing language at a relatively high rate, investigators found. The researcher also showed that demeaning language was used more often in medical records of Hispanic and Black patients, reaffirming previous research. Investigators noted that words chosen by clinicians can contribute to patients developing a negative attitude toward their healthcare provider, affecting follow-ups and overall treatment outcomes. This is particularly important after the passage of the 21st Century Cures Act, which mandates that patients have free access to their personal medical records, they added.

"No matter what type of specialty you're in, and no matter if you're a male or female clinician, you should choose your words carefully," study investigator Jyotishman Pathak, PhD, professor of psychiatry and of population health sciences, Weill Cornell Medicine, Cornell University, New York, told *Medscape Medical News*. In physician-patient encounters, especially with patients of lower socioeconomic status or less education, "there's already a power dynamic going on," Pathak added. "And if patients come across phrases that are perhaps demeaning and stigmatizing, it makes it even worse." The findings were presented at the American Psychiatric Association (APA) 2024 Annual Meeting.

**Artificial Intelligence–Based Algorithm**
Pathak and his colleagues used natural language processing based on artificial intelligence (AI) and machine learning to update a list of stigmatizing words put together by the National Institute of Drug Abuse's (NIDA) Words Matter campaign, which includes words like addict, abuse, dirty, junkie, and alcoholic. They developed a preliminary version of an algorithm and applied it to close to 1 million clinical notes from electronic health records of a random sample of 2700 patients diagnosed with OUD or substance use disorder (SUD) between 2010 and 2023 at Cornell. The patient encounters included visits to primary care providers, emergency room physicians, social workers, psychiatrists, psychologists, or other clinicians.

Researchers divided patients into those with evidence of stigmatizing language in their clinical notes (SL group) and those with no evidence of stigmatizing language (No SL group). About 85% of patients with OUD/SUD (n = 2279) had stigmatized language terms in 111,422 notes. The most common negative terms included abuser, addict, substance dependence, and alcoholic.

Individuals in the SL group tended to be older, and there were more people in the SL group than in the No SL group in each age category from ages 33 to 80 years. The SL group also had more women (34% vs 29%), Black patients (18% vs 15%) and Hispanic patients (23% vs 17%) than did the No SL group. Such results are consistent with what has been reported in other studies and patient surveys, noted Pathak. The study showed a greater percent of female healthcare providers in the SL group than in the No SL group (50% vs 42.4%), which is a new finding. It's not clear whether these female clinicians are older and were trained at an earlier era, said Pathak, who also noted the increased focus on diversity, equity, and inclusion today in medical schools.

Investigators also found more social workers in the SL group than in the No SL group (6% vs 0.2%). "We saw a very high use of stigma language in social worker notes," said Pathak, adding this was "surprising" and "disappointing. Patients are already very vulnerable, and you would expect that the language being used would have more empathy," he said.

Researchers found the opposite situation for the psychiatrists who made up 12% of the SL group and 26% of the No SL group. "We actually found that both psychiatrists and psychologists used less stigmatizing language in their clinical documentation," said Pathak. "It looks like they're more aware of what's the right terminology to use."

**Better Education Needed**

Commenting on the research for *Medscape Medical News*, Howard Y. Liu, MD, chair, Council on Communications, APA, and professor of adult, child, and adolescent psychiatry, University of Nebraska Medical Center, Omaha, Nebraska, said that the study is a reminder that terms like addict and drunk are still being used by professionals. "This can be hurtful to individuals living with a substance use disorder and can be a barrier to them seeking help" or being upfront about their drinking or drug use with their clinical team, said Liu.

**Very important for providers:** The study showed less use of stigmatizing language among psychiatrists and psychologists but more frequent use by social workers, which suggests to Lui that "across professions, we need to educate ourselves about person-first language. He also shared and that those in the education system should act as role models. We need to ensure that in community and public service clinics, as well as in academic health centers where future clinicians are trained, professors and peers are using person-first language and challenging stigmatizing language when it arises.

## SUGGESTED READINGS ON THIS TOPIC

Ashraf, I. Opioid Pharmacology: A Pharmacological Insight. Kindle Edition. 2014. ASIN : B00O5IO6YY.

Blanco C, Volkow ND. Management of opioid use disorder in the USA: present status and future directions. *Lancet*. 2019;393(10182):1760–1772. doi: 10.1016/S0140-6736(18)33078-

Carley, JA. Therapeutic Approaches to Opioid Use Disorder: What is the Current Standard of Care? Int J Gen Med.2021; 14: 2305–2311.

Cruz SL. Opioids: Pharmacology, Abuse, and Addiction. Springer. 2022. ISBN-10 : 3031099354

Leshner AI, Manche M. Medications for Opioid Use Disorder Saves Lives. National Academies Press. 2019.

Norton, M. The Pharmacist's Guide to Opioid Use Disorders. American Society of Health-System Pharmacists. 2018. ISBN-10 : 1585285862.

Payte JT, Zweben JE, Martin J. Opioid maintenance treatment. In Principles of Addiction Medicine. Chevy Chase, MD: *American Society of Addiction Medicine*; 2003: 751-766.

SAMHSA. Medications for Opioid Use Disorder - Treatment Improvement Protocol (Tip 63). 2018. ISBN-10 : 0359030904.

Simon, EJ. Opiates: Neurobiology. Lowinson, JH, Ruiz, P, Millman, RB, and Langrod, JG (editors), *Substance Abuse A Comprehensive Sourcebook*. Fourth Edition. Lippincott Williams & Wilkins. 2005.

Singh VM, Browne T, Montgomery J. The Emerging Role of Toxic Adulterants in Street Drugs in the US Illicit Opioid Crisis. Public Health Rep. 2020 Jan;135(1):6-10. doi: 10.1177/0033354919887741. Epub 2019 Nov 18. PMID: 31738861; PMCID: PMC7119254.

Stanford, M, Avoy, D. Professional Perspectives on Addiction Medicine: Understanding Opioid Addiction and the Functionality of

Methadone Treatment. *Santa Clara County Health & Hospital System*. 2007.

Strang J, Volkow ND, Degenhardt L, et al. Opioid use disorder. *Nat Rev Dis Primer*. 2020;6(1):3. doi: 10.1038/s41572-019-0137-5

Tvildiani, D. Opioids: Pharmacology, Clinical Uses and Adverse Effects. Nova Science Publishers, Inc. 2012. ISBN-10 : 1619421011.

Volkow ND, Jones EB, Einstein EB, Wargo EM. Prevention and treatment of opioid misuse and addiction: a review. *JAMA Psychiatry*. 2019;76(2):208–216. doi: 10.1001/jamapsychiatry.2018.3126

# CHAPTER 11. CANNABIS PHARMACOLOGY

## Key Concepts

$\Delta^9$-tetrahydrocannabinol(THC) Main psychoactive cannabinoid in cannabis.

Adiponectin — Hormone secreted by adipose (fatty) tissue involved in energy homeostasis. Enhances insulin sensitivity and glucose tolerance, as well as oxidation of fatty acids in muscle.

Cannabinoids — Also called phytocannabinoids, are commonly found in the marijuana plant of which there are over 60.

Cannabinoid receptors — The chemistry of the ECS is the endocannabinoids where they are released into synapse and bind to and activate distinct cannabinoid receptor. 2 types of cannabinoid receptors have been identified; $CB_1$ and $CB_2$. $CB_1$ receptors are found primarily in the brain and the $CB_2$ receptors are located mainly in immune cells and in peripheral tissues of the body in adipocytes (or "fat cells") that are associated with lipid and glucose metabolism.

Endocannabinoids — Endocannabinoid, is a word condensed from two other words; endogenous: from within, and cannabinoid: substances resembling the components within the C. sativa plant. The two major endocannabinoids are arachidonoyl ethanolamide (anandamide) and 2-arachidonoyl glycerol (2-AG).

| | |
|---|---|
| Endocannabinoid system | (ECS) is a physiological system consisting of cannabinoid receptors and corresponding chemical messengers that play a role in regulating body weight, glucose and lipid metabolism, pain, cognitive functioning and addiction. |
| Metabolic Syndrome | The Metabolic Syndrome is a cluster of conditions that occur together, increasing risk of heart disease, stroke and diabetes. Syndrome includes insulin resistance, hypertension, cholesterol abnormalities.. Patients are most often overweight or obese. |

# CHAPTER 11

## Cannabis Pharmacology

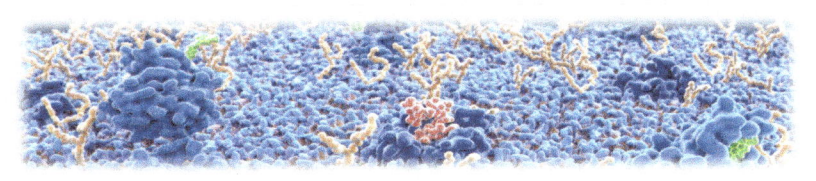

CANNABIS PHARMACOLOGY:
PHARMACODYNAMICS & PHARMACOKINETICS

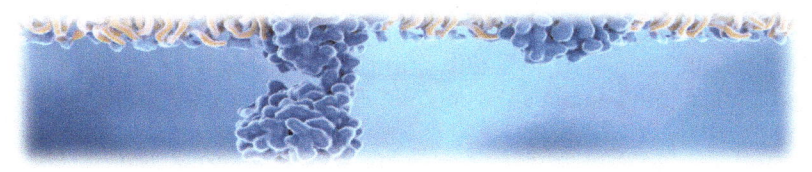

The therapeutic value of the cannabis plant has been referenced for approximately four millennia by a variety of sources and throughout different countries. While cannabis has been used medicinally for quite some time, it wasn't until rather recently that neuroscience research has discovered safer and more effective treatment possibilities. Only as recently as the 1990s, scientists found and were able to replicate receptor-proteins located on the surface of cells that are responsible for many of the actions of
$\Delta^9$-tetrahydrocannabinol (THC), the main psychoactive ingredient of cannabis. This new understanding has allowed scientists to develop a foundation for a cannabinoid pharmacology that can pave the way for more efficient cannabinoid-based medicines.

### About the Cannabis Plant

The marijuana plant, referred to as Cannabis sativa (*C. sativa*), is both a widespread illegal drug of abuse and a recognized medicinal plant. One of the challenges for neuroscience was to isolate the active components of the plant associated with potential therapeutic uses and at the same time try to develop cannabinoid-based medicines without any adverse effects. After four decades of research, there is a much greater understanding about the pharmacology of plant-derived cannabinoid compounds (called phytocannabinoids) and how they relate to the endogenous cannabinoids within the human body.

**Pharmacology of Cannabis**
There are more than 550 chemical compounds in cannabis, with more than 100 phytocannabinoids being identified. These cannabinoids work by binding to the cannabinoid receptors, as well as other receptor systems. Also within cannabis are the aromatic terpenes, more than 100 of which have been identified. Cannabis and its constituents have been indicated as therapeutic compounds in numerous medical conditions, such as pain, anxiety, epilepsy, nausea and vomiting, and post-traumatic stress disorder.

The two main cannabinoids are delta-9-tetrahydrocannabinol (THC) and cannabidiol (CBD). Delta-8-THC is similar in potency to THC but is present in only small concentrations. Cannabinol and cannabidiol (CBD) are the other major cannabinoids present. Cannabis potency has increased in the past decades, up from about 4% in the 1980s to an average of 15% today. Marijuana extracts, used in dabbing and edibles, can contain an average of 50% and up to 90% THC.

While most research has concentrated on evaluating the molecular and biochemical mechanisms of THC that underlie actions of the cannabinoids, these other compounds also play a role in the acute and long-term consequences of marijuana use.

Inhalation burning plant material (*pyrolysis*) is a very unique method of drug delivery into the system. First it provides rapid delivery of the drug into the bloodstream via the lung tissue such that the effects may be felt within minutes and last for 2 to 3 hours. Clinical psychopharmacology and toxicology illustrate this point all too well through studies of other plants that are smoked, such as tobacco and cocaine. When cannabis is smoked, THC in the inhaled smoke rapidly absorbs within seconds and is delivered to the brain quickly (as one would expect from a very lipophilic substance). Oral ingestion of THC is quite different than smoking. Some cannabis users prepare teas and other liquid solutions, and sometimes bake the marijuana in cookies to ingest the substance orally. However, maximum THC and blood cannabinoid levels are only reached after 1 to 3 hours. Thus, onset of the psychoactive effects is much slower after oral ingestion. However, burning cannabis releases over 100 compounds which can be carcinogenic.

## Cannabis Naturally In the Human Body?

Well, sort of. In the way the body has its own natural morphine (endorphins) that is are similar in chemistry to morphine from the opium plant; the body also has its own versions of chemical agents of the cannabis plant, called *endocannabinoids*. These chemical messengers help regulate processes of brain and body functions. Since science has now developed a more sophisticated understanding of the endocannabinoids, new medicines can be developed to treat a variety of health conditions including obesity, Type 2 diabetes, non-morphine analgesics, and addiction medicines, to name a few. In the not so distant future, it is plausible to expect that neuroscience research will discover novel medicinal ways to facilitate changes within the endocannabinoid system that can further help treat other conditions, from addiction and alcoholism, to epilepsy, pain, anxiety, and depression. In the 1990s, the discovery of specific cellular receptors of THC revealed a whole endogenous signaling system now referred to as the *endocannabinoid system* (figure below).

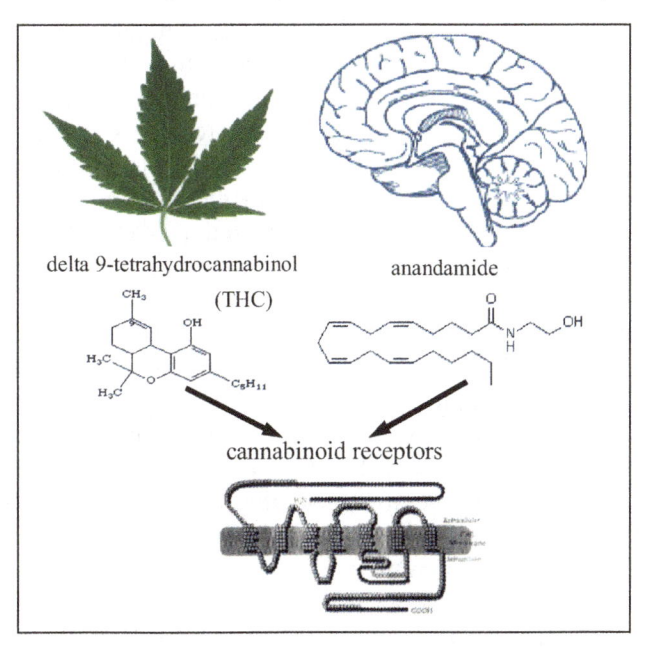

## Endocannabinoids

The Endocannabinoid System (ECS) is a physiological system consisting of cannabinoid receptors and corresponding chemical messengers that is believed to play an important role in regulating body weight, glucose and lipid metabolism, pain, movement, cognitive functioning and even addiction. The word, *endocannabinoid,* is a word condensed from two other words; *endogenous*: from within, and *cannabinoid*: substances resembling the components within the *C. sativa* plant. The two major endocannabinoids are anandamide and 2-arachidonoyl glycerol (2-AG). As their chemical names suggest, both are derived from arachidonic acid, which is also the precursor for the prostaglandins, which allows one to see the potential role of the ES in pain and inflammation treatments.

**Cannabinoid Receptors in the Brain and Body**

Basically, the chemistry of the ECS is the endocannabinoids where they are released into synapse and bind to and activate distinct cannabinoid receptor. To date, 2 types of cannabinoid receptors have been identified; $CB_1$ and $CB_2$. $CB_1$ receptors are found primarily in the brain and the $CB_2$ receptors are located mainly in immune cells and in peripheral tissues of the body in adipocytes (or "fat cells") that are associated with lipid and glucose metabolism.

It is the $CB_1$ receptor that is presumed to mediate all the CNS effects of the cannabinoids. The number of $CB_1$ receptors in the brain is large, comparable to the numbers of receptors for the monoamines, serotonin and dopamine. The large number of $CB_1$ receptors, called *receptor reserve*, tells us how a partial agonist like THC is able to produce a response. Namely, the more receptors in the system, the greater the likelihood of an activator-inhibitor interaction. Signal transduction studies have revealed that THC is not a very strong partial activator.

The distribution of $CB_1$ receptors within the brain is rather heterogeneous, with the largest concentrations found in basal ganglia, cerebellum, hippocampus, and the cerebral cortex. $CB_1$ receptor activation is particularly expressed in an area of the brain called the nucleus accumbens, a small subcortical area believed to be important in motivational processes that mediate the incentive value of food, and which may also play an important part in the establishment and maintenance of drug addiction.

CB1 receptors are also integral in initiating food intake and, when activated, will stimulate the ingestion of food. Research indicates that endocannabinoids may play a role in appetite control. This is achieved by modulating the expression and release of appetite suppressing and appetite stimulating neurotransmitters in the hypothalamus region of the brain.

The CB2 receptor is not expressed in the brain. It was originally detected in macrophages and is particularly abundant in immune tissues, where the largest concentrations have been detected in B-cells and natural killer cells. The functions of the CB2 receptor in the immune system are less clear. Most of the research studies seemed to suggest that the cannabinoids are primarily immunomodulatory in nature. That is, depending on dosage, some immune cells are suppressed while others are stimulated.

**General Effects of Cannabis**
Since cannabis inhalation exposes the user to many different compounds in addition to THC, the subjective effects of cannabis vary somewhat among individuals. The behavioral response to cannabis can be a function of dose, setting, experience, expectation of the user, cannabinoid content, and peripheral compounds that are produced as the cannabis is burned. Nevertheless, several behavioral effects are attributed to cannabis use, which are generally dose-dependent

Marijuana generally produces a *bi-phasic psychic reaction:* the euphoric *stimulant phase* and the sedative *depressive phase*. During the initial stimulant phase, short-term memory is impaired and appetite is usually suppressed. Users can easily lose their train of thought. Also during this phase, THC acts like a sympathomimetic, which can induce a panic reaction with symptoms of anxiety and paranoia.

Following the stimulant phase, drowsiness, lethargy and *anergy* (low energy) are common. Like drugs in the sedative-hypnotic class, REM sleep is inhibited and thus restful restoration is compromised. Unlike sedatives however, there is no REM rebound from THC use. During the depressive phase, appetite is often increased and at extremely high doses (greater than 12 mg), cannabis can produce memory impairment, confusion, disorientation and even delirium.

Some studies have documented impairment of a variety of cognitive and performance tasks involving memory, perception, learning, reaction time and motor coordination. The short term damage from marijuana use can also result in dysphoria, disorientation and panic attacks. Recent findings also indicate that long-term use of cannabis produces changes in the brain similar to those seen after long-term use of other major drugs of abuse. Mild cross-tolerance to effects of cannabis will occur in some individuals tolerant to CNS depressants including alcohol and opiates.

**Physiological Effects**
While cannabis produces euphoria in humans, in general, animals do not self-administer THC in controlled studies. Cannabinoids generally do not lower the threshold of electrical stimulation needed for animals to stimulate the brain reward system, as do other drugs with abuse potential. Researchers have found that THC changes the way in which sensory information gets into and is acted on by the hippocampus. This is a component of the brain's limbic system crucial for learning, memory, and integrating sensory experiences with motivations. Investigations have shown that neurons in the information processing system of the hippocampus and the activity of the nerve fibers are suppressed by THC. In addition, researchers have discovered that learned behaviors, which depend on the hippocampus, also deteriorate.

**Pulmonary Effects**
Cannabis smoking is associated with large airway inflammation, increased airway resistance, and lung hyperinflation, and those who smoke cannabis regularly report more symptoms of chronic bronchitis than those who do not smoke. Chronic bronchitis and pharyngitis have been associated with repeated exposure, with an increased frequency of pulmonary illness. These effects appear to be both similar and additive to those produced by tobacco smoking.

Cannabis smoke can be divided into two phases: the gas phase and the particulate or tar phase. Cannabis smoke contains several irritants and toxic agents like carbon monoxide, ammonia, hydrogen cyanide, acetone, acetaldehyde and toluene. During the gas phase, a number of these known carcinogens, including benzene and various *nitrosamines,* have been detected. Several poly-nuclear hydrocarbons such as benzoanthracene, benzopyrene, and a variety of naphthalenes, which are known carcinogens.

**Immune System**
According to the several research studies, there is a link between cannabis use, immune system, and viral infections (Maggirwar, SB. 2021). Research has suggested a link between cannabis, immune function, and viral infections. Cannabis use may be associated with adverse effects on immune function and, thereby, increase the risk of acquiring or transmitting infections such as HIV and HCV. However,

data are not sufficiently strong to suggest that cannabis use adversely affects the progression of viral diseases. Cannabis use is also associated with adverse respiratory/pulmonary complications such as chronic cough and emphysema, and the impairment of immune function. However, it is also evident that cannabis or its constituents, including THC and CBD, have some beneficial effects such as improving appetite and food intake in patients with HIV/AIDS and positive effects in patients with hepatic steatosis. Nevertheless, as suggested above, more research is needed to study the long-term effects of cannabis use on pulmonary/respiratory diseases, immune function and the risk of infection transmission, and the molecular/genetic basis of immune dysfunction in chronic cannabis users.

**Heart Rate and Blood Pressure Effects**
A consistent and sudden sympathomimetic effect of cannabis is a 20-100% increase in heart rate, lasting up to 3 hours. Cannabis also induces a dose-dependent tachycardia and orthostatic hypotension during the initial stimulant phase of the behavioral syndrome.

Research indicates that smoking cannabis with cocaine use has the potential to cause severe increases in heart rate and blood pressure beyond that of each drug by itself. In one study, experienced marijuana and cocaine users were given cannabis alone, cocaine alone, and then a combination of both. Each drug alone produced cardiovascular effects; but when they were combined, the effects were greater and lasted longer. The heart rate of the subjects in the study increased 29 beats per minute with cannabis alone and 32 beats per minute with cocaine alone. However, when the drugs were used together, the heart rate increased an average of 49 beats per minute, and the increased rate persisted for a longer time. In some situations, an individual may smoke cannabis and inject cocaine in addition to physically stressful activities, which may significantly increase an overload on the cardiovascular system.

**Effects of Heavy Cannabis Use on Learning and Social Behavior**
A study of college students has shown that critical skills related to attention, memory, and learning are impaired among people who use cannabis heavily, even after discontinuing its use for at least 24 hours. Researchers compared 65 "heavy users," who had smoked cannabis a median of 29 of the past 30 days, and 64 "light users," who had smoked a median of 1 of the past 30 days. After 19-24 hours of closely monitored abstinence from cannabis and other

drugs including alcohol, the undergraduates were given several standard tests measuring aspects of attention, memory, and learning. Compared to the light users, heavy cannabis users made more errors and had more difficulty sustaining attention, shifting attention to meet the demands of changes in the environment, and in registering, processing, and using information.

The findings suggest that greater impairment among heavy users is likely due to an alteration of brain activity produced by cannabis. Longitudinal research also indicates frequent use among young people below college age who have lower achievement, more deviant behavior, higher delinquency and aggression, poorer relationships with parents, and more associations with drug-using peers.

**Pregnancy**
All drugs of abuse can damage a mother's health during pregnancy, a time when she should take special care of herself. Drugs also interfere with proper nutrition and rest, which will hinder immune system functioning. Some studies have found that babies born to mothers who used marijuana during pregnancy were smaller than those born to mothers who did not use the drug. In general, smaller babies are more likely to develop health problems.

A nursing mother who uses marijuana also passes some of the THC to the baby through her breast milk. Research indicates that the use of marijuana by a mother during the first month of breast-feeding can impair the infant's motor development (control of muscle movement) and have other damaging effects.

**Risk of schizophrenia linked with cannabis use disorder**
Young men with cannabis use disorder have an increased risk of developing schizophrenia, according to a study led by researchers at the Mental Health Services in the Capital Region of Denmark and the National Institute on Drug Abuse (NIDA) at the National Institutes of Health. The study, published in *Psychological Medicine*(link is external), analyzed detailed health records data spanning 5 decades and representing more than 6 million people in Denmark to estimate the fraction of schizophrenia cases that could be attributed to cannabis use disorder on the population level.

Researchers found strong evidence of an association between cannabis use disorder and schizophrenia among men and women, though the association was much stronger among young men. Using statistical models, the study authors estimated that as many as 30% of cases of schizophrenia among men aged 21-30 might have been prevented by averting cannabis use disorder.

**Cannabis use and teen suicide**
A Columbia University study has found that teens who use cannabis recreationally are two to four times as likely to develop psychiatric disorders, such as depression and suicidality, than teens who don't use cannabis at all. The research, published in JAMA Open Network (May 3, 2023) also finds that casual cannabis use puts teens at risk for problem behaviors, including poor grades, truancy, and trouble with the law, which can have long-term negative consequences that may keep youth from developing their full potential in adulthood.

"Perceptions exist among youth, parents, and educators that casual cannabis use is benign," said lead study author Ryan Sultan, MD, assistant professor of clinical psychiatry, Department of Psychiatry, Columbia, and a pediatric and adult psychiatrist, New York-Presbyterian/Columbia University Irving Medical Center. "We were surprised to see that cannabis use had such strong associations to adverse mental health and life outcomes for teens who did not meet the criteria for having a substance use condition." The Columbia study is the first to identify that subclinical, or nondisordered, cannabis use—symptoms and behavior that do not meet the criteria for clinical disorder—has clear adverse and impairing associations for adolescents.

To conduct their research, Dr. Sultan and colleagues analyzed responses from a representative sample of respondents to the National Survey on Drug Use and Health which collects data on tobacco, alcohol, illicit drugs, and mental health annually. The cross-sectional study included approximately 70,000 adolescents between the ages of 12-17. The researchers found that more that 2.5 million U.S. teens—or about 1 in 10 –were casual cannabis users. More than 600,000 teens—roughly 1 in 40—met the criteria for cannabis addiction. To be considered to have cannabis use disorder, an individual must meet at least two of 11 criteria, which include an inability to reduce consumption, constant cravings, and relationship and social problems.

Additionally, nondisordered cannabis users were 2-2.5 times more likely to have adverse mental health outcomes and behavioral problems, compared to teens who didn't use cannabis at all. Teens with an addiction to cannabis were 3.5 to 4.5 times more likely to have these issues

**Immature brain regions put teens at elevated risk**
Numerous studies note that cannabis use can alter the development of the cerebral cortex, the brain's center of reasoning and executive function, posing a risk to young people whose brains have not matured. Marijuana use in adolescence is associated with difficulty thinking, problem-solving, and reduced memory, as well as a risk of long-term addiction.

Exposing developing brains to dependency forming substances appears to prime the brain for being more susceptible to developing other forms of addiction later in life, said senior study author Frances Levin, MD, Professor of Psychiatry at Columbia and addiction psychiatrist, New York-Presbyterian/Columbia University Irving Medical Center. Dr. Levin, who directs Columbia's Division of Substance Use Disorders, says mental health problems and cannabis use are closely linked. "Having depression or suicidality may drive teens to use cannabis as way to relieve their suffering," she said. "Concurrently, using cannabis likely worsens depressive and suicidal symptoms."

**Cannabis Use Disorder**
Cannabis Use Disorder is the continued use of cannabis in spite of the serious distress or impairment it causes. The strong desire to use the drug causes difficulties in controlling its use, and people with the disorder continue to use it even when there are harmful results. The buds, stems and seeds of the cannabis sativa plant contain amounts of Delta-9-tetrahydrocannabinol (THC), the most psychoactive compound found in the plant, according to the National Institute of Drug Abuse. According to the American Psychiatric Association (APA), most people who use cannabis begin in early adolescence or as young adults.

**DSM-5 Symptoms of Cannabis Use Disorder**
The Diagnostic and Statistical Manual of Mental Disorders, 5th Edition, which is published by the APA, provides the following criteria for Cannabis Use Disorder.
- Using cannabis for a minimum of one year with the presence of at least two of the following symptoms accompanied by serious impairment of functioning and agitation.
- Used in larger amounts over a longer time than what was intended.

- Repeatedly tried to stop or lessen the amount of cannabis used.
- Unusual amount of time is spent trying to get, use and/or recover from cannabis effects.
- Having cravings for cannabis, such as thoughts and images, dreams, and perceiving its smell because of an obsession with it.
- Keep on using cannabis even in light of the fact that it has negative consequences, such as others warning to leave the relationship or being left by a partner or friends, poor job performance and criminal charges.
- Using cannabis is more important than other areas of life—job, school, hygiene and responsibilities to family members and friends.
- Using cannabis and taking dangerous risks, such as driving a car.
- Using cannabis even though the person is aware of the physical and psychological problems he has because of it (lack of motivation, chronic cough).
- Builds a tolerance to cannabis—taking larger amounts to get the psychoactive effect experienced when it was first used.
- Cannabis is used to halt the symptoms of withdrawal.

The severity of Cannabis Use Disorder is separated into three categories depending on the number of symptoms the person displays, according to the APA.

- **Mild**. The disorder is considered mild if an individual displays two or three of the above symptoms.
- **Moderate**. For the disorder to be considered moderate, a person must exhibit four or five of the above symptoms.
- **Severe**. The diagnosis of severe Cannabis Use Disorder is when an individual shows six or more of the above symptoms.

**Vulnerability to Cannabis Use Disorder**
There are several risk factors for Cannabis Use Disorder, according to the DSM-5, including:
- Family history of chemical dependence.
- History of Conduct Disorder or Antisocial Personality Disorder.
- Low socio-economic status.
- History of tobacco smoking.
- Abusive family.
- Unpredictable family circumstances.

- Family members who smoke cannabis.
- Poor performance in school.
- Easy to get cannabis.
- Drug-tolerant culture.

Tolerance readily develops (after a day or two) to the behavioral and pharmacological effects of THC in both human and animal experimental models. In humans, tolerance develops to mood, memory, cardiovascular and autonomic effects. The mechanism of this tolerance is thought to be a desensitization of the THC receptor, perhaps by some alterations in its interaction with the second messenger. After exposure is stopped, tolerance is lost with similar rapidity.

**Treatment for Cannabis Use Disorder**
Many people won't go beyond the mild form of Cannabis Use Disorder and will commonly use cannabis in their teens and early 20s. As he gets older, a person has usually finished his education, is beginning a career and may be getting married and starting a family. With these responsibilities, the rewards they bring far outweigh the use of cannabis. The result is either stopping or reducing the use of cannabis with no impact on functioning.

However, others will continue to use cannabis frequently and in large amounts. Long-term use of cannabis is related to amotivation syndrome, which is a gradual shift into indifference and apathy—goals will be unmet, no new goals will be set, everyday tasks will be left unfinished and responsibilities will slowly be neglected. The impact of the long-term use will cause the quality of the person's life to be debilitated, and the person won't reach his full potential.

When a person seeks treatment for Cannabis Use Disorder, he has a great chance of stopping its use. Many people will realize that using cannabis is hindering them in achieving success; however, they're unable to stop on their own. They either enter treatment because of the criminal justice system or family members are pressuring them.

A serious roadblock in an individual with the disorder to find treatment is that, many times, they need to be convinced that it's causing problems. Often, the tolerant culture that accepts the use of cannabis, false information on the Internet and with other users, as well as the indifference that the cannabis use causes can be a barrier for the person to seek treatment.

Cannabis use disorders appear to be very similar to other substance use disorders, although the long-term clinical outcomes may be less severe. On average, adults seeking treatment for marijuana use disorders have used marijuana nearly every day for more than 10 years and have attempted to quit more than six times. People with cannabis use disorders, especially adolescents, often also suffer from other psychiatric disorders (*comorbidity*). Available studies indicate that effectively treating the mental health disorder with standard treatments involving medications and behavioral therapies may help reduce marijuana use, particularly among those involved with heavy use and those with more chronic mental disorders.

The following behavioral treatments are considered evidence-based, which means they produce better outcomes than no treatment at all, placebo, or general addictions counseling.
- **Cognitive-behavioral therapy**: A form of psychotherapy that teaches people strategies to identify and correct problematic behaviors in order to enhance self-control, stop drug use, and address a range of other problems that often co-occur with them.
- **Contingency management**: A therapeutic management approach based on frequent monitoring of the target behavior and the provision (or removal) of tangible, positive rewards when the target behavior occurs (or does not).
- **Motivational enhancement therapy**: A systematic form of intervention designed to produce rapid, internally motivated change; the therapy does not attempt to treat the person, but rather mobilize his or her own internal resources for change and engagement in treatment.
- **Rational Emotive Behavior Therapy:** Psychoeducation is used to challenge false beliefs individuals have about their cannabis use. This type of education provides factual information about the addiction. is treated with individual or group therapy following the model, which can help the person with the disorder to realize the dysfunctional thought patterns from its use and replacing them with adaptive thinking. People with the disorder will also learn to recognize, tolerate and manage their emotions instead of using cannabis to help manage their moods.
- **Medication-Assisted Treatments (combined with counseling):** Because sleep problems feature prominently in the cannabis withdrawal syndrome, studies are examining the effectiveness of medications that aid in sleep. Medications that

have shown promise in early studies or small clinical trials include the sleep aid zolpidem (Ambien®), an anti-anxiety/anti-stress medication called buspirone (BuSpar®), and an anti-epileptic drug called gabapentin (Neurontin®) that may improve sleep and, possibly, executive function. Other agents being studied include the nutritional supplement N-acetylcysteine and chemicals called FAAH inhibitors, which may reduce withdrawal by inhibiting the breakdown of the body's own endocannabinoids. Future directions include the study of substances called *allosteric modulators* that interact with cannabinoid receptors to inhibit THC's rewarding effects.

Lastly, there is some research on the use of a "replacement therapy" using CBD to treat the withdrawal and cravings and then initiating an individualized tapering plan.

**Cannabis Withdrawal Syndrome**
Nearly half of people who regularly use cannabis experience cannabis withdrawal syndrome when they try to stop, according to a meta-analysis published online in *JAMA Network Open* in April 2022. According to the *DSM-5*, symptoms of cannabis withdrawal syndrome may arise within seven days of quitting or reducing the use of cannabis and include irritability, aggression, nervousness, anxiety, problems with sleep, changes in appetite, depressed mood, and physical symptoms such as headaches, sweating, and nausea. "Cannabis withdrawal syndrome is clinically relevant and not something we should trivialize. It may be a reason people have difficulty quitting," lead author Anees Bahji, M.D., a psychiatry resident at Queen's University in Kingston, Ontario, told *Psychiatric News*. "The symptoms are terrible, which can set people up for a cycle where they try to make the symptoms go away by using cannabis again."

The DSM-5 diagnostic criteria for cannabis withdrawal include:
- Stopping cannabis use that has been heavy and prolonged (typically daily or almost daily for at least a few months)
- At least three of the below signs and symptoms begin within one week of stopping cannabis use
- Irritability, anger, aggression
- Nervousness or anxiety
- Difficulty sleeping
- Decreased appetite or weight loss
- Restlessness
- Depressed mood

- One or more of these physical symptoms causing significant discomfort: abdominal pain, shakiness/tremors, sweating, chills or fever, or headache

The signs and symptoms must be causing significant distress or impairing the ability to function in life, whether socially, at work, personal relationships, etc.

| | **DSM-5 Diagnostic Criteria for Cannabis Withdrawal Syndrome** |
|---|---|
| A. | Cessation of cannabis use that has been heavy and prolonged (i.e., usually daily or almost daily use over a period of a least a few months) |
| B. | 3 or more of the following signs and symptoms develop within approximately 1 week of Criterion A:<br>– Irritability, anger or aggression<br>– Nervousness or anxiety<br>– Sleep difficulty (insomnia, disturbing dreams)<br>– Decreased appetite or weight loss<br>– Restlessness<br>– Depressed mood<br>– At least one of the following physical symptoms causing significant discomfort: abdominal pain, shakiness/tremors, sweating, fever, chills, or headache |
| C. | The signs or symptoms from criterion B cause clinically significant distress or impairment in social, occupational or other important areas of functioning. |
| D. | The symptoms are not due to another medical condition and are not better explained by another mental disorder. |

DSM-5, Diagnostic and Statistical Manual of Mental Disorders

As with all drugs, the relative intensity of the withdrawal syndrome is dependent on the quantity, frequency, and duration of drug use. While a severe syndrome of physical dependence is not usually associated with cannabis withdrawal, the probability of developing some form of craving is great. The mechanism for these various withdrawal effects is unknown, but it is likely related to the unmasking of the desensitized receptors on drug cessation.

**Care for Patients Experiencing Cannabis Withdrawal Syndrome**

**Observation and monitoring**
Patients should be observed every three to four hours to assess for complications such as worsening anxiety and dissociation, which may require medication.

As cannabis withdrawal is usually mild, no withdrawal scales are required for its management.

**Management of cannabis withdrawal**
Cannabis withdrawal is managed by providing supportive care in a calm environment, and symptomatic medication as required.

**Follow-up care**
The preferred treatment for cannabis dependence is psycho-social care. Patients who have been using large amounts of cannabis may experience psychiatric disturbances such as psychosis; if necessary, refer patients for psychiatric care.

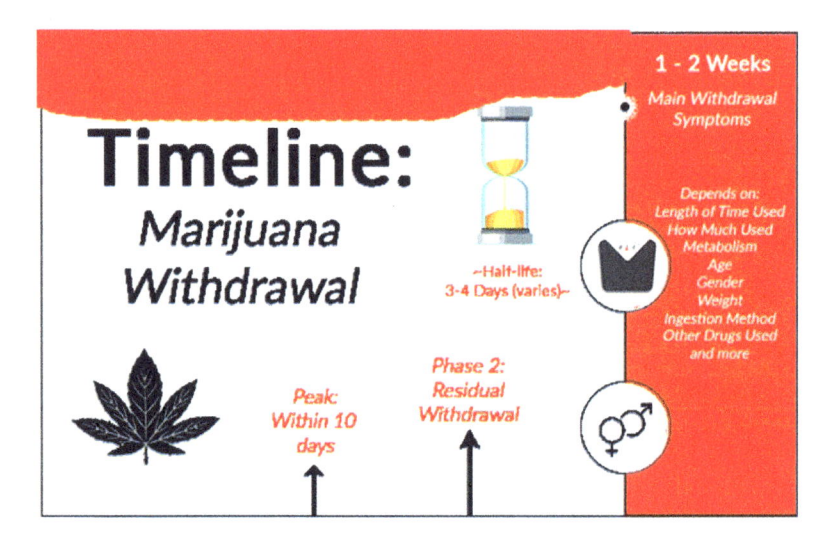

**Timeline: Marijuana Withdrawal**

~Half-life: 3-4 Days (varies)~

Peak: Within 10 days

Phase 2: Residual Withdrawal

1 - 2 Weeks
Main Withdrawal Symptoms

Depends on:
Length of Time Used
How Much Used
Metabolism
Age
Gender
Weight
Ingestion Method
Other Drugs Used
and more

**Toward Cannabinoid-Based Medicines**
The controversy over the issue of "medical marijuana" is actually all but over since medical research has made significant advances about the science of cannabinoid-based medicines. Synthetic analogs and other drugs acting on the human body's endogenous cannabinoid system are beginning to provide a myriad of potential therapeutic benefits attributed to marijuana, without the smoke, the contaminants, and the variable potency.

Just as nicotine is not tobacco, or taxol is not yew tree bark, and digoxin is not foxglove, cannabinoids are not marijuana. Research has cast new light on the function of the human endogenous cannabinoid system (ECS) and how cannabinoid-based medicines will be of significant therapeutic value in the not-so-distant future.

By using powerful new research tools, the varied functions of the EC system are being elucidated and the potential for the development of novel new medications is now being described. And, as the reader will discover, we are clearly moving beyond the limitations and problems associated with medical marijuana and moving toward cannabinoid-based medicines.

**Cannabinoid-Based Medicines (CbMs)**

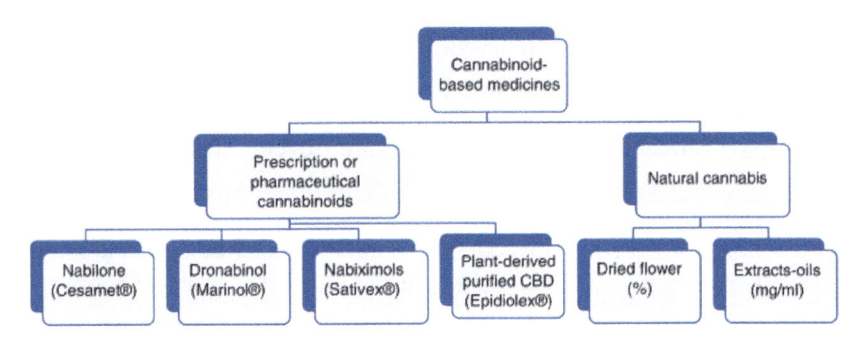

```
                    Cannabinoid-
                    based medicines
                   /               \
        Prescription or            Natural cannabis
        pharmaceutical              /         \
        cannabinoids          Dried flower   Extracts-oils
    /      |      |      \         (%)        (mg/ml)
Nabilone Dronabinol Nabiximols Plant-derived
(Cesamet®) (Marinol®) (Sativex®) purified CBD
                                (Epidiolex®)
```

Significant advances came when scientists discovered ways to more efficiently modify endocannabinoid activity indirectly, thereby avoiding abuse potential and unwanted side effects associated with THC. The most current pharmacological methods either decrease endocannabinoid activity by blocking the receptors where they exert their effect, or increase the action of endocannabinoids by inhibiting their breakdown, usually by blocking the enzymes that deactivate them.

As research progresses, scientists will be able to develop better approaches that will use the potential of the endocannabinoid system to treat more diseases and conditions. Cannabinoid-based medicines will more than likely act through the activity-inhibition mechanisms at selective cannabinoid receptor sites, through reuptake inhibition, and/or by targeting the degrading enzymes responsible for endocannabinoids.

In addition to appetite stimulation and suppression of nausea and vomiting, possible therapeutic uses of cannabinoid receptor agonists would include treatment of:

- postoperative pain, cancer pain, and neuropathic pain
- inflammatory disorders

- metabolic syndrome (obesity, high blood pressure, increased triglycerides, Type 2 diabetes)

Of all these potential indications, analgesia has probably received the most research attention. There is an increasing amount of evidence showing that the cannabinoid receptor system is an analgesic system. Research into pain medicines is allowing scientists to measure the specific effects of cannabinoids on various pain pathways. This system appears quite distinct from the endogenous opioid system, which indicates there are different types of pain and that certain pain types not responsive to opioid drugs might be better treated with cannabinoid-based medicines. While there is no drug as of yet with a selective pharmacologic profile, there are several distinct chemical classes of compounds known to interact with the $CB_1$ receptor.

In the 1970s, Pfizer pharmaceutical company launched a cannabinoid research program that resulted in the development of a cannabinoid analog, *levonantradol*, which was 1,000 times more potent than THC. Clinical trials showed efficacy for postoperative pain and chemotherapy-associated nausea and vomiting; however, side effects (sleepiness, dysphoria, dizziness, thought disturbance, and hypotension) were judged to be excessive, and the project was discontinued.

Marinol and Syndros, which contain dronabinol (synthetic THC), and Cesamet, which contains nabilone (a synthetic substance similar to THC), are approved by the FDA. Dronabinol and nabilone are used to treat nausea and vomiting caused by cancer chemotherapythe product is thought to exert its action by acting on cannabinoid receptors distributed throughout the central nervous system and in immune cells.

In 2005, Health Canada began using Sativex as a buccal spray for adjunctive analgesic treatment in adult patients with advanced cancer who experience moderate to severe pain during the highest tolerated dose of strong opioid therapy for persistent background pain.

Clinical trials data from a double-blind parallel group study showed that the addition of cannabinoid-based treatment to existing opioid and other analgesic medication significantly improved pain relief relative to placebo in patients with cancer pain not responding adequately to strong opioids. Furthermore, more than 40% of patients were able to achieve a clinically important reduction in pain.

In 2006 in the United Kingdom, rimonabant (Acomplia) was approved for use and is the first drug to target the endocannabinoid pathway by inhibiting the actions of anandamide and 2-AG on $CB_1$ receptors. Rimonabant had a very interesting mechanism of action in that it blocked $CB_1$ receptors within the ECS involved in obesity and weight control. The idea was that if you inhibit $CB_1$ receptors, it results in a decrease in appetite. Blocking $CB_1$ receptors also has direct actions on adipose tissue and the liver to improve glucose, fat and cholesterol metabolism improving insulin resistance, triglycerides and high-density lipoprotein cholesterol (HDL-C) and in some patients, blood pressure.

However, even though rimonabant had a novel mechanism of action, Sanofi-Aventis has withdrawn rimonabant from the market globally and it is no longer under development.

Acomplia was officially withdrawn in January 2009 due to the risks of dangerous psychological side effects, including suicidality. However, it nevertheless still showed the connection between $CB_1$ receptors and obesity, adiponectin levels, associated health consequences and a potential targeted treatment.

Approved in in 1985 and marketed in 2006, Nabilone (Cesamet® )is a synthetic cannabinoid and is primarily used to treat severe nausea and vomiting caused by cancer chemotherapy. It is for use only when other medications have been unable to control the nausea and vomiting.

**Future of Cannabinoid-Based Medicines:**
Obesity has reached global epidemic proportions with more than 1 billion adults overweight and at least 300 million of them recognized as clinically obese. Obesity is widely recognized as a major contributor to the global burden of chronic disease and disability and appears on the WHO list of Top 10 global health risks.

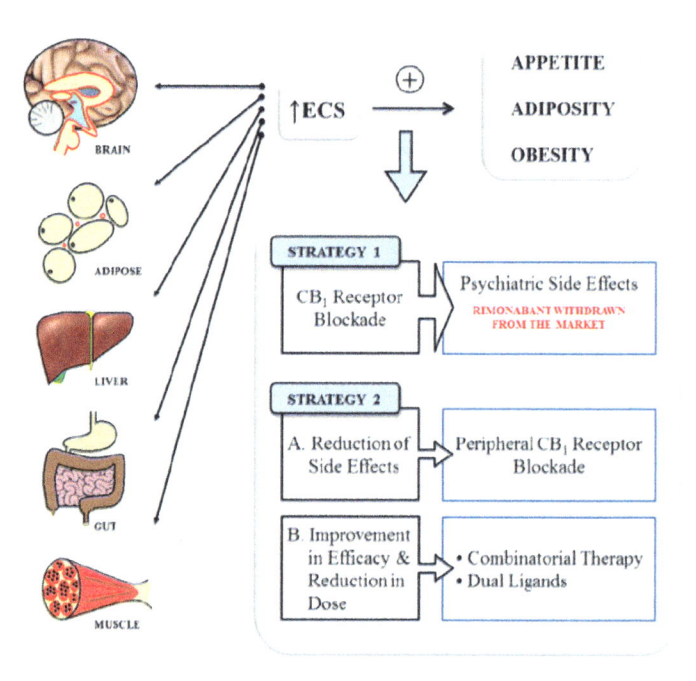

The combination of a sedentary lifestyle and a calorie-dense diet tends to disrupt the body's energy balance system, leading to obesity and the chronic over activity of the endocannabinoid system (ECS). Furthermore, research is showing how some chronic pathologic states, including obesity, lead to on-going over stimulation of the synthesis of endocannabinoids (or under-stimulation of their breakdown), resulting in over activation of the $CB_1$ receptors, which maintains or exacerbates the symptoms of these disorders.

In these situations of over activity, the ECS system is working beyond its normal range and the over stimulation seems to promote fat storage associated with insulin resistance, glucose intolerance, elevated triglycerides and low HDL cholesterol levels, all of which are risk factors for cardiovascular disease. $CB_1$ receptor blockade may be an effective treatment to modulate this overactive EC system resulting in the restoration of metabolic balance.

# SUGGESTED READINGS ON THIS TOPIC

Bahji A, Stephenson C, Tyo R, Hawken ER, Seitz DP. Prevalence of Cannabis Withdrawal Symptoms Among People With Regular or Dependent Use of Cannabinoids: A Systematic Review and Meta-analysis. *JAMA Netw Open.* 2020;3(4):e202370. doi:10.1001/jamanetworkopen.2020.2370

Cermak, Timmen L.. From Bud to Brain: A Psychiatrist's View of Marijuana. Cambridge University Press. 2020. ISBN-10 : 1108735738.

Cermak T, Stanford M.. (2023). Chapters on Neurodevelopmental Impact of Prenatal and Early Adolescent Cannabis Use and Resulting Neurocognitive Deficits and The Impacts of Cannabis on Adolescent Psychological Development. *Encyclopedia of Child and Adolescent Health.* Elsevier.

D'Souza, D.C., Ranganathan, M., Braley, G., Gueorguieva, R., Zimolo, Z., Cooper, T., Perry, E., and Krystal, J. Blunted Psychotomimetic and Amnesic Effects of $\Delta^9$-Tetrahydrocannabinol in Frequent Users of Cannabis. *Neuropharmacology* 1-12. (2008).

Freeman, T., et al. (2020). Cannabidiol for the treatment of cannabis use disorder: A phase 2a double-blind placebo-controlled, randomized, adaptive Bayesian trial. Lancet Psychiatry 7 (10): 865–874.

Gray, KK., et al. (2012) A double-blind randomized controlled trial of N-acetylcysteine in cannabis-dependent adolescents. American Journal of Psychiatry 169: 805–812

Jeffries, Shaun D.. Discovering the Endocannabinoid System: A New Frontier in Medical Science. Independently published. 2023. ASIN : B0BYRNM6HB.

Kendall, Dave.. Behavioral Neurobiology of the Endocannabinoid System. Springer. 2009. ISBN-10: 354088954X.

Maggirwar, SB. The Link between Cannabis Use, Immune System, and Viral Infections. Viruses. 2021 Jun; 13(6): 1099).

Mason, B., et al. (2012). A proof-of- concept randomized controlled study of gabapentin: Effects on cannabis use, withdrawal and executive function deficits in cannabis-dependent adults. Neuropsychopharmacology 37 (7): 1689–16.

Mechoulam, R et al. Identification of an endogenous 2-monoglyceride, present in canine gut, that binds to cannabinoid receptors. *Biochem Pharmacol*. 50:83-90. (1995).

Patel, Vinhood B.Neurobiology and Physiology of the Endocannabinoid System. Academic Press. 2023;. ISBN -10 : 0323908772.

Preedy, Victor R.. Handbook of Cannabis and Related Pathologies: Biology, Pharmacology, Diagnosis, and Treatment. Academic Press. 2017. ISBN-10 : 0128007567.
Russo, Ethan B. Cannabis and Cannabinoids: Pharmacology, Toxicology, and Therapeutic Potential. Routledge. 2002. ISBN-10 : 0789015080.

Shrier, L.A., Rhoads, A.M., Fredette, M.E., and Burke, P.J. (2014) Counselor in your pocket: Youth and provider perspectives on a mobile motivational intervention for marijuana use. Substance Use & Misuse 49 (1–2): 134–144.

Sultan RS, Zhang AW, Olfson M, Kwizera MH, Levin FR. Nondisordered Cannabis Use Among US Adolescents. *JAMA Netw Open*. 2023;6(5):e2311294. doi:10.1001/jamanetworkopen.2023.11294

Trash, Louis. Endocannabinoid System (ECS): Unlocking the Power of Natural Healing: Discovering the Therapeutic Potential of Cannabinoids and the ECS. MOBISOFT HOLDING NETHERLANDS B.V. 2023. ISBN-10 : 9403641002.

# CHAPTER 12. HALLUCINOGENIC DRUGS

# Key Concepts

| | |
|---|---|
| Anticholinergic effects | Urinary retention, constipation, dry mouth, confusional states, and tachycardia are the most common. The increase in heart rate is usually manifested as a sinus tachycardia that results from muscarinic blockade of vagal tone on the heart. |
| Anticholinergic Syndrome | A clinical syndrome resulting from antagonization of acetylcholine at the muscarinic receptor resulting in the inhibition of the transmission of parasympathetic nerve impulses. The central anticholinergic signs and symptoms include altered mental status, disorientation, delirium, agitation, somnolence, The peripheral anticholinergic syndrome includes hyperthermia, mydriasis, dry mucosa membranes, dry, hot and red skin, peripheral vasodilatation, tachycardia, and urinary retention. |
| Antimuscarinic effects | Antimuscarinics can cause tachycardia, or a higher than usual heart rate, when interfering with receptors that typically slow the heart rate. |
| Atropine | Atropine is a muscarinic antagonist. Excess doses of atropine may cause side effects such as palpitations, difficulty swallowing, hot dry skin, thirst, dizziness, restlessness, tremor, fatigue, and problems with coordination. As a medicine it is used to treat bradycardia (low heart rate), |

| | |
|---|---|
| | reduce salivation and bronchial secretions before surgery, and as an antidote for overdose of cholinergic drugs or mushroom poisoning. |
| Cholinergic system | The cholinergic system includes the neurotransmitter molecule, acetylcholine (Ach). It is an important system and a branch of the autonomic nervous system which plays a critical role in memory, digestion, control of heart beat, blood pressure, movement and many other functions. |
| Deliriant drugs | Atropine and scopolamine are classical muscarinic cholinergic antagonists that exert multiple CNS effects. Belonging to a group of deliriant hallucinogens, these drugs induce delirium-like hallucinations, hyperactivity, altered affective states and amnesia. |
| Dissociative drugs | Dissociative drugs can temporarily alter a person's mood, thoughts, and perceptions of reality. Among other health effects and safety concerns, people who use dissociative drugs report feeling strong emotions, ranging from intense happiness and a feeling of connectedness to fear, anxiety, and confusion. People who use these drugs also report experiencing intense or distorted visions or sensations. Drugs if this category include PCP, ketamine, dextromethorphan (DXM), and salvia. |
| Hallucinogens | Hallucinogens are psychoactive substances that powerfully alter perception, mood, and a host of cognitive processes. There are 3 |

| | |
|---|---|
| | primary categories: psychedelics, dissociative drugs and, deliriants. |
| Pharmacovigilance | A careful and critical approach to the use of new drugs, or the new use of established drugs is needed to ensure their use is safe and appropriate. |
| Scopolamine | As a medicine, scopolamine is a belladonna alkaloid with anticholinergic effects indicated for the treatment of nausea and vomiting associated with motion sickness and postoperative nausea and vomiting. Because scopolamine is able to pass the blood-brain barrier, it can cause hallucinations including delirium-like hallucinations, hyperactivity, altered affective states and amnesia. |

# CHAPTER 12

## Hallucinogenic Drugs

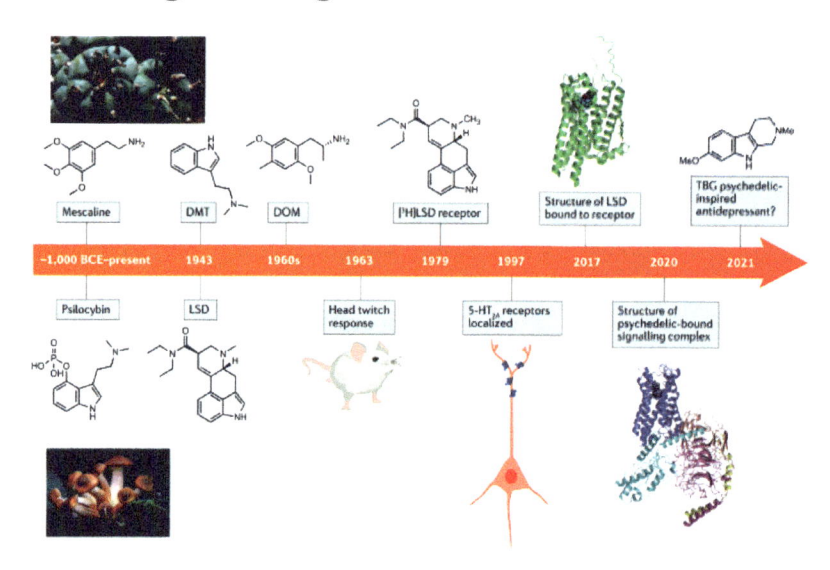

Technically by definition, hallucinogenic drugs alter and distort perceptions in space and time. An hallucination is a false perception, and these drugs produce exaggerated sensory phenomena including visual, auditory, and tactile hallucinations.

There are three categories of hallucinogenic drugs: psychedelics, dissociatives, and deliriants. 1) **Psychedelic drugs** include mescaline, psilocybin, and LSD; 2) **Dissociative drugs** include PCP, ketamine, dextromethorphan, and salvia distort sensory perceptions and can produce "out-of-body" type experiences. 3) **Deliriant drugs**, as Atropa Belladonna (aka, deadly nightshade) which contains atropine, and Datura stramonium (aka, jimson weed) which includes the chemicals of atropine, hyoscyamine, and scopolamine. Deliriants create false perceptions and confusions to a person's reality. The hallmarks of these classes of drugs are the changes to a person's perception they cause in their users.

The classic psychedelics exert primary activity as agonists at the 5-$HT_{2A}$ receptor (e.g., lysergic acid diethylamide (LSD), psilocybin, dimethyltryptamine (DMT) and mescaline). These drugs distort the perception of space and time, and produce exaggerated sensory phenomena in vision, hearing, and touch. The subjective effects associated with these drugs are determined by a number of factors such as setting, expectations, user's personality, mental health status. and dose. In some cases, adverse psychiatric effects occur including "bad trips", panic reactions and even a psychotic episode during intoxication.

While hallucinogenic drugs can have adverse consequences, their dependence potential, as measured by their reinforcing properties and neuroadaptive response, is low compared to other drugs. Somatic signs reflecting sympathetic arousal include dilated pupils, higher body temperature, increased heart rate and blood pressure, sweating, loss of appetite, sleeplessness, dry mouth, and tremors.

**Psychedelic Drugs**

**LSD**
LSD's psychedelic properties are a result of its actions on the serotonin neurotransmitter system. LSD is thought to stimulate the various receptor subtypes for serotonin, and has particular potency in activating the serotonin autoreceptor. To date, no evidence confirms that LSD supports self-administration in animal studies and there is no known lethal dose level for LSD. A similar activation of the serotonin system is seen with MDMA, a derivative of amphetamine and has both dopamine and serotonin stimulating properties. Unlike LSD, MDMA stimulates serotonin neurotransmission by blocking its reuptake into the presynaptic terminal. This action on serotonin gives MDMA psychedelic properties in addition to its amphetamine-like stimulating properties.

Further, there is no evidence that a withdrawal syndrome is associated with termination of chronic psychedelic drug use. The phenomenon of flashbacks, in which the perceptual changes associated with LSD spontaneously appear after drug cessation, are reported to occur in about 23 percent of regular users. It is still unclear whether flashbacks represent a withdrawal syndrome and are related to, or predictive of, hallucinogen dependence.

Most users of LSD voluntarily decrease or stop its use over time. LSD is not considered a drug with "abuse potential" since it does not act on the dopamine MLP system, the area for compulsive drug-seeking behaviors. However, like many drugs, LSD produces tolerance, so some users who take the drug repeatedly must take progressively higher doses to achieve the state of intoxication that they had previously achieved. This is an extremely dangerous practice, given the unpredictability of the drug.

Interestingly, rapid tolerance (called tachyphylaxis) develops soon with LSD and other psychedelics when they are repeatedly administered, and the extent of the tolerance is greater than with other drugs. The mechanism of LSD tolerance is unclear. Since LSD stimulates serotonin receptors and a typical response of receptors to continued activation is a desensitization process, it is possible that serotonin receptor desensitization plays a role.

**Psilocybin**
Psilocybin and psilocin are naturally occurring substances found in a variety of mushrooms but the species, *Psilocybe mexicana,* It was first isolated from its natural botanical source in the 1950s and then synthesized in the lab in 1961 by Dr. Albert Hoffman of LSD fame. Psilocybin is used primarily by oral ingestion of either the fresh or dried mushroom where it is well absorbed from the gastrointestinal (GI) tract. Initial effects can include nausea and vomiting due to the drug's rapid absorption from the GI tract. Psilocybin is serotonin-like and thus its hallucinogenic actions are related to its actions on brain serotonin systems.

An average 4mg dose can initiate the process of drug action characterized by physical and mental relaxation and some perceptual distortions. With increasing doses, hallucinations may take place. Autonomic effects are minimal and usually include mydriasis, elevated blood pressure and increased heart rate. The behavioral toxicity with psilocybin is similar to that observed with LSD, and includes symptoms of increased body temperature, anxiety, panic states, paranoia and depersonalization. There is no evidence that physical dependency is associated with psilocybin abuse and it is cross-tolerant with some of the other hallucinogens including LSD.

**Mescaline**
Like psilocybin, mescaline is a naturally occurring hallucinogen. Mescaline is the chief psychoactive ingredient of peyote cactus (*peyotl*) common to Southwest United States and Mexico. Most of the plant grows underground with only a small top being visible above ground. This top, or crown, is cut into small pieces and dried into "mescal buttons" which are then ingested orally.

A dose of 3 mg/kg will produce euphoria whereas a dose of 5 mg/kg will produce active hallucinations lasting 6 to 12 hours. Mescaline does not get metabolized (biotransformed) in the liver, and the far majority of the drug gets excreted unchanged by the kidney. The absence of liver biotransformation probably accounts for the drug's long duration of action. As an adrenergic substance, mescaline will produce all of the classic sympathomimetic effects including pupillary dilation, increased heart rate and blood pressure, elevated body temperature, EEG arousal and tremors. Toxic doses (greater than 500 mg) can produce convulsions and death due to respiratory depression.

The CNS effects of mescaline produce a profound sensory and psychic alteration much like LSD. Toxic doses can produce a psychotic reaction with paranoia, delusions and extreme panic states. However, the low potency of mescaline, as compared with other hallucinogens, makes the occurrence of behavioral toxic overdose very rare. As with many of the other hallucinogens, physical dependence is not seen although tolerance does develop slowly with repeated use.

Mescaline is cross-tolerant to both LSD and psilocybin, although it seems odd that an adrenergic substance like mescaline could produce cross-tolerance to serotonergic compounds. However, even though mescaline contains a catechol structure, and therefore is an adrenergic substance, it must also affect serotonin nerve fibers to produce some of its hallucinogenic properties; this is probably the connection it has with LSD and psilocybin.

**Dissociative drugs**

**Phencyclidine (PCP)**
Phencyclidine is representative of a unique class of drugs that includes the anesthetic Ketamine. PCP was developed as an injectable anesthetic in the 1950s. However, phencyclidine anesthesia is quite dissimilar to that produced by typical anesthetics. It produces a dissociative state in which patients are generally unresponsive and perceive no pain. Patients are amnesic for the surgery and CNS depression seen with other general anesthetics is absent. The delirium that often occurs on emergence from PCP anesthesia curtailed PCP's use as an anesthetic in humans. It is still sometimes used as a veterinary anesthetic, but is no longer marketed in the United States.

At sub-anesthetic doses, PCP produces behavioral effects common to several other drugs including amphetamines, barbiturates, opiates, and psychedelics. Given its wide range of behavioral effects, PCP's broad neurochemical action in the brain is not surprising. PCP antagonizes the actions of the excitatory amino acid neurotransmitter glutamate at the N-methyl-D-aspartate (NMDA) receptor, one of the receptor subtypes for glutamate. Glutamate is found throughout the brain and increases the flow of calcium (Ca+) ions into cells to cause excitatory actions.

The NMDA receptor controls the Ca+ ion channel acted on by glutamate and binding of PCP to the receptor blocks calcium entry into the cell. It is likely that the diverse behavioral effects of PCP are due to the fact that glutamate is widely distributed in the brain and regulates the activity of a number of other neurotransmitter systems. PCP also affects brain dopamine systems in ways similar to amphetamine.

The subjective effects of PCP administration can vary dramatically depending on a user's personality, who may experience vastly different reactions during different drug-taking episodes. In most cases, low doses produce euphoria, feelings of unreality, distortions of time, space and body image, and cognitive impairment. Higher doses produce restlessness, panic, disorientation, paranoia, and fear of death. As with its use as an anesthetic, PCP often causes amnesia to occur beginning immediately after the drug is taken until its effects begin to wear off. PCP is often associated with violent behavior in users but laboratory studies indicate that it does not increase aggressive behavior in animals. The violence often associated with PCP use is likely to be due to a combination of its ability to block pain and its stimulant and hallucinogenic actions.

The mechanism of action of PCP's reinforcing effects remain unclear. Part of PCP's behavioral effects are similar to dopamine-stimulating drugs like amphetamine and its administration potentiates the sedating properties of alcohol and barbiturates. As previously mentioned, PCP blocks the action of glutamate at the NMDA receptor. All of these actions may be relevant to the production of its reinforcing effects.

Animals who received repeat PCP administration have shown to develop tolerance to many of its effects. The magnitude of the tolerance, however, is less than what is seen with most other drugs of abuse. Systematic studies of PCP tolerance in humans have been few, but chronic PCP users report that after regular use they increase the amount of PCP smoked by at least twice. Some evidence from animal studies also suggests that sensitization may develop to PCP under certain conditions.

A withdrawal syndrome occurs in animals that have been chronically administered PCP. It is characterized by signs of CNS hyperexcitability such as twitches, tremors and susceptibility to seizures. A PCP withdrawal syndrome in humans is observed upon cessation of drug use. Symptoms of depression, confusion, disorientation, memory deficits, drug craving, increased appetite, and increased need for sleep have been reported to occur between 1 week and up to 8 months after termination of chronic PCP use. It is not clear why the long duration of post-acute withdrawal symptoms occur in some individuals.

**Ketamine**
Ketamine (esketamine, Ketalar, Ketaset) is a dissociative anesthetic which means that when administered at a certain dose, it leaves the patient semiconscious and in an analgesic state where any discomfort that may be experienced is not "associated" with the body. The site where ketamine binds is the sigma opioid receptor within the opioid peptide system. The substance is also a noncompetitive antagonist at the glutamate - NMDA receptor.

Because PCP is its parent compound, ketamine produces similar effects as those already described for PCP. Interestingly, ketamine has become one of the several illegal club drugs that are abused by a younger group. As an abused drug in this class of club drugs, it has a street name of "K", or "Special K'. In this context, ketamine (usually stolen from a medical clinic or pharmaceutical company and distributed on the street), is prepared in a liquid form for injection or in a powder form for snorting.

**Dextromethorphan**
DXM (dextromethorphan) is a cough-suppressing ingredient found in a variety of over-the-counter cold and cough medications, usually sold in the form of a liquid, tablets or gel caps. Like PCP and Ketamine, dextromethorphan is a dissociative anesthetic, meaning DXM effects can include hallucinations.

DXM may produce euphoria and mind-altering effects when taken in quantities greater than the recommended treatment dose. People who misuse DXM describe different "plateaus" ranging from mild distortions of color and sound to visual hallucinations and "out-of-body" sensations, and loss of motor control. Common DXM effects can include confusion, dizziness, double or blurred vision, slurred speech, impaired physical coordination, abdominal pain, nausea and vomiting, rapid heartbeat, drowsiness, numbness of fingers and toes, and disorientation.

**Salvia Divinorum**
*Salvia divinorum* is a perennial herb in the mint family that is abused for its hallucinogenic effects. Its psychedelic effects include perceptions of bright lights, vivid colors, shapes, and body movement, as well as body or object distortions. May also cause fear and panic, uncontrollable laughter, a sense of overlapping realities, paranoia, and hallucinations. Users typically experience rapid onset of intense hallucinations that can impair judgment and disrupt sensory and cognitive functions. Adverse physical effects may include: Loss of coordination, dizziness, and slurred speech.

Salvinorin A the active component of Salvia, is most active when vaporized and inhaled. Chemically, Salvinorin A is a psychotropic terpenoid. The grouping of psychoactive plants containing terpenoid essential oils includes Salvia Divinorum, Wormwood (Absinthe), and Cannabis Sativa (tetrahydrocannabinols, THC). A dose of 200 to 500 micrograms produces profound hallucinations when smoked. Its' effects in the open field test in mice and loco motor activity tests in rats are similar to mescaline. Salvinorin A's action in the brain are not well elucidated. However, recent tissue testing (in vitro assays) have suggested that Salvinorin A may act at the kappa opiate receptor site, but functional assays are lacking to determine the exact mechanism of action of this drug substance.

**Deliriants**
Deliriant drugs, such as atropine and scopolamine, induce characteristic hyperactivity and dream-like hallucinations and form a separate group of hallucinogens known as "deliriants".

There are two principal psychoactive substances within deliriant drugs that act as antagonists within acetylcholine systems: atropine and scopolamine. These chemicals produce their effects by essentially blocking certain cholinergic (muscarine) receptor sites in the brain. Atropine and scopolamine come from plants including deadly nightshade (Atropa belladonna), mandrake (Mandragora officinarum), henbane and datura (Datura stramonium). Because atropine and scopolamine block actions within the acetylcholine system, their effects include an *anticholinergic syndrome* of sorts. Blocking of the muscarinic postsynaptic receptors in the acetylcholine system produces an inhibition of secretion of various body fluids. Low perspiration and dry mouth are characteristic of this effect. Other symptoms of anticholinergic effects include tachycardia (racing heart), extreme elevation of body temperature, and dilated (widening) pupils.

The toxic behavioral effects of the deliriant drugs include delirium-like hallucinations, hyperactivity, altered affective states and amnesia, confusion, drowsiness, impaired concentration and other symptoms resembling a toxic psychosis. These drugs do not produce sensory effects, and therefore are not popular recreational drugs. Medicine has had a lengthy history of applying therapeutic dose ranges of these substances for a variety of conditions. For example, because scopolamine blocks cholinergic-muscarinic receptors, it can causes dryness in the nose, throat and mouth and thus has a role in treating cold and flu symptoms as a decongestant.

**Effects of Hallucinogens on the mind and body**
The National Institute of Drug abuse (NIDA) conducts research on the short- and long-term health effects of psychedelic and dissociative drugs to better inform health decisions and policies related to their use. While research is ongoing, scientific studies have revealed important information about how these drugs work:

- **Effects vary widely.** Effects of psychedelic and dissociative drugs may be difficult to predict and depend on many factors. These include the amount taken and potency (concentration and strength), as well as a person's unique biology, age, sex, personality, mood, expectations, mindset—commonly called "set"—and environment, or "setting." Using psychedelic and dissociative drugs that contain contaminants or using them in combination with other substances may also produce effects not associated with using these drugs alone.
- **Psychedelic and dissociative drugs temporarily alter thought patterns, mood, and perceptions of reality.** People who use these substances report feeling strong emotions, ranging from intense happiness and a feeling of connectedness to fear, anxiety, and confusion. Many people who use psychedelic drugs, such as psilocybin and LSD, report seeing vibrant shapes, colors, and scenes and reliving vivid memories. People who use dissociative drugs, such as ketamine and PCP, describe experiencing distorted vision and hearing.

- **Dissociative drugs can make people feel "detached."** Many people who use dissociative drugs report feeling as though they are floating or are disconnected from their body.
- **People may experience adverse health effects.** Physical side-effects of these substances, such as headache, nausea, or changes in heart rate, are generally not life-threatening. However, illicitly manufactured or processed drugs may be contaminated with colorless and odorless fentanyl or other dangerous substances that can cause serious adverse events, including overdose and death. Psychedelic or dissociative drugs may also produce adverse or debilitating psychological effects such as fear or anxiety.
- **Using psychedelic and dissociative drugs has been linked to dangerous behavior and injuries.** People using these drugs may have impaired thought processes and perception that cause them to behave in unusual and sometimes dangerous ways. This may lead to injuries and other safety issues, particularly if there is not another individual present who can help prevent or respond to an emergency.

**Psychedelics In Medicine**
In clinical research settings around the world, renewed investigations are taking place on the use of psychedelic substances for treating illnesses such as addiction, depression, anxiety and posttraumatic stress disorder (PTSD). Since the termination of a period of research from the 1950s to the early 1970s, most psychedelic substances have been classified as "drugs of abuse" with no recognized medical value. However, controlled clinical studies have recently been conducted to assess the basic psychopharmacological properties and therapeutic efficacy of these drugs as adjuncts to existing psychotherapeutic approaches.

Central to this revival is the re-emergence of a paradigm that acknowledges the importance of set (i.e., psychological expectations), setting (i.e., physical environment) and the therapeutic clinician–patient relationship as critical elements for facilitating healing experiences and realizing positive outcomes. The public is often well-versed in the potential harms of psychedelic drugs, but much of this knowledge is from cases involving patients who used illicit substances in unsupervised nonmedical contexts (Tupper, KW, 2015).

The U.S. Food and Drug Administration (FDA) has approved the ketamine derivative esketamine (under the brand name Spravato®) as a treatment for severe depression in patients who do not respond to other treatments. The FDA has also granted Breakthrough Therapy Designation for two formulations of psilocybin being studied as potential medical treatments for depression. Several other psychedelics are being investigated for their therapeutic potential, but this research is in the early stages and these substances are not legally available outside of limited, experimental settings. In June 2023, the FDA released a draft guidance to help researchers design safe studies that will yield interpretable results to support future study and applications for psychedelics.

From the MedPage Today article, in 2023, there were several medicinal psychedelics for psychiatric conditions showing benefits in major depression, bipolar depression, PTSD, and anorexia.

The phase IIa trial, an investigational N,N-dimethyltryptamine treatment -- commonly known as the hallucinogen **DMT** -- significantly reduced depressive symptoms by 7.4 points more than placebo ($P=0.02$) at 2 weeks after treatment when using the Montgomery-Asberg Depression Rating Scale (MADRS). The antidepressant effects were seen within just a week after a 21.5-mg infusion of the agent, dubbed SPL026, was administered with supportive therapy. Since this trial, several other psychedelics have made their way down the developmental pipeline, showing a wide range of psychiatric therapeutic effects.

In August 2023, another phase II trial from Raison CL, et al published in JAMA June 2023, showed that just a single dose of **psilocybin** significantly improved depression symptoms and functional disability in patients with major depressive disorder. Here, a 25-mg dose of synthetic psilocybin -- found in Psilocybe mushrooms, commonly known as "magic mushrooms" -- resulted in a sustained 12.3-point (95% CI -17.5 to -7.2) greater improvement versus active niacin placebo in MADRS score on day 43. With this treatment, which was co-administered with psychological support, patients had a significant improvement in symptoms as early as the second day.

Of note, psilocybin didn't just work well for major depressive disorder. In July, the same single synthetic dose of the psychedelic was found to be safe and tolerable in a phase I study of women with anorexia. Only 10 women were enrolled in the early-stage trial, which reported significant improvements in psychopathology, but no changes in body mass index. Later in the year, psilocybin eased symptoms of treatment-resistant bipolar depression in a trial of 15 people. MADRS scores decreased by 24 points at 3 weeks in participants with bipolar type II disorder, and 11 patients even met remission criteria. "Psychedelics have the potential to ease the suffering of many patients with difficult-to-treat mood disorders, and some folks with a cyclical mood disorder could benefit," study author Scott T. Aaronson, MD, of the Sheppard Pratt Health System in Baltimore, told *MedPage Today* in early December.

Other trials this year also highlighted psilocybin's therapeutic effects on treatment-resistant depression -- with or without the aid of traditional antidepressants -- and depression for patients with cancer.

## MDMA, Ketamine

In September 2023, positive findings from a late-stage trial highlighted MDMA's therapeutic effects on post-traumatic stress disorder (PTSD) symptoms. Building on phase II findings released in 2021, adding MDMA pharmacotherapy to psychotherapy significantly improved PTSD symptoms compared with placebo with psychotherapy (least squares mean change -23.7 vs -14.8). The compound, which was granted a breakthrough therapy designation in 2017, also significantly improved clinician-rated functional impairment in a diverse patient population.

"The hope is that MDMA and psychedelics in general might have a signal in not just PTSD and depression ... but in other mental health disorders as well," study author Jennifer M. Mitchell, PhD, of the University of California San Francisco, told *MedPage Today* in the fall. "The objective will be to evaluate all of the psychedelics in each of these different disorders to determine how far the therapeutic efficacy reaches."

Because of the successes observed in phase II and III trials, MAPS Public Benefit Corporation announced in mid-December that it submitted a new drug application to the FDA, asking for priority review. If approved, the Drug Enforcement Administration would be required to reschedule MDMA, making it available for prescription medical use, the developer said.

While not a classic psychedelic in the traditional sense, ketamine also continued to prove its therapeutic benefits throughout 2023. According to a recent study by Anand A, et al published in JAMA May 2023, ketamine worked just as well as electroconvulsive therapy -- the "gold standard" for treatment-resistant depression. Following a 3-week treatment period, 55.4% of the patients in the ketamine group and 41.2% of those in the electroconvulsive therapy group had a treatment response, a 14.2% difference (95% CI 3.9-24.2).

In IV form, ketamine is only FDA approved as a sedative, analgesic, and general anesthetic. Esketamine (Spravato) nasal spray is approved alongside an oral antidepressant for treatment-resistant depression. "Ketamine's effectiveness, in the aggregate results, looks a bit better than electroconvulsive therapy for major depression not associated with psychotic features," lead investigator Amit Anand, MD, director of Psychiatry Translational Clinical Trials at Mass General Brigham in Boston, told at the APA annual meeting.

## Pharmacovigilance: Evaluating the Safety and Effectiveness of a Medicine

When a new drug, or a new use for an existing drug, is launched, it typically has not been as widely tested as other available therapies, and there is often insufficient good-quality published evidence to be able to judge safety and effectiveness. The safety profile cannot be fully assessed, because only a limited number of patients will have been exposed to the drug by the time of licensing. This presents a dilemma for innovative physicians who seek to provide their patients with the best available therapeutic intervention, without exposing them to dangerous consequences of unforeseen effects.

Obviously, some fundamental questions about the drug safety and effectiveness profile must be known and include these markers:

- The dose-response relationship. Ability to determine the optimal dosing and frequency given the diagnosis and patient health profile (i.e. age, gender, ethnicity, gender, preexisting physical; and mental health conditions, other medications prescribed, prior treatment history, etc.)

- Indications for use. Ability to determine that the use of the drug for a diagnosis is safe and appropriate. Perhaps even more importantly, the ability to determine when the drug would be contraindicated because of potentially dangers toxic interactions with other drugs the patient is taking for other preexisting health conditions.

To address this problem, physicians can use the STEPS (Safety, Tolerability, Effectiveness, Price, and Simplicity) mnemonic to provide an analytic framework for making better decisions about a new drug's appropriate place in therapy.

A key element is to base this evaluation on patient-oriented evidence rather than accept disease-oriented evidence (which may be misleading), while avoiding inappropriate reliance on studies that report only noninferiority results or relative risk reductions. The primary question to ask for each new drug prescribing decision is, "Is there good evidence that this new drug is likely to make my patient live longer or better compared with the available alternatives?" (Pegler, S. 2010.).

## SUGGESTED READINGS ON THIS TOPIC

Anand A, et al "Ketamine versus ECT for nonpsychotic treatment-resistant major depression" N Engl J Med 2023; DOI: 10.1056/NEJMoa2302399.

Miller, RL. Psychedelic Medicine: The Healing Powers of LSD, MDMA, Psilocybin, and Ayahuasca. Park Street Press. 2017. ISBN-10 : 1620556979.

National Institute of Drug Abuse (NIDA). Psychedelic and Dissociative Drugs
https://nida.nih.gov/research-topics/psychedelic-dissociative-drugs

Pegler S, Underhill J. Evaluating the safety and effectiveness of new drugs. Am Fam Physician. 2010 Jul 1;82(1):53-7. PMID: 20590071.

Raison CL, Sanacora G, Woolley J, et al. Single-Dose Psilocybin Treatment for Major Depressive Disorder: A Randomized Clinical Trial. *JAMA*. 2023;330(9):843–853. doi:10.1001/jama.2023.14530

Tupper KW, Wood E, Yensen R, Johnson MW. Psychedelic medicine: a re-emerging therapeutic paradigm. CMAJ. 2015 Oct 6;187(14):1054-1059. doi: 10.1503/cmaj.141124. Epub 2015 Sep 8. PMID: 26350908; PMCID: PMC4592297.

Winkelman, MJ. Advances in Psychedelic Medicine: State-of-the-Art Therapeutic Applications. Praeger. 2019. ISBN-10 : 1440864101.

# CHAPTER 13. INHALANTS

## Key Concepts

| | |
|---|---|
| Aliphatic nitrites | Organic inhalants like cyclohexyl nitrite, amyl nitrite and butyl nitrite (now illegal). |
| Gases | Household or commercial inhalants including propane, aerosols and sprays. |
| Peripheral Neuropathy | Peripheral neuropathy causes pain and numbness in the hands and feet. The pain is described as tingling or burning, while the loss of sensation often is compared to the feeling of wearing a thin stocking or glove. |
| Inhalants | Inhalants are a diverse group of volatile substances whose chemical vapors can be inhaled to produce psychoactive effects. While other abused substances can be inhaled, the term "inhalants" is used to describe substances that are rarely, if ever, taken by any other manner. A variety of products common in the home and workplace contain substances that can be inhaled to get high; however, people do not typically think of these products (e.g., spray paints, glues, and cleaning fluids) as drugs because they were never intended to be ingested by people. |
| Kaposi's sarcoma | Kaposi's sarcoma is a form of skin cancer that can involve internal organs. It is most often found in patients with acquired immunodeficiency syndrome (AIDS) and can be fatal. |
| Solvents | A group of inhalants including paint thinners, gas, glues, and various household or industrial cleaners. |

# CHAPTER 13

# Inhalants

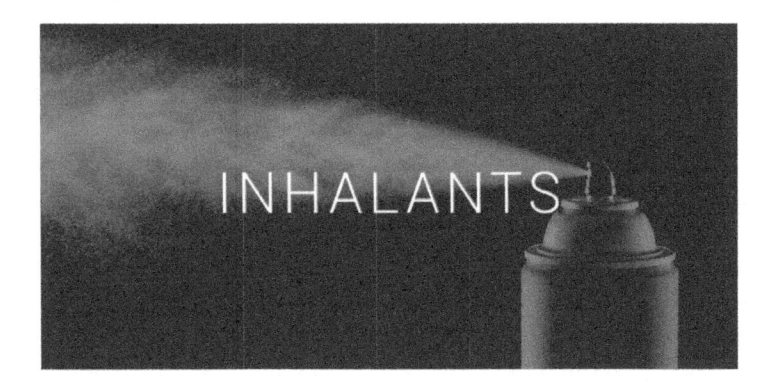

Although other substances that are misused can be inhaled, the term *inhalants* refers to the various substances that people typically take *only* by inhaling. The inhalants are a diverse group of substances that include glues, aerosols, refrigerants, cleaning fluids, cements, lighter fluid, marker pens, gasoline, volatile anesthetics, fingernail polish, bottled fuel gas, paint, paint remover, and room deodorizers.

Inhalants fall into four general categories: solvents, gases, nitrates and aerosols. Industrial or household **solvents** include paint thinners, degreasers (dry-cleaning fluids), gasoline, glues, art supplies, felt-tip-marker fluid, and electronic contact cleaners. **Gases** used in household or commercial products include cigarette lighters and propane tanks, whipping cream aerosol (whippets), refrigerant gases, household aerosol propellants and other associated solvents such as spray paints, hair or deodorant sprays, and fabric protector sprays. Also included in this category are medical anesthetic gases such as ether, chloroform, halothane, and nitrous oxide (laughing gas). Aliphatic (organic) **nitrites** include cyclohexyl nitrite, which is available to the general public; amyl nitrite, which is available only by prescription; and butyl nitrite, which is now an illegal substance. **Aerosols** are sprays that contain propellants and solvents. They include spray paints, deodorant and hair sprays, vegetable oil sprays for cooking, and fabric protector sprays.

Evidence from research studies suggests that a number of commonly abused volatile solvents and anesthetic gases have neurobehavioral effects and mechanisms of action similar to those produced by CNS depressants, which include alcohol and medications such as sedatives and anesthetics.

Inhaled chemicals are absorbed rapidly into the bloodstream through the lungs and are quickly distributed to the brain and other organs. Within seconds of inhalation, the user experiences intoxication along with other effects similar to those produced by alcohol. Alcohol-like effects may include slurred speech; the inability to coordinate movements; euphoria; and dizziness. In addition, users may experience lightheadedness, hallucinations, and delusions.

Because intoxication lasts only a few minutes, abusers frequently seek to prolong the high by inhaling repeatedly over the course of several hours, which is a very dangerous practice. With successive inhalations, abusers can suffer loss of consciousness and possibly even death. At the least, they will feel less inhibited and less in control. After heavy use of inhalants, abusers may feel drowsy for several hours and experience a lingering headache. (NIDA. 2020. https://nida.nih.gov/publications/research-reports/inhalants/how-are-inhalants)

Sniffing highly concentrated amounts of the chemicals in solvents or aerosol sprays can directly induce heart failure and death. This is especially common from the abuse of fluorocarbons and butane-type gases. High concentrations of inhalants also cause death from suffocation by displacing oxygen in the lungs (and thus in the central nervous system) so that breathing ceases. Other irreversible effects caused by inhaling specific solvents can be permanent. Hearing loss can be caused by toluene (paint sprays, glues, dewaxers) and trichloroethylene (cleaning fluids). Peripheral neuropathies (limb spasms) can result from taking hexane (glues and gasoline) and nitrous oxide (whipping cream or gas cylinders).

Central nervous system brain damage can also result from toluene (paint sprays, glues and dewaxers). Finally, bone marrow damage can be caused by sniffing gasoline (benzene). There are also serious but potentially reversible effects. Liver and kidney damage can result from substances containing toluene and chlorinated hydrocarbons (correction fluid and dry cleaners). Blood oxygen depletion can be very hazardous, caused by organic nitrites ("poppers," "bold" and "rush") and methylene chloride (varnish removers and paint thinners).

According to NIDA research, although people are exposed to volatile solvents and other inhalants in the home and in the workplace, many do not think of inhalable substances as drugs because most of them were never meant to be used in that way. Inhalants can be breathed in through the nose or the mouth in a variety of ways, such as;
- "sniffing" or "snorting" fumes from containers;
- spraying aerosols directly into the nose or mouth;
- "bagging" — sniffing or inhaling fumes from substances sprayed or deposited inside a plastic or paper bag;
- "huffing" from an inhalant-soaked rag stuffed in the mouth; and
- inhaling from balloons filled with nitrous oxide.

Young people are likely to abuse inhalants, in part because inhalants are readily available and inexpensive. Sometimes children unintentionally misuse inhalant products that are found around the house in household products. Parents, therefore, should see that these substances are monitored closely so that they are not inhaled by young children.

The chemicals found in solvents, aerosol sprays, and gases can produce a variety of additional effects during or shortly after use. These effects are related to inhalant intoxication and may include belligerence, apathy, impaired judgment, and impaired functioning in work or social situations; nausea and vomiting are other common side effects. Exposure to high doses can cause confusion and delirium. In addition, inhalant abusers may experience dizziness, drowsiness, slurred speech, lethargy, depressed reflexes, general muscle weakness, and stupor. For example, research shows that toluene can produce headache, euphoria, giddy feelings, and the inability to coordinate movements (NIDA. 2020)

Inhaled nitrites dilate blood vessels, increase heart rate, and produce a sensation of heat and excitement that can last for several minutes. Other effects can include flush, dizziness, and headache.

Inhalant abusers risk an array of other devastating medical consequences. The highly concentrated chemicals in solvents or aerosol sprays can induce irregular and rapid heart rhythms and lead to fatal heart failure within minutes of a session of prolonged sniffing. This syndrome, known as "sudden sniffing death," can result from a single session of inhalant use by an otherwise healthy young person.

Sudden sniffing death is associated particularly with the abuse of butane, propane, and chemicals in aerosols. Death from inhalants is usually caused by a very high concentration of fumes. Even when using aerosol or volatile products for their legitimate purposes (painting or cleaning), it is wise to do so in a well-ventilated room or better yet, outdoors. Amyl and butyl nitrites have been associated with Kaposi's sarcoma (KS), the most common cancer reported among AIDS patients. Early studies of KS showed that many people with KS had used volatile nitrites. Researchers are continuing to explore the hypothesis of nitrites as a factor contributing to the development of KS in HIV-infected people.

Inhalant abuse also can cause death by—
- **asphyxiation** — from repeated inhalations that lead to high concentrations of inhaled fumes, which displace available oxygen in the lungs;
- **suffocation** — from blocking air from entering the lungs when inhaling fumes from a plastic bag placed over the head;
- **convulsions or seizures** — from abnormal electrical discharges in the brain;
- **coma** — from the brain shutting down all but the most vital functions;
- **choking** — from inhalation of vomit after inhalant use; or
- **fatal injury** — from accidents, including motor vehicle fatalities, suffered while intoxicated.

Based on independent studies performed over a 10-year period in three different states, the number of inhalant-related fatalities in the United States is approximately 100–200 per year (NIDA. 2020).

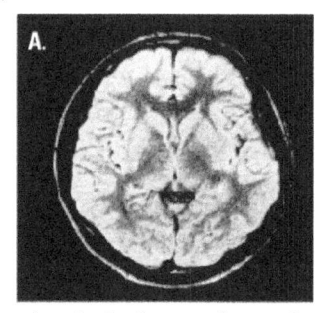

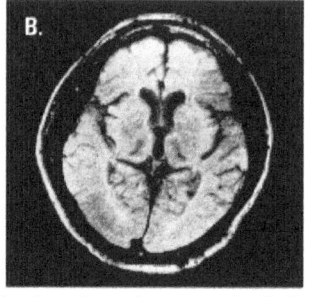

*Compared with the brain of an individual with no history of inhalant abuse (A), that of a chronic toluene abuser (B) is smaller and fills less of the space inside the skull (the white outer circle in each image). Courtesy of Neil Rosenberg, M.D., NIDA Research Report (NIH 05-3818).*

Sustained chronic use of inhalants can lead to pathology including kidney, liver, and bone marrow suppression following benzene and chlorinated hydrocarbon exposure; cardiotoxic effects following haolgenated hydrocarbon exposure, lead encephalopathies in gasoline inhalation, neurodegenerative changes in toluene users, and peripheral neuropathies in hexane users.

| ABUSED INHALANT SUBSTANCES ||
| Product | Chemical Ingredients |
|---|---|
| **Aerosols**<br>Spray paint, hair sprays, deodorants, medical sprays, asthma mists | Toluene, butane, propane, fluorocarbons, hydrocarbons |
| **Adhesives**<br>Model airplane glue, rubber cement, polyvinylchloride cement | Toluene, ethylacetate, hexane, methylethyl ketone, trichloroethylene |
| **Solvents And Gases**<br>Nail polish remover, paint remover, paint thinner, correction fluid, and thinner, fuel gas, cigarette lighter fluid, gasoline | Acetone, ethylacetate, toluene, methylene chloride, methanol, esters, trichloroethylene, trichloroethane, propane, butane, isopropane, mixed hydrocarbons |
| **Cleaning Agents**<br>Dry cleaning fluid, spot remover, degreaser | Xylene, petroleum distillates, chlorohydrocarbons tetrachloroethylene, tricholoroethane |

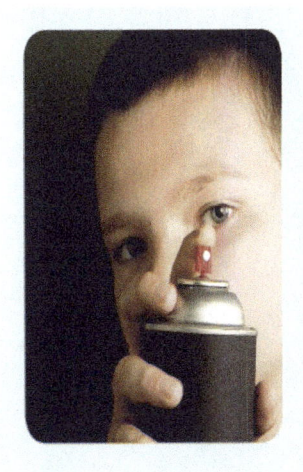

## How Can Inhalant Abuse Be Recognized?

Early identification and intervention are the best ways to stop inhalant abuse before it causes serious health consequences. Parents, educators, family physicians, and other health care practitioners should be alert to the following signs:

- Chemical odors on breath or clothing
- Paint or other stains on face, hands, or clothes
- Hidden empty spray paint or solvent containers, and chemical-soaked rags or clothing
- Drunk or disoriented appearance
- Slurred speech
- Nausea or loss of appetite
- Inattentiveness, lack of coordination, irritability, and depression

## SUGGESTED READINGS ON THIS TOPIC

Bowen, S.E.; Batis, J.C.; Paez-Martinez, N.; and Cruz, S.L. The last decade of solvent research in animal models of abuse: Mechanistic and behavioral studies. *Neurotoxicol Teratol* 28(6):636-647, 2006.

Fung, H.L., and Tran, D.C. Effects of inhalant nitrites on VEGF expression: A feasible link to Kaposi's sarcoma? *J Neuroimmune Pharmacol* 1(3):317-322, 2006.

Hall, M.T.; Edwards, J.D.; and Howard, M.O. Accidental deaths due to inhalant misuse in North Carolina: 2000-2008. *Subst Use Misuse* 45(9):1330-1339, 2010.

Lubman, D.I.; Yücel, M.; and Lawrence, A.J. Inhalant abuse among adolescents: Neurobiological considerations. *Br J Pharmacol* 154(2):316-326, 2008.

NIDA. 2022. https://nida.nih.gov/publications/research-reports/inhalants

# CHAPTER 14. METHODS OF DRUG TESTING

## Key Concepts

| | |
|---|---|
| Blood drug testing | Healthcare providers mainly use this type of test in emergencies. It's also typically used to detect alcohol (ethanol) levels because it can provide a precise level. |
| Breath drug testing | This is primarily used to detect recent alcohol consumption. The result is called a breath alcohol concentration (BrAC). Officials often use it to estimate a person's blood alcohol content (BAC). However, BrAC can sometimes overestimate or underestimate the BAC. Recent research has focused on the potential use of breath testing for detecting cocaine, marijuana, benzodiazepines, amphetamines, opioids, methadone and buprenorphine. |
| Creatinine | Creatinine is a metabolic byproduct of protein metabolism, which normally appears in urine in relatively constant quantities over a 24-hour period with regular liquid consumption. |
| False Positives | Defined as a drug free sample falsely being reported as showing positive for drugs. |
| Gas chromatography–mass spectrometry | (GC-MS) A test that is able to detect small quantities of a substance and confirm the presence of a specific drug and is the most accurate, sensitive, and reliable method of testing. |

| | |
|---|---|
| Hair follicle drug testing | A hair sample can provide information on substance use over time. Scalp hair has a detection window of three months, while slower-growing body hair has a detection window of up to 12 months. The results can vary based on the characteristics of each person's hair. Hair testing can detect the use of cocaine, phencyclidine (PCP), amphetamines, opioids and 3,4-Methylenedioxymethamphetamine (MDMA). |
| Prescription drug testing | Perspiration testing involves wearing an absorbent pad on the skin that's collected and tested after a certain amount of time. The results provide information on how much of a substance the person consumed over the entire time that they wore the pad. Perspiration testing gives a detection window of hours to weeks. |
| Urine Toxicology Screens | (UTS) medical testing for urinary metabolites of recreational drugs. Two types are mainly used: immunoassay and gas chromatography–mass spectrometry (GC-MS). UTS are most commonly used to detect alcohol, amphetamines, benzodiazepines, opioids, cocaine and cannabinoids (THC) and phencyclidine (PCP). |
| Immunoassays | A UTS that uses antibodies to detect the presence of specific drugs or metabolite. Immunoassay techniques are used in many home-testing kits or point-of-care screenings. |

# CHAPTER 14

# Methods of Drug Testing

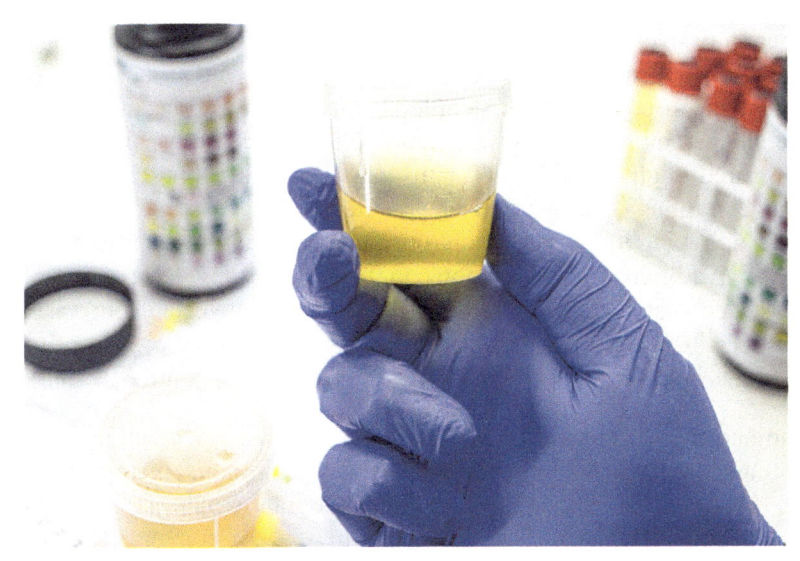

According to the National Library of Medicine, broadly defined, drug testing uses a biological sample to detect the presence or absence of a drug or its metabolites. This process can be completed in a variety of settings and with a variety of techniques. Many drug screening immunoassays were initially designed for use in the workplace as a drug screening tool for employees. As these tests have become cheaper, more readily available, and easier to use, these tests are now standard in many clinical laboratories. Despite their prevalence, many physicians, therapists counselors, and providers do not understand how these tests function and their associated limitations. Despite the drawbacks, drug testing plays an essential role in the clinical setting because clinical examination, patient self-reporting, and collateral reporting will often underestimate the actual incidence of substance use. The use of drug screens is also becoming increasingly important in the management of patients with chronic pain and in the treatment of substance use disorders.

The most commonly tested-for substances are amphetamines, cannabinoids, cocaine, opiates, and phencyclidine (PCP). These drugs are also referred to as the "NIDA five" as these were the five drugs that were recommended for drug screening of federal employees by the

National Institute on Drug Abuse (NIDA). This responsibility now falls on the Substance Abuse and Mental Health Services Administration (SAMHSA). There are now expanded drug screens that include testing for oxycodone, methadone, buprenorphine, and fentanyl, among many other drugs.

There are several biological samples that can be used for testing. These include blood or serum, sweat, hair, oral fluid, and urine. The most commonly used biological sample is urine, as it is non-invasive, and the concentration of a given xenobiotic is generally higher when compared to other samples. This usually results in a higher sensitivity. Concentrations of drugs and metabolites also tend to be high in the urine, allowing longer detection times than concentrations in the serum allow. Additional considerations include how long a xenobiotic (a substance that is foreign to the body) remains detectable in various matrices. It is important to consider these aspects in the context of why testing is being performed (McNeil SE, Chen RJ, Cogburn M. 2023).

Immunoassays remain the most common and easily accessible form of testing. More advanced methods, particularly in confirmatory testing, are available and include gas chromatography/mass spectrometry (GC/MS) and liquid chromatography/mass spectrometry (LC/MS). These advanced methods tend to have higher specificity and sensitivity as compared to immunoassays, but are more expensive and require specialized equipment and training

Two types of urine toxicology screens (UTS) are typically used; immunoassay and gas chromatography–mass spectrometry (GC-MS). Immunoassays, which use antibodies to detect the presence of specific drugs or metabolites, are the most common method for the initial screening process. Advantages of immunoassays include large-scale screening through automation and rapid detection.

Forms of immunoassay techniques include cloned enzyme donor immunoassay; enzyme-multiplied immunoassay technique (EMIT), a form of enzyme immunoassay; fluorescence polarization immunoassay (FPIA); immunoturbidimetric assay; and radioimmunoassay (RIA). In addition, immunoassay techniques are used in many home-testing kits or point-of-care screenings.

The main disadvantage of immunoassays is obtaining false-positive results when detection of a drug in the same class requires a second test for confirmation. Results of immunoassays are always considered presumptive until confirmed by a laboratory-based test for the specific drug (eg, GC-MS or high-performance liquid chromatography). Yet even GC-MS can fail to identify a positive specimen (eg, hydromorphone, fentanyl) if the column is designed to detect only certain substances (eg, morphine, codeine).

Gas chromatography–mass spectrometry is considered the criterion standard for confirmatory testing. The method is able to detect small quantities of a substance and confirm the presence of a specific drug (eg, morphine in an opiate screen). It is the most accurate, sensitive, and reliable method of testing; however, the test is time-consuming, requires a high level of expertise to perform, and is costly. For these reasons, GC-MS is usually performed only after a positive result is obtained from immunoassay.

**Urine Testing**
Results of a urine test show the presence or absence of specific drugs or drug metabolites in the urine. Metabolites are drug residues that remain in the system for some time after the effects of the drug have worn off. A positive urine test does not necessarily mean the subject was under the influence of drugs at the time of the test. Rather, it detects and measures use of a particular drug within the previous few days.

The following is a summary of the analytical methods used by laboratories to detect the presence of drugs or their metabolites in urine.

**Immunoassays**
These tests are most commonly used to screen samples. In the event that drugs or their metabolites are detected, then the sample is normally tested again using an even more sensitive test such as Gas Chromatography and Mass Spectrometry (GCMS). Immunoassays work on the principle of antigen-antibody interaction. Antibodies are chosen which will bind selectively to drugs or their metabolites. The binding is then detected using either enzymes, radioisotopes or fluorescent compounds.

- **EMIT.** The Enzyme Multiplied Immunoassay Technique. It uses an enzyme as the detection mechanism. It is the cheapest, simplest to perform and the most widely used of the immunoassays. Unfortunately, it is also the easiest to fail and more worryingly, the least accurate: giving a 4-34% false positive rate.

- **RIA** (Radio Immunoassay) is manufactured by Roche Diagnostics. It is similar to EMIT but uses a radioactive isotope such as iodine instead of an enzyme. However, because it involves using radioactive substances, it is less popular than EMIT. This is a highly sensitive form of testing mainly used by the military.
- **FPI** (Fluorescence Polarization Immunoassay) is manufactured by Abbott Laboratories. Fluorescent compounds mark the selective binding of antibodies to drugs and their metabolites. It is highly sensitive and highly specific.

**Thin Layer Chromatography**
This procedure involves the addition of a solvent to the sample causing the drugs and their metabolites to travel up a porous strip leaving color spots behind. As each different substance travels a specific distance, the strip can then be compared with known standards. This test gives no quantitative information, it merely indicates the presence of drugs or their metabolites. Furthermore, it relies on the subjective judgement of a technician and requires considerable skill and training. It is not widely used.

**Gas Chromatography and Mass Spectrometry**
These are the most precise tests for identifying and quantifying drugs or their metabolites in the urine. They are usually used as a confirmation test following a positive result on an Immunoassay. It involves a two-step process, whereby *Gas Chromatography* separates the sample into its constituent parts and *Mass Spectometry* identifies the exact molecular structure of the compounds. The combination of Gas Chromatography and Mass Spectrometry is considered to be the definitive method of establishing the presence of drugs or their metabolites in the urine. However, the equipment necessary to perform it is extremely expensive and this is reflected in the price for testing each sample. Occasionally problems do arise with poor calibration of the equipment.

Although urine is most commonly tested, occasionally laboratories use one of the following methods to detect the presence of drugs or their metabolites:

**Hair Testing**
Analysis of hair may provide a much longer "testing window" for the presence of drugs and drug metabolites, giving a more complete drug-use history that goes back as far as 90 days. Like urine testing, hair

testing does not provide evidence of current impairment, only past use of a specific drug. Hair testing cannot be used to detect alcohol.

**Perspiration Testing**
Another type of drug test consists of a skin patch that measures drugs and drug metabolites in perspiration. The patch, which looks like a large adhesive bandage, is applied to the skin and worn for some length of time. A gas-permeable membrane on the patch protects the tested area from dirt and other contaminants. The sweat patch is sometimes used in the criminal justice system to monitor drug use by parolees and probationers, but so far it has not been widely used in workplaces or schools.

**Saliva Testing**
Traces of drugs, drug metabolites, and alcohol can be detected in oral fluids, the generic term for saliva and other material collected from the mouth. Oral fluids are easy to collect—a swab of the inner cheek is the most common way. They are harder to adulterate or substitute, and collection is less invasive than with urine or hair testing. Because drugs and drug metabolites do not remain in oral fluids as long as they do in urine, this method shows more promise in determining current use and impairment.

**Alcohol Breathalyzers**
Unlike urine tests, breath-alcohol tests do detect and measure current alcohol levels. The subject blows into a breath-alcohol test device, and the results are given as a number, known as the Blood Alcohol Concentration, which shows the level of alcohol in the blood at the time the test was taken. In the U.S. Department of Transportation regulations, an alcohol level of 0.04 is high enough to stop someone from performing a safety-sensitive task for that day.

**Blood Testing**
Although expensive and intrusive, blood testing is the most accurate confirmation of drug use. Since blood testing accurately detects the presence of the drug or its metabolites at the time of testing, the results from this type of test are the best indication of current intoxication. Blood testing for the use of drugs is primarily used in accident investigations or for health/life insurance medicals. Cannabinoids can be detected up to six hours after consumption by testing blood; after that, the metabolite concentration falls rapidly, and cannabinoids are not detectable in the blood after 22 hours.

**Standard Test Panels**

A standard panel typically includes amphetamine, methamphetamine, cocaine, benzodiazepines, barbiturates, phencyclidine (PCP), opioids, and cannabinoids (THC).

**Urine Toxicology Screens**
Urine is most commonly tested because it is the main excretory route for drugs and their metabolites. Furthermore, the drugs remain detectable for much longer and asking for a urine sample is less intrusive than a blood sample. Although drugs can be detected in saliva and perspiration, the detection time is much shorter than urine and laboratories tend not to use these tests for this reason. Finally, hair testing is uncommon because it is expensive and in any case often requires a urine test for confirmation.

**Urine Creatinine**
The urine creatinine level is useful, when performed with a drug screen, as an indicator of specimen *validity.*

Creatinine is a metabolic byproduct of protein metabolism, which normally appears in urine in relatively constant quantities over a 24-hour period with regular liquid consumption. Therefore, urine creatinine can be used as an indicator of urine water content. Greater than normal intake of water will increase the urine water content (lowering the creatinine level) consequently diluting the amount of drug in urine. Conversely, a limited intake of water can lead to an abnormally concentrated urine specimen (as occurs with dehydration) resulting in elevated creatinine levels. The urine becomes more dilute when a person drinks larger amounts of water.

Most normal urine samples will have a creatinine value between 20 and 350 mg/dl (milligrams per deciliter). A specimen with a urine creatinine level less than 20 mg/dl is considered "dilute". Among urine samples submitted for employment related drug testing, about two percent are found to be dilute. On the other hand, eight percent of those urine specimens submitted for court-directed drug testing have a creatinine level under 20 mg/dl.

A quality laboratory will measure the urine creatinine level on every specimen tested and report when the specimen is dilute. Accordingly, when the urine is more dilute, there is a lower concentration of drugs. It is recommended that negative drug test results be disqualified when the specimen has a creatinine level less than 20 mg/dl. Conversely, a positive result on a dilute specimen should not be disqualified, because this shows that the drug was in such high concentrations that it was detected even though the urine is dilute.

**Urine Creatinine Interpretation**
The levels at which creatinine may be considered dilute (<20 ml/dL) or abnormally dilute (<=5 mg/dL) are based on the critical points that the Substance Abuse and Mental Health Services Administration (SAMSHA) has set as decision points for interpreting dilute or substituted urine specimens.

< 20 mg/dL  **Dilute urine specimen** - most likely due to increased water intake. Can be a result of short-term water loading (flushing) in an attempt to dilute any drug below testing cutoff concentrations.

<=5 mg/dL  **Abnormally dilute** - specimen showing an excessively low creatinine value. May be indication that the specimen is not consistent with normal human urine.

**Note**  The above interpretations are general guidelines. Other physiological conditions may account for low creatinine concentrations such as diabetes, kidney disease or use of prescription diuretics.

Individuals being drug tested and those responsible for urine testing programs are very aware that specimens submitted for testing are vulnerable to adulteration or tampering. Although collection procedures may be in place to ensure specimen integrity, donors have shown considerable ingenuity in their efforts to defeat the testing process. Possible methods of avoiding drug use detection include the addition of adulterants to the specimen, the substitution of someone else's urine and specimen dilution. Both specimen adulteration and specimen substitution are difficult to accomplish during an observed collection.

Additionally, the presence of adulterants in a urine specimen has the same implications as the presence of drugs. As a result, the most common way to mask drug use is by "internal" dilution. This is done by excessive water consumption or by taking diuretics such as herbal teas.

Some donors deliberately drink large quantities of fluids for medical reasons or because they think it is a healthy habit. If a donor consistently provides a dilute specimen they should be reminded that it is their responsibility to provide a specimen suitable for testing and failure to do so might be considered "Refusal to Test". They should reduce their liquid consumption and limit their use of caffeine and herbal teas. Most people will comply unless they are attempting to mask their drug use.

The best way to minimize the percentage of dilute urine specimens is by using a random collection program. Unannounced specimen collection presents the donor with little time to prepare. Another good practice is to get a first morning voiding if possible, since this specimen often is more concentrated. People diluting their urine by drinking large amounts of liquids cannot continue this practice indefinitely. By increasing the frequency of collection you are likely to catch these individuals off guard.

An effective additive need only fool the screening test, since the specimen would then never progress to GCMS confirmation. Some additives are more effective than others and some are more easily detected. For example, bleach, liquid soap, salt, oven cleaner, vinegar and glutaraldehyde can indeed cause a false negative EMIT screening test, but when too much is added, they also interfere with the test to the extent that the laboratory is alerted to an invalid specimen. Therefore, there is a measure of luck associated with the successful use of these products. One must use just enough additive to hide the positive result, but not so much that that the laboratory is alerted.

Observed collection provides the first line of defense against specimen tampering. Additionally, laboratories now routinely test each specimen for creatinine to identify diluted specimens. Those specimens with a low creatinine level are further tested for specific gravity. When specimen adulteration is suspected on the basis of color, odor or an EMIT screen alert, a more comprehensive battery of tests for adulterants is employed. This includes tests for oxidants, nitrites, glutaraldehyde, chromate, and surfactant (soap). As drug users expand their cover-up techniques, laboratories continue to develop more sophisticated countermeasures.

The table below describes common adulterants and the "red flags" that a laboratory can use to suspect their presence. Further procedures, such as test for nitrites, oxidants and specific gravity may be used to confirm.

| Product | Adulterant | Red Flags |
|---------|------------|-----------|
| Bleach | Oxidant | EMIT Alert |
| Klear | Nitrate | GC/MS Negative |
| Whizzies | Nitrite | GC/MS Negative |
| Urine Aid | Glutaraldehyde | GC/MS Negative |
| Urine Luck | Chromate | GC/MS Negative |
| CarboClean | Diuretic (flushing) | Creatinine Low |
| Golden Seal | Diuretic (flushing) | Creatinine Low |
| Soap | Surfactant | EMIT Alert |

**Detectable Time Periods**

It varies from person to person according to age, gender, metabolism and general state of health; also the analytical method, the type of drug, the quantity and frequency of its use influence the detection time. These drug detection times are based on urine analysis. Drug detection times for hair follicle testing tend to be higher, whereas detection times for blood, saliva and perspiration testing tend to be lower.

See chart next page

| SUBSTANCE | APPROXIMATE DETECTION PERIOD |
|---|---|
| Alcohol (UAC) | + = recent drinking (< 8 hours)<br>- = no recent drinking |
| **NOTE**: Urine Alcohol Concentration (UAC): The presence of alcohol in the urine indicates alcohol intake within about the preceding 8 hours. Concentration of alcohol depends on how long the urine has been in the bladder and makes any urine quantitative measure difficult to interpret. ||
| Amphetamines | 2-5 days |
| Barbiturates | Short acting 2 days, Long acting 3-4 weeks |
| Benzodiazepines<br>  therapeutic<br>  chronic abuse | <br>2 – 4 days<br>up to 4 weeks |
| **NOTE**: Clonazepam (Klonipin) is a long half-life benzodiazepine that can be detected for approximately 3 weeks ||
| Cannabinoids (THC)<br>  single use<br>  moderate use (4/wk)<br>  heavy use (daily)<br>  chronic heavy use | <br>3 days<br>3 – 5 days<br>10 days<br>up to 36 days |
| Cocaine | 2-4 days |
| Codeine | 1 - 3 days |
| Euphorics (MDMA) | 2-4 days |
| Ketamine (Special K) | 5-7 days |
| LSD | 1 – 2 days (immunoassay) |
| Methadone | 2 - 3 days |
| Methamphetamine | 2 - 3 days |
| Morphine | 1 - 3 days |
| Phencyclidine (PCP)<br>  single use<br>  moderate use (4/wk)<br>  heavy use (daily)<br>  chronic heavy use | <br>3 days<br>5 – 10 days<br>10 -20 days<br>up to 30 days |
| Phenobarbital | 10-20 days |
| Propoxyphene | 6 hrs - 2 days |
| Steroids Anabolic (oral) | 14-28 days |
| Steroids Anabolic (parentally) | 1-3 months |
| **SOURCE:** *Principles of Addiction Medicine 3rd Edition* , (Graham, A.W., Schultz, T.K., Mayo-Smith, M.F., Ries, R.K., Wilford, B.B., Eds). American Society of Addiction Medicine, 2003. ||

## Drug Testing - False Positives

In drug testing, a false positive is defined as a drug free sample falsely being reported as showing positive for drugs. This can occur for a number of reasons including: improper laboratory procedure, mixing up samples, incorrect paperwork and, albeit rarely, passive inhalation. But the most common cause of drug testing false positives are dilute urine samples. Another big reason of drug testing false positives is cross reactants. A cross reactant is a substance which because of its similar chemical structure to a drug or its metabolite can cause a false positive result.

The following substances may cause cross reactivity on an Immunoassay screen but are unlikely to be mistaken on a Gas Chromatography/Mass Spectrometry test:

**Ibuprofen**
Ibuprofen is a common pain reliever and anti-inflammatory which even in low doses used to cause a false positive for marijuana/cannabis on the EMIT test. The EMIT has been changed to use a different enzyme to eliminate these drug test false positives. But recent evidence suggests that Ibuprofen taken in very high doses, along with other anti-inflammatories such as Naproxen will still interfere with the EMIT test.

**Decongestants and Cold Remedies**
Ephedrine and pseudoephedrine (and Phenylpropanolamine some time ago) are both substances found in many over-the-counter cold remedies. They can result in a drug test false positive for amphetamines on the EMIT test. Antitussives, to suppress coughs, such as dextromethorphan and pyrilamine may cause a drug test false positive for opiates.

**Antidepressants**
Aside from when this class of drugs is specifically tested for, some of them, including amitriptyline, can test positive for opiates for up to three days after use. Even quinine in tonic water may cause a positive result for opiates.

**Poppy Seeds**
Poppy seeds which are usually found on bread contain traces of morphine and can lead to positives for opiates. Codeine, which is found in many pain relievers, may cause a false positive for morphine or heroin because of its similar chemical structure.

**Antibiotics**
Certain newly developed antibiotics including amoxicillin and ampicillin have been reported to cause false positives for cocaine.

**DHEA**
This treatment developed for use by AIDS patients will cause a false positive for anabolic steroid use.

**Enzymes**
A small fraction of the population excrete large amounts of certain enzymes in their urine which may produce a positive drug test. The enzymes in question are endogenous lysozyme and malate dehydrogenate, which according to research may run as high as 10% of positive samples.

**Melanin**
Melanin is the pigment which protects skin and hair from UV light. It is also very similar in chemical structure to THC (Tetrahydrocannabinol, the active component in cannabis) and some data exists claiming it causes false positives for cannabis. Unfortunately, an equal amount of data suggests that there is no link whatsoever.

**One more word about drug tests: Words Matter!**
Drug test results are not "dirty" or "clean". If one is dirty, the need a shower. If one is clean, they do not need a shower. Testing methods result in either negative or positive findings.

**Therapeutic Drug Testing: Clinical Evaluation of Response to Treatment (CERT)**

Drug screening and testing – described here as the *Clinical Evaluation of Response to Treatment* (CERT) is a vital aspect of addictions treatment that has great potential for either helping or hindering patient response to treatment and progress in recovery. Yet, there are no manuals for programs to follow when it comes to the therapeutic use of drug testing and how to use it in a patient-centered manner that can enhance the therapeutic alliance between counselor and patient. Clinics and programs are provided relatively little specific guidance from federal, state, or accreditation authorities in this regard.

Consequently, treatment programs can tend to follow procedures based on tradition, staff convenience, or licensing compliance requirements. Monetary constraints also are a concern, but there often is acceptance of whatever CERT approaches are most readily available, rather than adopting more compelling patient-centered strategies.

As with most chronic illnesses, the patient's response to treatment and their care plan goals can be inconsistent initially. This is also common in the treatment of substance use disorders. CERT can have an important role in monitoring patients' progress during treatment and also as an early-warning method for monitoring how well the chosen counseling techniques are working to help the patient accomplish the goals of their care plan.

In short, effective CERT policies and practices respond to clinical questions, such as:
- How is the patient responding to their treatment plan?
- Is the current level of care sufficient?
- Which drugs are new or continuing problems?
- Has a formerly stable patient run into trouble?
- Howe effective is my counseling approach with this particular patient?

**Monitoring, Screening, Testing Defined**
In health care, "monitoring" is an ongoing process allowing oversight of a patient's response to and progress during treatment. In this regard, monitoring for continued or episodic drug use while the patient is in treatment should not be a form of adversarial surveillance merely to detect misbehavior and rules breaking by the patient. Rather, it is one important way of assessing a patient's clinical situation, progress in recovery, and if the care plan should be revisited and modified from its original version.

CERT can also be used to advocate for the patient and to help encourage or maintain healthy behavioral changes. CERT must be further divided into monitoring assessments that are designed either for screening or testing purposes. These terms are sometimes used interchangeably in the literature yet, distinctions between screening and testing are important from perspectives of clinic operations, costs, and patient benefits.

**CERT Advantages:**
- Positive UA results are seen as continued symptoms of a health condition and the diagnosis.
- An objective measure of continued use on which to base new clinical decisions.
- Provides important data to help counselors re-evaluate their patient's stage of change and to revise the care plan goals accordingly.
- Allows counselors to titrate (adjust or modify) the strength of the counseling "dose" accordingly based on patient's response to treatment.

- Increases patient interaction with the treatment program on a regular basis.
- Can serve as a basis for patient-staff dialogue and relationship building.
- Can be a measure of patient progress in treatment and response to care plan.
- Is one aspect of a larger continuous quality improvement effort that is patient-centered and based on an individualized treatment plan.

**CERT Disadvantages:**
- If misused, it can create a climate of distrust and antagonism.
- May be humiliating for patients and staff.
- The quality and quantity of CERT information can be limiting.
- Misinterpreted results can negatively affect the therapeutic alliance.
- Laboratory errors jeopardize patient-staff relationships.
- Extra staff time required.
- Added costs are involved.

In simplest terms, CERT can serve as an objective measure of a patient's ability to reduce or eliminate substance use disorder. However, this alone should not be expected to either bring about or enforce change. Drug testing should primarily be a tool for counselors to gauge the effectiveness of the choice in counseling methods as well as the relevance of the treatment plan to the patient. Treatment programs are expected to offer treatment in a climate of trust that nurtures efforts by patients to improve and change their lives. If CERT creates an atmosphere of tension, control, power, or punishment, then trust and patient growth are smothered – consequently, monitoring might become a waste of effort, time, and money. These disadvantages can be managed when creating an effective CERT program that is patient-centered and will ultimately improves outcomes. Properly applied, objective data about substance use can serve to strengthen staff-patient bonds by enhancing mutual respect and confidence.

CERT results should not be the only means of detecting substance use problems and programs need to be very cautious about making decisions affecting patients' lives based solely on drug test reports. It was recognized long ago that placing too much reliance on drug screen or test results – whether positive or negative – can depersonalize a program to the point of working against all other aspects of rehabilitation. And again, CERT is really for the staff's information about whether or not the approach being used to help their patients is sufficient and helping or not. It is critical feedback to inform the counselor of the efficacy of their treatment decisions and directions.

CERT is intended to assign a qualitative outcome: either a result is positive, drug is present in sufficient amounts that can be clearly detected by the screen; or it is negative, below the standard level of detection or absent. Some researchers have contended that determining the exact quantitative amount of illicit substances in specimens during CERT, which is possible with many laboratory drug-identification tests,, can provide important information about the frequency and patterns of drug use.

Others – most prominently the National Drug Court Institute – have strongly argued that this is unreliable and has more potential for harm than good; in particular, drug concentrations in a specimen should not be misinterpreted as implying a lot of or a little drug use and are of no value for understanding a patient's actual involvement in substance abuse

**Why Not Just Ask Patients?**
Since CERT is limited in terms of the information that can be objectively obtained, communication with the patient for information-gathering purposes assumes a critical role in the therapeutic relationship. There is good evidence suggesting that asking patients about their substance use, along with CERT data, provides a powerful approach, even when the responses differ from each other, which encourages the counselor to explore "discrepancies" that can be incorporated into the Motivation Interviewing process.

Patient-history taking is an essential component of the therapeutic process, yet it can require skill and experience. Ideally, CERT simply confirms what has already been determined during individual discussions with and clinical observations of the patient.

**Enhancing Self-reports**
- The patient should not be significantly intoxicated at the time of the interview.
- The setting should be nonthreatening, nonjudgmental, and generally encourage honest
  reporting. It is the beginning of the development of the therapeutic alliance between counselor and patient.

- The counselor should have a good rapport with the patient and be able to communicate
  Clearly and in a way that the patient understands.
- The patient should be assured of confidentiality.
- Questions should be clearly worded and open-ended.

**Putting CERT into Practice**
Unless they are properly conducted, CERT practices have a potential for turning helpful and caring therapeutic relationships into adversarial struggles between patients and staff. Treatment programs have used positive CERT reports for negatively modifying patient privileges including discharging patients from treatment. When CERT is used primarily as a basis for punitive actions, barriers are created between patients and clinic staff; consequently, patients might be expected to respond accordingly in a negative fashion. Research evidence on outcomes does not support the value of punishments for promoting change during treatment and such aversive control techniques may significantly increase treatment dropout rates and continued compulsive use, or worse.

From a more positive perspective, a properly designed CERT program with accurate record- keeping can be used as documentation of the patient's progress with treatment. These data can help to advocate on behalf of patients (with their permission) in family, workplace, judicial, and other situations in which a patient's progress in recovery might be questioned. Furthermore, there is an extensive body of evidence in the field of "contingency management" supporting the value of reward reinforcements in promoting the attainment of various worthwhile recovery goals during treatment, including decreases in substance abuse measured via CERT.

An effective CERT strategy can help reduce or eliminate continued compulsive substance use by including a sufficient frequency of random assays, primarily urinalyses, coupled with immediate feedback to patients that can be best facilitated by on-site drug screening.

**Addressing Tampering**
Occasionally a client may attempt to conceal drug use by tampering with a urine specimen. At the time the suspect specimen is submitted, the client should be taken into a private setting and told that there is some uncertainty about the specimen. Staff members should not be accusatory and should attempt to make the client comfortable. However, staff persons should avoid tension-relieving jokes that might

communicate the wrong message about the purpose or importance of urine specimen collection and testing. Tampered urine specimens usually indicate substance use.

Clients who alter their specimens rarely admit it. Specimen tampering is a critical concern in treatment and may signal a relapse. Drug use combined with denial may reflect a breakdown of the therapeutic process. If a client attempts to alter more than one specimen sample, it may be necessary to observe the client giving another sample immediately and on subsequent testing occasions until the client's abstinence is reasonably verified. Doing so should be viewed as a last resort to establish the client's drug use and to encourage truthfulness.

If a situation warrants observing urine collection, the counselor should consult with a supervisor for approval and direction. The counselor should follow the agency's policy and procedures for observing urine collection. Observing urine specimen collection is uncomfortable for staff members and may be humiliating for the client.

Urine collection procedures should be explained to the client at the first individual session including the possibility that urine collections may be observed occasionally. An observed urine collection procedure is a last resort for clients who are having difficulties in the recovery process. It is important to view this procedure as a therapeutic activity. In many cases, drug testing can move clients back on track and prompt them to tell the truth about drug use.

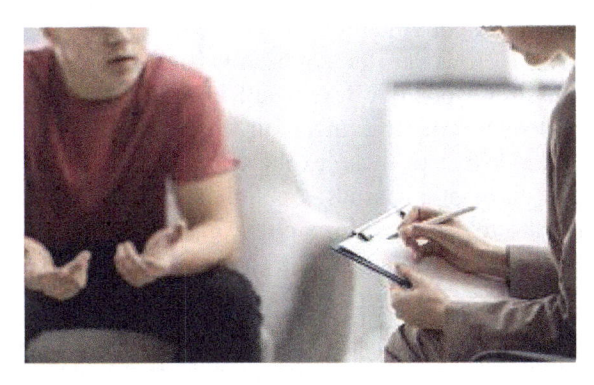

**Addressing a Positive Urine Test**

A positive drug test is a significant event in treatment. It might mean one use, or it might indicate a return to chronic use. In response to a positive result, the counselor should take the following steps:

- Reevaluate the period surrounding the test. Were there other indications of a problem such as missed appointments, unusual behavior, discussions in treatment sessions or groups, or family reports of unusual activity?
- Give the client an opportunity to explain the result, for example, by stating, "I received a positive result from the lab on your urine test from last Monday. Did anything happen that weekend you forgot to tell me about?"
- Avoid discussion about the validity of the results (e.g., the lab could have made an error; the bottle might have been mixed up with another client's).
- Consider temporarily increasing the frequency of testing to determine the extent of use.
- Reinforce a client's honesty if he or she admits to use, and stress the therapeutic importance of the admission. This interaction may result in admissions of other instances of substance use that had gone undetected.
- Collaborate with corrections or court staff as appropriate.

Sometimes a client responds to the news of a positive urine test with a partial confession of drug involvement, for instance, that he or she was at a party and was offered drugs but did not use them. These partial confessions are often the closest the client can get to actually admitting drug use. Occasionally a client reacts angrily to notification of positive test results. Typically, the client may accuse the counselor of lack of trust and display indignation at the suggestion of drug use.

These reactions can be convincing and may cause a counselor initially to react defensively. However, the counselor calmly should inform the client that discussing a positive test result is necessary for treatment and that the counselor's questioning is in the client's best interest. If the client is unresponsive to these explanations, the counselor should attempt to move on to other issues. At some other time, the topic of truthfulness may be revisited and the client given another opportunity to discuss the urine test result.

In general, a client should not be discharged from treatment because of a positive drug test or Breathalyzer results. If there are repeated positive test results, however, it may be necessary for the counselor to review the treatment plan and to increase the frequency of sessions. For example, the counselor should review the treatment plan with the client and to evaluate the goals. More individual sessions could be scheduled for a client who is not responding to the initial treatment plan with its level of care and frequency of sessions. If a client continues to have positive drug tests, the counselor may be required to refer the client to a higher level of care as undertreating the severity level of the client's SUD should be avoided.

Even if the client denies drug or alcohol use, the counselor must proceed as if there was use. Lapses should be analyzed with the client (possibly in an individual session), and a plan for avoiding relapse reformulated. It may become necessary to assess the need for residential treatment.

The counselor's confidence in and certainty of the test results are critical at this point and may be instrumental in inducing an honest explanation from the client of what has been happening. If the urine testing process succeeds in documenting out-of-control drug use and establishes the need for increasing the intensity of outpatient treatment or considering residential treatment, it has served a valuable function.

**Summary of CERT Essentials in Clinical Practice**
- There is little advantage in substance-use monitoring unless it is known in advance how results will be used therapeutically in a patient-centered approach to CERT.
- Properly educate staff about CERT procedures so that their benefits and limitations can be appreciated.
- Frequent, unexpected (random) on-site screening with immediate feedback to the patient is conducive to therapeutic effect and behavioral change.
- Obtain urine specimens in a treatment atmosphere that conveys trust and dignity; rather than punishment and power. Take patient's denials of drug use seriously and investigate the possibility of false-positive results.
- Screening results should be combined with patient self-reports of substance use for greatest accuracy.
- CERT alone is rarely enough to convince a patient to reduce use or remain abstinent. Positive reinforcements can have vital roles.
- Punishment is usually ineffective; rather, care plan review and revise, casework, counseling, and other interventions are needed when substance abuse continues.
- Even the most complete CERT data tell just part of a patient's real progress in recovery.

- Behavioral, psychological, and socioeconomic problems cannot be directly detected by CERT.
- Over-reliance on CERT can go against other aspects of treatment. It is important to remember that programs' primary focus should be on individual patient needs rather than on a screen or test results alone.

## SUGGESTED READINGS ON THIS TOPIC

Barceloux, DG. Medical Toxicology of Drug Abuse: Synthesized Chemicals and Psychoactive Plants. Wiley. 2012. ISBN-10 : 0471727601.

Graham, A.W., Schultz, T.K., Mayo-Smith, M.F., Ries, R.K., Wilford, B.B., Eds. Principles of Addiction Medicine 3rd Edition. American Society of Addiction Medicine, 2003.

McNeil SE, Chen RJ, Cogburn M. Drug Testing. [Updated 2023 Jul 29]. In: StatPearls [Internet]. Treasure Island (FL): StatPearls Publishing; 2024 Jan-. Available from: htttps://www.ncbi.nlm.nih.gov/books/NBK459334/

Substance Abuse and Mental Health Services Administration Center for Substance Abuse Treatment. Counselor's Treatment Manual. HHS Publication No. (SMA) 13-4152.

Substance Abuse and Mental Health Services Administration (SAMHSA) Clinical Drug Testing in Primary Care (TAP 32). 2013.

# CHAPTER 15
# SCHIZOPHRENIA: SYMPTOMS, CAUSES AND TREATMENTS

## Key Concepts

| | |
|---|---|
| Akathisia | A movement disorder characterized by a feeling of inner restlessness and a compelling need to be in constant motion. Akathisia is often a side effect of certain drugs. |
| Anosognosia | A neurological condition in which the patient is unaware of their psychiatric condition. It can affect the patient's conscious awareness of deficits involving judgment, emotions, memory, executive function, language skills, and motor ability. |
| Anterograde Amnesia | A condition in which events that occurred after the onset of amnesia cannot be recalled and new memories cannot be formed. |
| Antipsychotic | A class of medications originally developed to reduce the frequency and severity of psychotic episodes. The newer atypical or second-generation antipsychotics are now also used to treat bipolar disorder or more severe depression. Many people who take these medications don't have psychotic symptoms. |
| Catatonia: | A state of profound lack of movement and language, often including odd or unusual physical and verbal responses to stimuli. Sometimes alternates with periods of agitation and overexcitement. Can be associated |

| | |
|---|---|
| | with bipolar disorder, unipolar depression, schizophrenia, and other psychiatric and medical conditions. |
| Comorbid (co-occurring) | Any medical condition that presents (co-occurs) along with and often independent from another condition. People who have bipolar disorder can have other comorbid conditions — such as attention deficit hyperactivity disorder (ADHD), alcoholism, or anxiety disorder — that complicate the diagnosis and treatment of bipolar disorder. |
| Decompensation | A relapse to the return of symptoms that had previously been under control. |
| Delusions | An unshakable belief in something untrue. These irrational beliefs defy normal reasoning, and remain firm even when overwhelming proof is presented to dispute them. |
| Differential diagnosis | The process of distinguishing between two or more diseases or conditions that feature identical or similar symptoms. A doctor commonly performs a differential diagnosis to rule out other possibilities. |
| Executive function | The ability to organize, sort, and manage internal and external stimuli and generate adaptive and effective responses. Many psychiatric disorders weaken executive functioning, often leading to impaired judgment and uninhibited speech or behavior. |
| Extrapyramidal Syndrome | Abnormalities of movement related to injury of to injury of motor pathways other than the pyramidal tract. |

| | |
|---|---|
| Hallucinations | False or distorted sensory experiences that appear to be real perceptions. These sensory impressions are generated by the mind rather than by any external stimuli, and may be seen, heard, felt, and even smelled or tasted. |
| Neuroleptic Malignant Syndrome | A rare, potentially life-threatening disorder that is usually precipitated by the use of medications that block the dopamine. Most often, the drugs involved are those that treat psychosis. The syndrome results in dysfunction of the autonomic nervous system, the branch of the nervous system responsible for regulating such involuntary actions as heart rate, blood pressure, digestion, and sweating. Muscle tone, body temperature, and consciousness are also severely affected. |
| Neuroleptics | Tranquilizing drugs, especially one used in treating mental disorders. |
| Neuroplasticity | The ability of the nervous system to adapt in response to internal and external stimuli or events. Some treatments for bipolar disorder appear to affect the capacity for change and growth in the nervous system. |
| Orthostatic Hypotension | Also called postural hypotension — is an abnormal decrease in blood pressure that occurs when standing up from sitting or lying down. It may lead to fainting. |
| Psychotropic | A psychoactive drug or psychotropic substance is a drug that acts primarily upon the central nervous system |

| | |
|---|---|
| | where it produces an altering effect on perception, emotion, or behavior |
| Psychosis | A symptom or feature of mental illness typically characterized by radical changes in personality, impaired functioning, and a distorted or non-existent sense of objective reality. |
| Schizoaffective disorder | A psychiatric disorder in which symptoms of bipolar disorder and schizophrenia are both present. |
| Schizophrenia | A psychiatric disorder in which thought becomes dissociated from sensory input and emotions and is accompanied by hallucinations and delusional thinking. Thinking or cognitive skills are also often affected and day-to-day function can be severely impaired. Bipolar is sometimes misdiagnosed as schizophrenia. |
| Tardive Dyskinesia | Tardive dyskinesia is a mostly irreversible neurological disorder of involuntary movements caused by long term use of antipsychotic or neuroleptic drugs. |

# CHAPTER 15

# Schizophrenia: Symptoms, Causes and Treatments

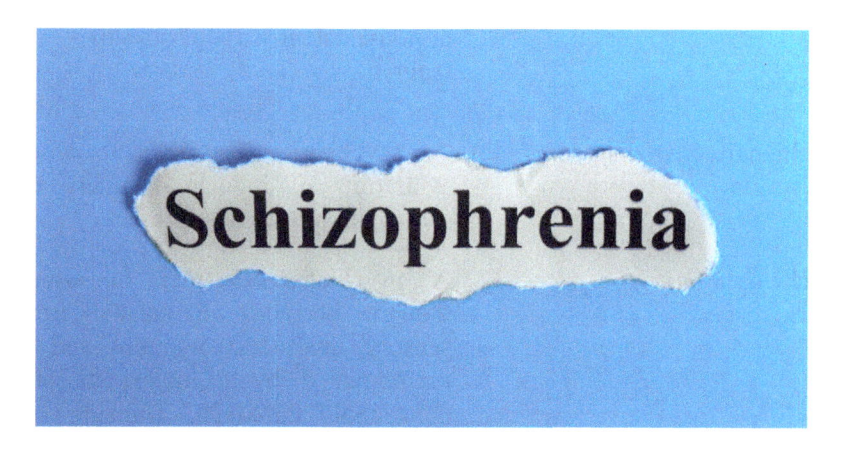

This chapter focuses on schizophrenia, as it can co-occur with substance use disorders, and the pharmacotherapy treatments available to help improve the quality of life for patients suffering from either of these diagnoses. As for any kind of medication, psychiatric medications, also called *psychotropics,* do not produce the same effect in everyone. Some people may respond better to one medication than another and some may need larger dosages than others. Some people experience side effects where others do not. Age, sex, body size, body chemistry, physical illnesses and other medications are some of the factors that can influence a medication's effect. Psychotropics can increase the effectiveness of other kinds of treatment including counseling and counseling helps with patient compliance in taking their medications.

## SCHIZOPHRENIA

The field of epidemiology is a branch of science that looks at how often conditions and diseases affect different groups of people and why. Healthcare experts can then use this information to plan and figure out ways to prevent or manage diseases.

An estimated 1% of people around the world live with schizophrenia, a type of psychosis, which means the person can't always tell the difference between what is real and what is a thought inside their head. The condition affects how the person thinks, feels, and acts. It sometimes runs in families, and experts say part of the reason may lie with family genes. The number of new cases per year is about 1.5 per 10,000 people.

By comparison, look at other health conditions and percentages as provided by the Center for Disease Control (CDC).

| | |
|---|---|
| Schizophrenia: 1% | ADHD: 5% |
| Diabetes: 11.6% | OCD: 1.2% |
| Seizure Disorder: 1.2% | Coronary Heart Disease: 5% |
| Depressive Disorders: 8.3% | Personality Disorders: 9% |
| PTSD: 3.5% | |

Most clinicians understand schizophrenia as a spectrum disorder rather than a single diagnosis, meaning that there are several symptoms and levels of severity not all the same for the diagnosis and can vary person to person. According to National Institute of Mental Health (NIMH), schizophrenia is a serious mental illness that affects how a person thinks, feels, and behaves. People with schizophrenia may seem like they have lost touch with reality, which can be distressing for them and for their family and friends. The symptoms of schizophrenia can make it difficult to participate in usual, everyday activities, but effective treatments are available. Many people who receive treatment can engage in school or work, achieve independence, and enjoy personal relationships.

Psychotic behavior is characterized by a loss of connectedness with reality. A person may develop bizarre ideas or false beliefs about reality (*delusions*). These may be based on false perceptions of reality (*hallucinations*). These are termed a *thought disorder*. People with psychosis may hear "voices" in their heads or have strange and illogical ideas (i.e., believing that others can track their thoughts or that they are someone famous in the world).

The person may develop poor hygiene, not bathing or changing clothes, and unable to coherently communicate. They often are initially unaware that their condition is actually an illness. These behaviors are symptoms of a psychotic illness such as schizophrenia. Psychosis can also be caused by drugs (stimulants and hallucinogens), by medications (steroids) or could be part of depression. Antipsychotic medications can help these symptoms. Antipsychotic medications affect neurotransmitters) that allow communication between cells. Two such neurotransmitters, dopamine and serotonin, are thought to be associated with some of the symptoms of schizophrenia.

Schizophrenia can range in severity from the incoherent patient who remains institutionalized to a responsible productive individual who is stabilized on medication. Although much has been learned in the past 40 years, scientists still do not know exactly what causes schizophrenia, and there is no cure.

Individuals with schizophrenia are unable to think coherently anti often misinterpret the meaning of events. Consequently, they are often incapable of caring for themselves and living independently. Moreover, many live in continual fear and distress, threatened by hallucinations and plagued by paranoid delusions. The psychotic state consists of bizarre behavior, an inability to think coherently or comprehend the environment, and most importantly, an inability to recognize the presence of these abnormalities.

**Risk Factors for Schizophrenia.** Some of the risk factors for schizophrenia are:

**Genetics.** Genes and the environment both play a role. But the chances of getting schizophrenia may be more than six times higher if one of the parents, siblings, or another close relative has it. Neuroscience thinks there may be a link between schizophrenia and your genes -- a chemical code you inherit from your parents that lives in every cell in your body. This code helps determine everything from eye color and height to parts of your personality.

In some cases, a change in a single gene -- scientists know of at least 10 different possible ones -- can raise the risk for schizophrenia by anywhere from four to 50 times, depending on the gene. In other cases, the cause may be the deletion of a certain set of genes. Although treatment is available, research suggests that as many as 30% of people with schizophrenia can be classified as treatment-resistant, indicating a critical need to identify new ways to treat this serious mental disorder. In one of the largest genetic studies of its kind researchers funded by the National Institute of Mental Health identified variations in 10 genes that significantly raise the risk for schizophrenia—information that could help identify new treatment targets (Singh T, et al. 2022).

For example, rare variants have now been identified that confer extraordinarily high risk for schizophrenia. Functional study of these variants may yield insights into the molecular and cellular impairments that ultimately give rise to psychosis. By restricting investigation to a single variant, etiologic heterogeneity is vastly reduced, which may lead to better discrimination of causal mechanisms. To date, the strongest identified single genetic risk factor for schizophrenia is the 3q29 deletion. The "3q29 deletion" cuts 21 specific genes and raises the risk by 40 times. Only about one in 100 people get schizophrenia. But of the 100 people with the 3q29 deletion, about 40 will get schizophrenia (Purcell RH, et al;. 2023).

Schizophrenia runs in families, and thus the argument for a genetic component; but how it is transmitted still remains unclear. Researchers have been intrigued by theories linking nutritional and immunological deficiencies to development of schizophrenia. It has been reported that schizophrenic patients do have immune system abnormalities, but researchers don't agree on what these include. Schizophrenia is a devastating disease, but some individuals do get better. A summary of 25 studies in which schizophrenic patients were followed for 10 years showed that 50% recover or improve to the point they can work and live on their own or improved somewhat but required a support network, and 15% did not improve and remained hospitalized, and 10% died, usually by suicide (Solmi M, et al. 2022).

**Environment.** Risk could also be increased if exposed to certain viruses or to malnutrition before birth (prenatal damage) especially during the first and second trimesters in the womb. Some research also suggests a link between autoimmune disorders and people developing psychosis. An autoimmune disorder is a condition in which the immune system begins to attack healthy cells by mistake. Some research ties living in a city or town to a higher risk for schizophrenia. Researchers aren't sure what things in an urban environment might raise someone's odds of getting the disorder. But they think the higher risk applies to people whose genes already raise their odds of developing schizophrenia.

**Brain chemicals.** Problems with some of the chemicals the brain makes, including certain neurotransmitters, may play a role in schizophrenia (i.e the dopamine hypothesis). As you know from prior chapters, neurotransmitters are chemicals that inform the brain cells to communicate with each other. Networks of neurons are probably involved, too.

**Drug use.** Recent research suggests that taking mind-altering drugs as a teen or a young adult increases the risks for schizophrenia (National Institute of Drug Abuse. 2023). The link between schizophrenia and pot use is stronger the earlier in life someone starts smoking marijuana, the more heavily they use it, and the higher the amount of THC (the mind-altering ingredient that gets you high).

The symptoms of schizophrenia are observed within a wide range of cognitive and emotional dysfunction classified as either positive or negative symptoms. **Psychotic symptoms** include hallucinations (primarily auditory), delusions, bizarre behavior and thought and movement disorders. **Negative symptoms** include flat affect (expressionless demeanor), loss of motivation, loss of interests and isolation. **Cognitive symptoms** that include problems in attention, concentration, and memory. These symptoms can make it hard to follow a conversation, learn new things, or remember appointments. A person's level of cognitive functioning is one of the best predictors of their day-to-day functioning.

For some, they can also experience a condition called, ***anosognosia*** which is where the person can't recognize health conditions or problems that they have. Experts commonly describe it as "denial of deficit" or "lack of insight." It falls under the family of agnosias, all of which happen when the brain can't recognize or process what the body's senses tell it. Anosognosia is incredibly common with certain mental health conditions affecting between 50% and 98% of people with schizophrenia and about 40% of people with bipolar disorder.

The brain keeps track of what's going on with the body using a "self-image." If there is an injury, the body updates the self-image to reflect that, and it will keep updating as the body heals. When structural brain damage causes anosognosia, neuroradiological findings typically show damage to the right parietal or right temporoparietal region. Less common areas of damage include the thalamus, basal ganglia, or left parietal region

Because that person's mind can't update their self-image, they can't process or recognize that they have a health problem.

That's what makes this condition different from the kind of denial described by the Kübler-Ross model (commonly known as the five stages of grief). A person in denial rejects or avoids accepting reality because it's unpleasant or distressing. A person with anosognosia can't recognize the problem at all.

Because they can't recognize they have a medical problem, people with this condition often don't see the need to care for that problem. In more severe cases, they actively avoid or resist treatment.

## DSM-5 Criteria for Schizophrenia

- Two or more of these symptoms must be present for at least one month (can be less if being successfully treated)
  And at least one symptom must be either (1), (2), or (3)
  - (1) Hallucinations
  - (2) Delusions (can be either bizarre or nonbizarre)
  - (3) Disorganized speech (e.g., frequent derailment or incoherence)
  - (4) Grossly disorganized or catatonic behavior
  - (5) Negative symptoms (e.g., affective flattening, alogia or avolition).
- Continuous disturbance for 6 months (attenuated symptoms, residual symptoms)
- Social or occupational dysfunction (or both) for significant portion of the time
- Notes: Catatonia can also be used as a specifier for any other diagnosis

Alterations in brain biochemistry have been associated with some cases of psychotic and negative symptoms of schizophrenia. For example, theories on the biochemical basis for schizophrenia have produced some interesting causal explanations for the disorder by inferring specific alterations in certain neurotransmitter. These biochemical alterations are summarized as follows:

- Increased D2 receptor site abnormalities (psychotic symptoms)
- Decreased dopamine function (negative symptoms)
- Increased norepinephrine function (psychotic symptoms)
- Decreased serotonin function (psychotic symptoms)

The most prominent theory of schizophrenia, one that has outlasted most others, is the *dopamine hypothesis.* This theory has a pharmacological foundation that tests true to research. That is, drugs that increase dopamine activity (dopamine agonists such as amphetamine, cocaine, L-dopa and methylphenidate) can produce a paranoid state in normal persons. The same drugs when given to schizophrenics sometimes exacerbate the symptoms, increasing psychosis and thought disturbances. On the other hand, drugs that block certain dopamine receptors (antagonists such as neuroleptics and naloxone) seem to ease some of the symptoms of schizophrenia. Dysregulation of the dopamine system is central to many models of the pathophysiology of psychosis in schizophrenia. However, emerging evidence suggests that this dysregulation is driven by the disruption of upstream circuits that provide afferent control of midbrain dopamine neurons. Furthermore, stress can profoundly disrupt this regulatory circuit, particularly when it is presented at critical vulnerable prepubertal time points (Sonnenschein S, et al. 2020.).

**Antipsychotic Medications**

**ANTIPSYCHOTICS**
TREAT SCHIZOPHRENIA & BIPOLAR DISORDER

1ST GEN (TYPICAL)
E.g. HALOPERIDOL
* ↑ EFFECTIVE
* ↑ RISK of ADVERSE EFFECTS
PRESCRIBED LESS OFTEN

2ND GEN (ATYPICAL)
E.g. ARIPIPRAZOLE
* ↓ SIDE EFFECTS
FIRST-LINE THERAPY

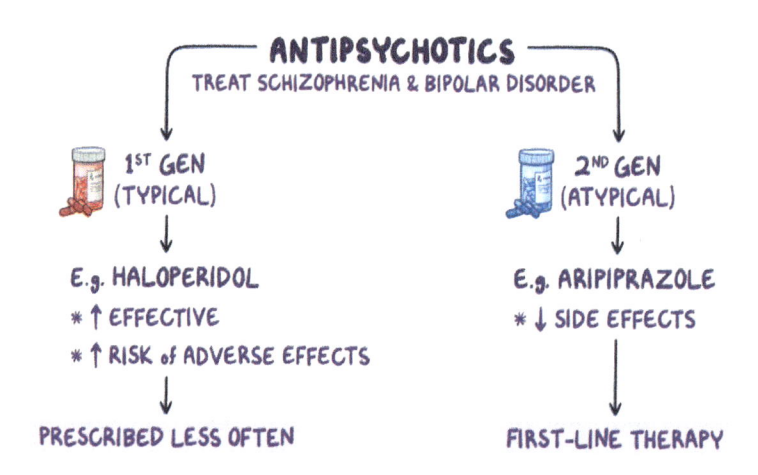

Antipsychotic medications can help make psychotic symptoms less intense and less frequent. These medications are usually taken every day in a pill or liquid forms. Some antipsychotic medications are given as injections once or twice a month. Importantly, people respond to antipsychotic medications in different ways. It is important to report any side effects to a health care provider. Many people taking antipsychotic medications experience side effects such as weight gain, dry mouth, restlessness, and drowsiness when they start taking these medications. Most side effects of antipsychotic medications are mild and many will decrease or disappear after a few weeks of treatment. These include drowsiness, rapid heartbeat, and dizziness when changing position (orthostatic hypotension). Some people gain weight while taking medications. Some may develop diabetes (Type 2) and can also have elevated cholesterol. Other side effects may include a decrease in sexual interest, problems with menstrual periods or skin rashes.

Long-term treatment of schizophrenia with one of the older antipsychotic drugs may cause the side effect of tardive dyskinesia (TD). This is a condition characterized by involuntary movements, most often involving the tongue. The risk of this side effect has been reduced with the newer medications. However, there is a higher incidence of TD in women, and the risk can increase with age. Other side effects can include pseudo-Parkinson's, akathisia and restless leg syndrome.

**Several Commonly Used Antipsychotic Medications** (BY GENERIC/TRADE NAME)
- Aripiprazole/Abilify
- Aripiprazole lauroxil/Aristada
- Asenapine/Saphris
- Brexpiprazole/Rexulti
- Cariprazine/Vraylar
- Clozapine/Clozaril
- Iloperidone/Fanapt
- Lumateperonee/Caplyta
- Lurasidone/Latuda
- Olanzapine/Zyprexa
- Olanzapine/samidorphan/Lybalvi
- Paliperidone (Invega Sustenna)
- Paliperidone palmitate/Invega Trinza
- Quetiapine/Seroquel
- Risperidone/Risperdal
- Ziprasidone/Geodon

**Add-on Treatments**
Along with antipsychotic drugs, the prescriber may prescribe a mood stabilizer or antidepressant. Mood stabilizers include: Lamotrigine (Lamictal), Lithium, Carbamazepine (Tegretol) and, Valproic acid (Depakote).

The most frequently prescribed types of antidepressants are called selective serotonin reuptake inhibitors (SSRIs). They include: Citalopram (Celexa), Fluoxetine (Prozac), Paroxetine (Paxil, Pexeva), Sertraline (Zoloft) and, Escitalopram (Lexapro)

**Psychosocial treatments**
Psychosocial treatments help people find solutions to everyday challenges and manage symptoms while attending school, working, and forming relationships. These treatments are often used together with antipsychotic medication. People who participate in regular psychosocial treatment are less likely to have symptoms reoccur or to be hospitalized. Examples of this kind of treatment include cognitive behavioral therapy, behavioral skills training, supported employment, and cognitive remediation interventions. It is also common for people with schizophrenia to have problems with drugs and alcohol. A treatment program that includes treatment for both schizophrenia and substance use is important for recovery because substance use can interfere with treatment for schizophrenia and vice versa.

**Facts and Statistics About Schizophrenia**

Schizophrenia is complex. The following facts from the National Institute for Mental Health (NIMH) and the National Alliance on Mental Illness (NAMI) can help bring a more in-depth understanding:
- It's uncommon for people under age 12 and over age 40 to receive a diagnosis of schizophrenia. The average age of onset is typically late teens to early 20s for men, and ages 25 to 30 for women.
- A person's chance of developing schizophrenia is more than 6 times higher if they have a close relative, like a parent or sibling, with the condition.
- A combination of genetics and environmental factors may cause schizophrenia.
- African Americans are likelier to get misdiagnosed with schizophrenia because clinicians often overemphasize positive symptoms of the condition and underemphasize mood symptoms consistent with major depression.
- Schizophrenia ranks in the top 15 leading causes of disability worldwide.
- People with schizophrenia often have other health conditions, such as heart disease, liver disease, and diabetes.
- People with schizophrenia may also have other mental health conditions, such as:

- - Substance use disorders
  - Post-traumatic stress disorder
  - Obsessive-compulsive disorder
  - Major depressive disorder
- Schizophrenia can't be detected with a lab test. A mental health care professional makes the diagnosis by evaluating symptoms and the patient's history.
- People with schizophrenia have a substantially elevated risk of suicide.
- Stigma associated with schizophrenia can cause social isolation and discrimination, which create barriers to accessing healthcare, education, housing, and employment.

**Lesser-known facts**
These more nuanced facts may help you empathize and understand some of the profound layers of schizophrenia:
- Many people living with schizophrenia don't think they have the condition called, *anosognosia*.
- Delusions that a person living with schizophrenia might experience may include thinking they are famous, the FBI is after them, or they have special or magical powers.
- While the delusions feel real to someone with schizophrenia, they may be aware that others don't believe their delusions. Neuroscientists refer to this as a meta-awareness of the delusion.
- People with schizophrenia can do work. Research finds that participating in a vocational training intervention program helped those living with schizophrenia-spectrum disorders increase their work motivation and improve work outcomes.
- Taking drugs like methamphetamines or LSD can cause a person to experience psychotic symptoms.
- Taking mind-altering drugs as a teenager or young adult can increase the risk of developing schizophrenia, according to Research findings.
- Using cannabis can contribute to ongoing episodes of psychosis.
- People living with schizophrenia in the United States live an estimated average 28.5 years fewer than others.
- Humor, metaphors, and emotions seems to be more difficult to process for people living with schizophrenia.
- During emergencies like natural disasters and war, people living with schizophrenia are at risk of experiencing neglect, abandonment, homelessness, abuse, and exclusion.

## SUGGESTED READINGS ON THIS TOPIC

Abel T, Nickl-Jockschat T. The Neurobiology of Schizophrenia. Academic Press. 2016. **ISBN-10 :** 0128018291

*American Psychiatric Association. Diagnostic and statistical manual of mental disorders (5th ed.). 2013. Arlington, VA: American Psychiatric Association.*

Bitter I. Managing Negative Symptoms of Schizophrenia. Oxford University Press. 2020. **ISBN-10 :** 0198840128

Cooke A. Understanding Psychosis and Schizophrenia: Why people sometimes hear voices, believe things that others find strange, or appear out of touch with reality, and what can help. BPS Books 2020. **ISBN-10 :** 1854337483

Lieberman, JA. Malady of the Mind: Schizophrenia and the Path to Prevention. Scribner. 2023. **ISBN-13 :** 978-1982136420

Lieberman J. The American Psychiatric Association Publishing Textbook of Schizophrenia. Amer Psychiatric Pub Inc. 2019. **ISBN-10 :** 1615371729

Marcopulos BA, Kurtz MM. Clinical Neuropsychological Foundations of Schizophrenia (American Academy of Clinical Neuropsychology. Psychology Press. 2012. **ISBN-10 :** 1848728778

NIDA. 2023, May 4. Young men at highest risk of schizophrenia linked with cannabis use disorder . Retrieved from https://nida.nih.gov/news-events/news-releases/2023/05/young-men-at-highest-risk-schizophrenia-linked-with-cannabis-use-disorder on 2024, June 2

National Alliance of Mental Health. Website accessed January 22, 2024.
https://www.nami.org/About-Mental-Illness/Mental-Health-Conditions/Schizophrenia

National Institute of Mental Health (NIMH). Schizophrenia Causes, Symptoms, Signs, Diagnosis and Treatments. CreateSpace Independent Publishing Platform. 2012.
**ISBN-10 :** 1469986744

Purcell RH, Sefik E, Werner E, King AT, Mosley TJ, Merritt-Garza ME, Chopra P, McEachin ZT, Karne S, Raj N, Vaglio BJ, Sullivan D, Firestein BL, Tilahun K, Robinette MI, Warren ST, Wen Z, Faundez V, Sloan SA, Bassell GJ, Mulle JG. Cross-species analysis identifies mitochondrial dysregulation as a functional consequence of the schizophrenia-associated 3q29 deletion. Sci Adv. 2023 Aug 18;9(33):eadh0558. doi: 10.1126/sciadv.adh0558. Epub 2023 Aug 16. PMID: 37585521; PMCID: PMC10431714.

Singh, T., Poterba, T., Curtis, D., Akil, H., Al Eissa, M., Barchas, J. D., Bass, N., Bigdeli, T. B., Breen, G., Bromet, E. J., Buckley, P. F., Bunney, W. E., Bybjerg-Grauholm, J., Byerley, W. F., Chapman, S. B., Chen, W. J., Churchhouse, C., Craddock, N., Cusick, C. M., DeLisi, L., … Daly, M. J. (2022). Rare coding variants in ten genes confer substantial risk for schizophrenia. *Nature, 604*(7906), 509–516.

Solmi, M., Radua, J., Olivola, M. *et al.* Age at onset of mental disorders worldwide: large-scale meta-analysis of 192 epidemiological studies. *Mol Psychiatry* **27**, 281–295 (2022). https://doi.org/10.1038/s41380-021-01161-7

Sonnenschein SF, Gomes FV and Grace AA (2020) Dysregulation of Midbrain Dopamine System and the Pathophysiology of Schizophrenia. *Front. Psychiatry* 11:613. doi: 10.3389/fpsyt.2020.00613

Steggles G. Schizophrenia: A Contemporary Introduction. Routledge. 2024.
**ISBN-10 :** 1032560398

Yeiser, B. Mind Estranged: My Journey from Schizophrenia and Homelessness to Recovery.  Bethany Yeiser; one edition (July 10, 2014). **ISBN-13 :** 978-0990345220
Yeiser, B. Awakenings: Stories of Recovery and Emergence from Schizophrenia.  Bethany Yeiser (February 9, 2024) **ISBN-10 :** 0990345246

Wilson R. Schizophrenia: Understanding Schizophrenia, and how it can be managed, treated, and improved. Ingram Publishing. 2020.
**ISBN-10 :** 1761032259

# CHAPTER 16
# BIPOLAR DISORDER: SYMPTOMS, CAUSES AND TREATMENTS

## Key Concepts

| | |
|---|---|
| Anticonvulsants | A class of medications to prevent seizures including valproate (Depakote) and carbamazepine (Tegretol), are also useful in treating mania. |
| Bipolar Disorder | A psychiatric condition characterized by extreme mood states of mania and depression. A person may have bipolar disorder even if they have experienced only one of the extreme mood states, making diagnosis very challenging. |
| Bipolar I | A type of bipolar disorder characterized by at least one full-blown manic episode that doctors can't attribute to another cause, such as a medication or substance abuse. A bipolar I diagnosis doesn't require an episode of major depression, although periods of mania often alternate with periods of depression. |
| Bipolar II | A type of bipolar disorder characterized by at least one major depressive episode that doctors can't attribute to another cause, along with one or more hypomanic episodes. The depression tends to be chronic and is usually more problematic than the hypomania. Some people with bipolar II develop a full manic episode, which changes the diagnosis to bipolar I. |

| | |
|---|---|
| Cyclothymia | Sometimes referred to as *bipolar lite*, a muted form of bipolar that nevertheless interferes with a person's life. It involves multiple episodes of hypomania and depressive symptoms that don't meet the criteria for mania or major depression. Symptoms must last for at least two years, (one year in children and teens) during which time there are no more than two symptom-free months. |
| Hypomania | An elevated mood that doesn't qualify as full-blown mania but typically involves increased energy, less need for sleep, clarity of vision, and a strong creative drive. |
| Mania | An extremely elevated mood typically characterized by euphoria, excessive energy, impulsivity, nervousness, impaired judgment, irritability, and a decreased need for sleep. |
| Manic-depression | Another name (older) for bipolar disorder. Manic episode: A period of elevated mood, either euphoric or irritable, typically characterized by impulsivity, nervousness, impaired judgment, irritability, and a decreased need for sleep. The period must last at least one week (or shorter if it leads to hospitalization). |
| Manic episode | A period of elevated mood, either euphoric or irritable, typically characterized by impulsivity, nervousness, impaired judgment, irritability, and a decreased need for sleep. The period must last at least one week (or shorter if it leads to hospitalization). |

| | |
|---|---|
| Mood disorder | A psychiatric condition that results in persistently disrupted moods and/or mood regulation. |
| Pressured speech | Urgent, non-stop talking that's difficult to interrupt. Pressured speech is a characteristic of hypomania and mania. |
| Rapid cycling | A state in which mood alternates between depression and mania more than four times in a year. |
| Unspecified bipolar | Unspecified bipolar and related disorders: A type of bipolar disorder listed in the *DSM-IV* that's characterized by hypomanic, manic, or depressive symptoms that cause problems in function, don't fit into any of the other bipolar categories, and can't be attributed to unipolar depression. |

# CHAPTER 16

# Bipolar Disorder: Symptoms, Causes and Treatments

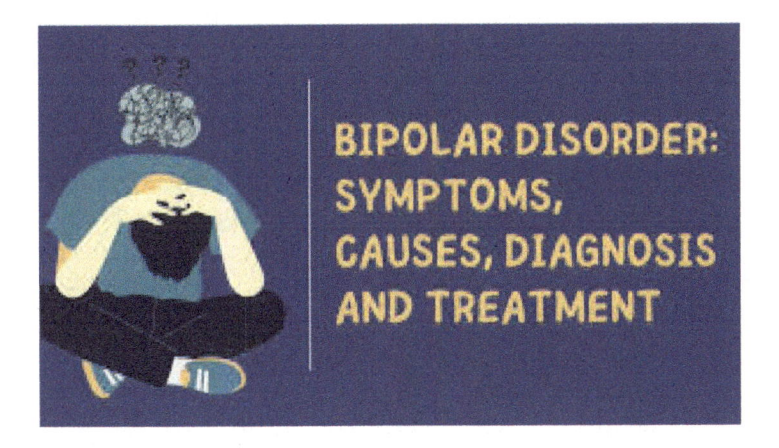

**BIPOLAR DISORDER**

Bipolar disorder (formerly called manic-depressive illness or manic depression) is a mental illness that causes unusual shifts in a person's mood, energy, activity levels, and concentration. These shifts can make it difficult to carry out day-to-day tasks. Bipolar disorder is a category that includes three main diagnoses: bipolar I, bipolar II, and cyclothymic disorder. All three types involve clear changes in mood, energy, and activity levels. These moods range from periods of extremely "up," elated, irritable, or energized behavior (known as manic episodes) to very "down," sad, indifferent, or hopeless periods (known as depressive episodes). Less severe manic periods are known as hypomanic episodes (NIMH. 2023).

1. **Bipolar I disorder** is defined by manic episodes that last for at least 7 days (nearly every day for most of the day) or by manic symptoms that are so severe that the person needs immediate medical care. Usually, depressive episodes occur as well, typically lasting at least 2 weeks. Episodes of depression with mixed features (having depressive symptoms and manic symptoms at the same time) are also possible. Experiencing four or more episodes of mania or depression within 1 year is called "rapid cycling."

Bipolar I disorder is diagnosed when a person experiences a manic episode. During a manic episode, people with bipolar I disorder experience an extreme increase in energy and mood changes, including feeling extremely happy or uncomfortably irritable. Some people with bipolar I disorder also experience depressive or hypomanic episodes, and most people with bipolar I disorder also have periods of neutral mood.

**Symptoms:**

**Manic Episode**
A manic episode is a period of at least one week when a person is extremely high-spirited or irritable most of the day for most days, possesses more energy than usual, and experiences at least three of the following changes in behavior:
- Decreased need for sleep (e.g., feeling energetic despite significantly less sleep than usual.
- Increased or faster speech.
- Uncontrollable racing thoughts or quickly changing ideas or topics when speaking.
- Distractibility.
- Increased activity (e.g., restlessness, several projects at the same time).
- Increased risky or impulsive behavior (e.g., reckless driving, spending sprees, sexual promiscuity).

These behaviors must represent a change from the person's usual behavior and be clear to friends and family. Symptoms must be severe enough to cause dysfunction in work, family, or social activities and responsibilities. Symptoms of a manic episode commonly require hospital care to ensure safety. During severe manic episodes, some people also experience disorganized thinking, false beliefs, and/or hallucinations, known as psychotic features.

**Hypomanic Episode**
A hypomanic episode characterized by less severe manic symptoms that need to last only four days in a row rather than a week. Hypomanic symptoms do not lead to the major problems in daily functioning that manic symptoms commonly cause.

**Major Depressive Episode**
A major depressive episode is a period of at least two weeks in which a person experiences intense sadness or despair or a loss of interest in

activities the person once enjoyed and at least four of the following symptoms:
- Feelings of worthlessness or guilt.
- Fatigue.
- Increased or decreased sleep.
- Increased or decreased appetite.
  Restlessness (e.g., pacing) or slowed speech or movement.
- Difficulty concentrating.
- Frequent thoughts of death or suicide.

2. **Bipolar II disorder.** To diagnose bipolar II disorder, the person must have at least one major depressive episode and at least one hypomanic episode.. With bipolar II, it is common that people return to their usual functioning between episodes. People with bipolar II disorder often first seek treatment as a result of their depressive episodes, since hypomanic episodes often feel pleasurable and can even increase performance at work or school. The hypomanic episodes are less severe than the manic episodes in bipolar I disorder. People with bipolar II disorder frequently have other mental illnesses such as an anxiety disorder or substance use disorder, the latter of which can exacerbate symptoms of depression or hypomania.

Treatments for bipolar II are similar to those for bipolar I: medication and psychotherapy. The most commonly used medications are mood stabilizers. Antidepressants are used cautiously for the treatment of bipolar-associated depression and continued only for a short time after the depression gets better as they increase the risk of switching depression into hypomania and mania. If depressive symptoms are severe and medication is not effective, electroconvulsive therapy (ECT) is a consideration.

3. **Cyclothymic disorder** (also called cyclothymia) is a milder form of bipolar disorder involving mood swings with hypomania and depressive symptoms that occur frequently. The recurring hypomanic and depressive symptoms are not intense enough or do not last long enough to qualify as hypomanic or depressive episodes. People with cyclothymia experience emotional ups and downs but with less severe symptoms than bipolar I or II disorder.

Cyclothymic disorder symptoms include the following:

- For at least two years, many periods of hypomanic and depressive symptoms, but the symptoms do not meet the criteria for hypomanic or depressive episodes.
- During the two-year period, the symptoms (mood swings) have lasted for at least half the time and have never stopped for more than two months.

Treatment for cyclothymic disorder can involve medication and talk therapy. For many people, talk therapy can help with the stresses of mood swings. Keeping a mood journal can be an effective way to observe patterns in mood fluctuation. People with cyclothymia may start and stop treatment over time.

Bipolar disorder occurs in up to 2.5% of the population, but the prevalence is much higher among first-degree relatives of individuals with bipolar or schizophrenia disorder. Individuals with bipolar disorder experience mood swings that are less severe in intensity. During what is known as a hypomanic episode, a person may experience elevated mood, increased self-esteem, and a decreased need for sleep. Unlike a manic episode, these symptoms are not so severe as to impact daily functioning or cause psychotic symptoms.

Bipolar disorder is often diagnosed during late adolescence (teen years) or early adulthood. Sometimes, bipolar symptoms can appear in children. Although the symptoms may vary over time, bipolar disorder usually requires lifelong treatment. Following a prescribed treatment plan can help people manage their symptoms and improve their quality of life.

**Causal Risk Factors for Bipolar Disorder**
The cause of bipolar disorder is not entirely known. Researchers are studying possible causes of bipolar disorder. Most agree that there are many factors that are likely to contribute to a person's chance of having the disorder. Genetic, neurochemical and environmental factors probably interact at many levels to play a role in the onset and progression of bipolar disorder. The current thinking is that this is a predominantly biological disorder that occurs in a specific part of the brain and is due to a malfunction of the neurotransmitters. As a biological disorder, it may lie dormant and be activated spontaneously or it may be triggered by stressors in life. Although, no one is quite sure about the exact causes of bipolar disorder, researchers have found these important clues:

**Genetic factors in Bipolar Disorder**
Some research suggests that people with certain genes are more likely to develop bipolar disorder. Research also shows that people who have a parent or sibling with bipolar disorder have an increased chance of having the disorder themselves. Many genes are involved, and no one gene causes the disorder. Learning more about how genes play a role in bipolar disorder may help researchers develop new treatments.

- Bipolar disorder tends to be familial, meaning that it "runs in families." About half the people with bipolar disorder have a family member with a mood disorder, such as depression.
- A person who has one parent with bipolar disorder has a 15 to 25 percent chance of having the condition.
- A person who has a non-identical twin with the illness has a 25 percent chance of illness, the same risk as if both parents have bipolar disorder.
- A person who has an identical twin (having exactly the same genetic material) with bipolar disorder has an even greater risk of developing the illness about an eightfold greater risk than a nonidentical twin.

Studies of adopted twins (where a child whose biological parent had the illness is raised in an adoptive family untouched by the illness) has helped researchers learn more about the genetic causes vs. environmental and life events causes.

**Neurochemical Factors in Bipolar Disorder**
Some studies show that the brains of people with bipolar disorder differ in certain ways from the brains of people who do not have bipolar disorder or any other mental disorder. Learning more about these brain differences may help scientists understand bipolar disorder and determine which treatments will work best. At this time, health care providers base the diagnosis and treatment plan on a person's symptoms and history, rather than brain imaging or other diagnostic tests.

Bipolar disorder is primarily a biological disorder that occurs in a specific area of the brain and is due to the dysfunction of certain neurotransmitters in the brain. These chemicals may involve neurotransmitters like norepinephrine, serotonin and probably many others. As a biological disorder, it may lie dormant and be activated on its own or it may be triggered by external factors such as psychological stress and social circumstances.

## Environmental Factors in Bipolar Disorder

- A life event may trigger a mood episode in a person with a genetic disposition for bipolar disorder.
- Even without clear genetic factors, altered health habits, alcohol or drug abuse, or hormonal problems can trigger an episode.
- Among those at risk for the illness, bipolar disorder is appearing at increasingly early ages. This apparent increase in earlier occurrences may be due to underdiagnosis of the disorder in the past. This change in the age of onset may be a result of social and environmental factors that are not yet understood.
- Although substance abuse is not considered a cause of bipolar disorder, it can worsen the illness by interfering with recovery. Use of alcohol or tranquilizers may induce a more severe depressive phase.

Bipolar disorder is recurrent, meaning that more than 90% of the individuals who have a single manic episode will go on to experience future episodes. Roughly 70% of manic episodes in bipolar disorder occur immediately before or after a depressive episode. Treatment seeks to reduce the feelings of mania and depression associated with the disorder, and restore balance to the person's mood.

A manic episode is characterized by extreme happiness, hyperactivity, little need for sleep and racing thoughts, which may lead to rapid speech. A depressive episode is characterized by extreme sadness, a lack of energy or interest in things, an inability to enjoy normally pleasurable activities and feelings of helplessness and hopelessness.

On average, someone with bipolar disorder may have up to three years of normal mood between episodes of mania or depression.

| Bipolar 1 Disorder | Bipolar 1 Disorder | |
|---|---|---|
| >1 manic episode | >1 hypomanic episode | >1 major depressive episode |
| A. Distinct period of mood disturbance.<br>B. Manic symptoms as described in DSM-5.<br>C. Severe mood disturbance.<br>D. Not attributable to a substance or other medical condition. | A. Distinct period of mood disturbance.<br>B. Manic symptoms as described in DSM 5 under Hypomanic episode.<br>C. Unequivocal/uncharacteristic change in functioning.<br>D. A and B above are observable by others.<br>E. Less severe than a manic episode.<br>F. Not attributable to a substance or other medical condition. | A. Depressive symptoms as described in the DMS 5 under Major Depressive episode.<br>B. Symptoms cause clinically significant distress or impairment in social, occupational or other important areas of functioning.<br>C. Not attributable to a substance or other medical condition. |

Those with bipolar disorder often describe their experience as being on an emotional roller coaster. Cycling up and down between strong emotions can keep a person from having anything approaching a "normal" life. The emotions, thoughts and behavior of a person with bipolar disorder are often experienced as beyond one's control. Friends, co-workers and family may sometimes intervene to try and help protect their interests and health. This makes the condition exhausting not only for the sufferer, but for those in contact with her or him as well.

**Bipolar cycling** can either be rapid, or more slowly over time. Those who experience rapid cycling can go between depression and mania as often as a few times a week (some even cycle within the same day). Most people with bipolar disorder are of the slow cycling type — they experience long periods of being up ("high" or manic phase) and of being down ("low" or depressive phase). Researchers do not yet understand why some people cycle more quickly than others.

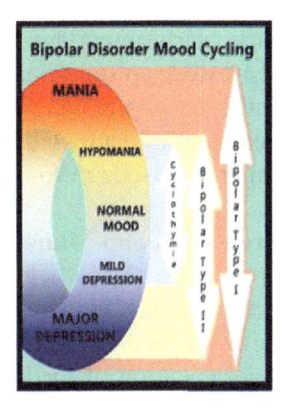

Living with bipolar disorder can be challenging in maintaining a regular lifestyle. Manic episodes can lead to family conflict or financial problems, especially when the person with bipolar disorder appears to behave erratically and irresponsibly without reason. During the manic phase, people often become impulsive and act aggressively. This can result in high-risk behavior, such as repeated intoxication, extravagant spending and risky sexual behavior.

**Bipolar disorder and other conditions**
According to the National Institute for Mental Health (NIMH), many people with bipolar disorder also have other mental disorders or conditions such as anxiety disorders, eating disorders, ADHD or substance use disorders. Sometimes people who have severe manic or depressive episodes also have symptoms of psychosis, which may include hallucinations or delusions. The psychotic symptoms tend to match the person's extreme mood. For example, someone having psychotic symptoms during a depressive episode may falsely believe they are financially ruined, while someone having psychotic symptoms during a manic episode may falsely believe they are famous or have special powers. Looking at a person's symptoms over the course of the illness and examining their family history can help a counselor or

psychotherapist determine whether the person has bipolar disorder along with another disorder - co-occurring disorders.

Identifying the first episode of mania or depression and receiving early treatment is essential to managing bipolar disorder. In most cases, a depressive episode occurs before a manic episode, and many patients are treated initially as if they have major depression. Usually, the first recognized episode of bipolar disorder is a manic episode. Once a manic episode occurs, it becomes clearer that the person is suffering from an illness characterized by alternating moods. Because of this difficulty with diagnosis, family history of similar illness or episodes is particularly important. People who first seek treatment as a result of a depressed episode may continue to be treated as someone with unipolar depression until a manic episode develops. Ironically, treatment of depressed bipolar patients with antidepressants can trigger a manic episode in some patients.

**Treatment and Management**

Treatment can help many people, including those with the most severe forms of bipolar disorder. An effective treatment plan usually includes a combination of medication and psychotherapy. The most common types of medications that health care providers prescribe include mood stabilizers and atypical antipsychotics. Mood stabilizers such as lithium or valproate can help prevent mood episodes or reduce their severity. Lithium also can decrease the risk of suicide.

Although bipolar depression is often treated with antidepressant medication, a mood stabilizer must be taken as well—taking an antidepressant without a mood stabilizer can trigger a manic episode or rapid cycling in a person with bipolar disorder. Because people with bipolar disorder are more likely to seek help when they are depressed than when they are experiencing mania or hypomania, it is important for health care providers to take a careful medical history to ensure that bipolar disorder is not mistaken for depression.

Although bipolar depression is often treated with antidepressant medication, a mood stabilizer must be taken as well—taking an antidepressant without a mood stabilizer can trigger a manic episode or rapid cycling in a person with bipolar disorder.

**Mood Stabilizers** (BY GENERIC/TRADE NAME)
- lithium carbonate/Eskalith, Lithane, Lithobid
- lithium citrate/Cibalith-S
- carbamazepine/Tegretol
- divalproex sodium (valproic acid) / Depakote
- lamotrigine/Lamictal
- topimarate/Topamax

**Anti-mania Medications** (BY GENERIC/TRADE NAME)
- All second-generation (atypical) antipsychotics

Medicines for Bipolar depression
- Fluoxetine combined with olanzepine/Symbax
- Lumateperone/Caplyta
- Lurasidone/Latuda
- Quetiapine/Seroquel

**Psychosocial treatments**
Psychotherapy can be an effective part of treatment for people with bipolar disorder. Psychotherapy helps people identify and change troubling emotions, thoughts, and behaviors. This type of therapy can provide support, education, and guidance to people with bipolar disorder and their families. Cognitive behavioral therapy (CBT) is an important treatment for depression, and CBT adapted for the treatment of insomnia can be especially helpful as part of treatment for bipolar depression.

Because bipolar disorder can cause serious disruptions in a person's daily life and create stressful family situations, family members may also benefit from professional resources, particularly mental health advocacy and support groups. From these sources, families can learn strategies for coping, participating actively in the treatment, and obtaining support. Treatment may also include newer therapies designed specifically for the treatment of bipolar disorder, including interpersonal and social rhythm therapy (IPSRT) and family-focused therapy (NIMH. 2023).

**Other treatment options**
Some people may find other treatments helpful in managing their bipolar symptoms:
- **Electroconvulsive therapy (ECT)** is a brain stimulation procedure that can help relieve severe symptoms of bipolar

disorder. Health care providers may consider ECT when a person's illness has not improved after other treatments, or in cases that require rapid response, such as with people who have a high suicide risk or catatonia (a state of unresponsiveness).
- **Repetitive transcranial magnetic stimulation** (rTMS) a type of brain stimulation that uses magnetic waves to relieve depression over a series of treatment sessions. Although not as powerful as ECT, rTMS does not require general anesthesia and has a low risk of negative effects on memory and thinking.
- **Light therapy** is the best evidence-based treatment for seasonal affective disorder (SAD) and many people with bipolar disorder experience seasonal worsening of depression or SAD in the winter. Light therapy may also be used to treat lesser forms of seasonal worsening of bipolar depression.

Unlike specific psychotherapy and medication treatments that are scientifically proven to improve bipolar disorder symptoms, complementary health approaches for bipolar disorder, such as natural products, are not based on current knowledge or evidence

## SUGGESTED READINGS ON THIS TOPIC

Bipolar disorder: assessment and management. Bipolar disorder: assessment and management. London: National Institute for Health and Care Excellence (NICE); 2023. (NICE Guideline, No. 185.) Available from: https://www.ncbi.nlm.nih.gov/books/NBK547001/

Centers for Disease Control (CDC). Mental Illness Prevalence. Accessed website March 2024. https://search.cdc.gov/search/?query=mental%20illness&dpage=1

Jain A, Mitra P. Bipolar Disorder. StatPearls Publishing LLC. 2024. Available from: https://www.ncbi.nlm.nih.gov/books/NBK558998. Accessed March 2024.

Jones S and Bentall R. The Psychology of Bipolar Disorder: New developments and research strategies. Oxford University Press. **ISBN:** 9780198530091

Lakshmi NY and Maj M. Bipolar Disorder: Clinical and Neurobiological Foundations. Wiley Publishers. 2010. ISBN: 978-0-470-72198-8

Miklowitz DJ and Gitlin MJ. Clinician's Guide to Bipolar Disorder. The Guilford Press. 2015. **ISBN-10 :** 1462523684

Mondimore, FM. The Concise Guide to Bipolar Disorder (A Johns Hopkins Press Health Book). Johns Hopkins University Press; 1st edition (October 11, 2022).
**ISBN-13 :** 978-1421444031

Strakowski SM, et al. Bipolar Disorder. Oxford University Press. 2020.
**ISBN:** 9780190908096

Weyandt L. Clinical Neuroscience: Foundations of Psychological and Neurodegenerative Disorders. Routledge. 2018. **ISBN-10 :** 1138630756

Yildiz A, Ruiz P, and Nemeroff C. The Bipolar Book: History, Neurobiology, and Treatment. Oxford University Press. 2015. **ISBN:** 9780199300532

Young AH and Juruena MF. Bipolar Disorder: From Neuroscience to Treatment. Springer. 2021.

# CHAPTER 17
# CLINICAL DEPRESSION: SYMPTOMS, CAUSES AND TREATMENTS

## Key Concepts

| | |
|---|---|
| **Anhedonia** | The inability to feel pleasure. |
| **Antidepressants** | Medications that are used to treat depression. There are different types of antidepressants, including: selective serotonin reuptake inhibitors (SSRIs), serotonin and norepinephrine reuptake inhibitors (SNRIs), tricyclic antidepressants, monoamine oxidase inhibitors (MAOIs), and atypical antidepressants. |
| **Antidepressant Withdrawal Syndrome** | A condition that happens when someone stops taking antidepressants. It can cause symptoms such as trouble sleeping, nausea, poor balance, flu-like symptoms, or anxiety. |
| **Anxiety disorder** | A chronic condition that causes anxiety so severe it interferes with your life. Some people with depression also have overlapping anxiety disorders. |
| **Atypical Depression** | A subtype of depression marked by excessive sleepiness, increased appetite, and a mood that can improve in response to positive events. Despite what its name might suggest, atypical depression isn't rare or unusual; it just differs from "typical" depression |
| **Avolition** | A lack of initiative or motivation to accomplish tasks. |

| | |
|---|---|
| **Chronic Depression** | A type of depression that causes symptoms that last at least two years. |
| **Co-Occurring Disorders.** | Having a mental health condition and also a drug or alcohol issue at the same time. |
| **Deep Brain Stimulation** | A procedure that involves implanting electrodes in the brain to produce electric impulses that stimulate specific areas. It may be used to treat some forms of depression that have not responded to other treatments. |
| **Depression** | A mental health condition that causes symptoms such as sadness, feelings of worthlessness, excessive guilt, or a lack of interest in daily activities. It can affect a person's work, sleep, appetite, and social life, according to the National Institute of Mental Health (NIMH). |
| **Dysphoric mood** | Low mood that may include dissatisfaction, restlessness, or depression. |
| **Dysthymia** | A type of chronic, low-grade depression that is less severe than clinical major depression. It can also last for years. Dysthymia may not disable a person, but it prevents one from functioning normally or feeling well. Modern diagnostic systems include "dysthymia" with "chronic major depression" (that is, a major depressive episode lasting 2 years or more in an adult or 1 year or more in children and adolescents) under the general term "persistent depressive disorder." |

| | |
|---|---|
| **Electroconvulsive therapy** | A treatment for depression performed under general anesthesia that uses an electric current to create a brief, controlled seizure. It is safe and often effective for treatment resistant depression. |
| **Hypersomnia** | Excessive daytime sleeping or sleepiness. |
| **Hyperthyroidism.** | A condition when the thyroid doesn't produce enough thyroid hormone. This can lead to symptoms of depression, fatigue, weight gain, and other health problems. |
| **Phototherapy** | Therapy consisting of exposure to light that is brighter than indoor light and mimics sunlight. It may help treat some forms of depression. |
| **Major Depressive Disorder** | A depressive disorder that lasts two weeks or more and significantly interferes with someone's daily life. Symptoms might include feelings of hopelessness, fatigue, and low energy. |
| **Monoamine oxidase inhibitors(MAOIs)** | A group of medicines sometime prescribed to treat severe depression. MAOIs increase the concentration of chemicals responsible for sending information between nerves in particular regions of the brain, which may lead to better mental functioning. |
| **Neurofeedback** | A type of therapy used for depression that teaches a person to alter their brain activity through intensive brain training exercises. |
| **Postpartum depression** | affects women who have recently given birth. Many new mothers experience a brief episode of mild mood changes known as the "baby |

blues," but some will have postpartum depression, a much more serious condition that requires active treatment and emotional support.

**Repetitive Transcranial Magnetic Stimulation (rTMS)**
A type of treatment that uses a magnet to target and stimulate certain areas of the brain through the skull. It's used to help depression and anxiety.

**Seasonal Affective Disorder**
Depression that happens seasonally, usually starting in fall or winter and ending in spring or early summer. It is often treated with phototherapy, which is regular exposure to special lights.

**Situational Depression**
An often short lived type of depression that develops after a traumatic or stressful event. Also known as *reactive depression.*

**Drug-Induced Depressive Disorder**
A condition characterized by depressive symptoms that occur during or soon after a person takes a certain medication or substance or experiences withdrawal from a certain medication or substance. Example: methamphetamine.

**Trigger**
A situation or event that provokes symptoms of depression.

**Vagus Nerve Stimulation**
A procedure for treatment-resistant depression. The vagus nerve connects the brain to the body and is thought to be involved in regulating mood.

# CHAPTER 17

# Clinical Depression: Symptoms, Causes and Treatment

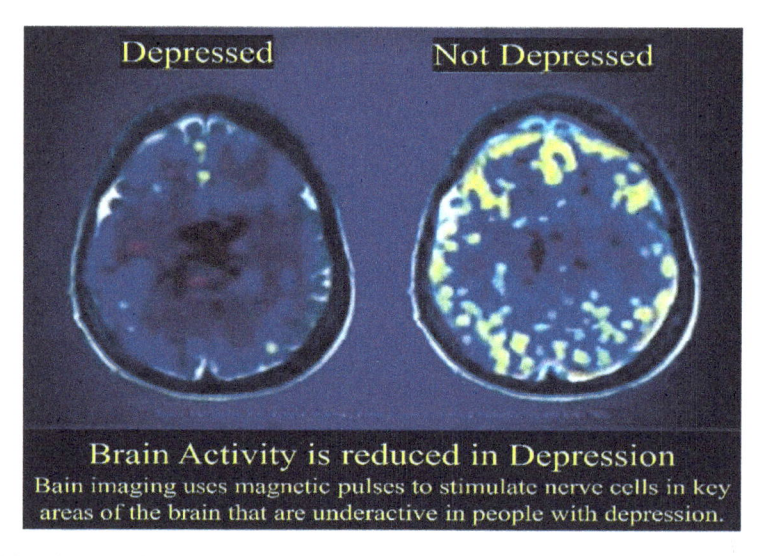

**Brain Activity is reduced in Depression**
Bain imaging uses magnetic pulses to stimulate nerve cells in key areas of the brain that are underactive in people with depression.

This chapter focuses on clinical depression, as it too co-occurs often with substance use disorders. Clinical depression is the more severe form of depression, also known as major depression or major depressive disorder (MDD). It isn't the same as depression caused by a loss, such as the death of a loved one, or a medical condition, such as a thyroid disorder.

Clinical depression is one of the most common mental disorders in the United States. It has a lifetime prevalence of about 5 to 17 percent, with the average being 12 percent. The prevalence rate is almost double in women than in men - 10.3% in females compared to males 6.2%. And, the prevalence of adults with a major depressive episode was highest among individuals aged 18-25 (18.6%). Source: Substance Abuse and Mental Health Services Administration. 2022.

For some individuals, major depression can result in severe impairments that interfere with or limit one's ability to carry out major life activities .To describe a major depressive episode a person must either have a depressed mood or a loss of interest or pleasure in daily activities consistently for at least a 2-week period. This mood must represent a change from the person's normal mood. Social, occupational, educational or other important functioning must also be negatively impaired by the change in mood.

Depressive disorders are twice as common in women as in men, although both sexes suffer its effects. Long-term use of stimulants, such as methamphetamine and cocaine has been identified as causing or aggravating depression. Alcohol dependence frequently causes depressive symptoms as well. However psychosocial effects such as stigma, poverty and isolation associated with drug use may also be highly relevant.

Depression can also co-occur with other medical disorders such as cancer, heart disease, stroke, Parkinson's disease, Alzheimer's and diabetes. In such cases, the depression is often overlooked and is not treated. Antidepressants are not stimulants, but rather reduce the symptoms of depression and help people feel the way they did before they became depressed.

Per the DSM-5, other types of depression falling under the category of depressive disorders are:
- Persistent depressive disorder, formerly known as dysthymia
- Disruptive mood dysregulation disorder
- Premenstrual dysphoric disorder
- Substance/medication-induced depressive disorder
- Depressive disorder due to another medical condition
- Unspecified depressive disorder

The table below shows the DSM-5 diagnostic criteria for major depressive illness.

| Table 1 DSM-5 Diagnostic Criteria for Major Depressive Disorder[3] |
|---|
| For a diagnosis of major depressive disorder, 5 or more of the following symptoms must be present nearly every day for at least a 2-week period (at least one of the symptoms is either depressed mood or anhedonia). Symptoms must impair functioning and cannot be secondary to another drug or illness.<br>• Depressed mood most of the time and on most days (e.g., feels sad, appears tearful)<br>• Anhedonia (e.g., decreased interest or pleasure in activities)<br>• Significant change in weight (e.g., weight loss, weight gain)<br>• Sleep disturbances (e.g., insomnia, hypersomnia)<br>• Psychomotor fluctuations (e.g., psychomotor agitation or retardation)<br>• Changes in energy levels (e.g., fatigue, loss of energy)<br>• Excessive guilt or feelings of worthlessness<br>• Difficulties concentrating<br>• Recurrent thoughts of death or suicidal thoughts (e.g., active or passive suicidal ideation with or without a plan)<br>Peripartum onset specifier: Onset of symptoms occurs during pregnancy or within 4 weeks after childbirth. Episodes can present with psychotic features. |

These theories for the cause of major depressive disorder are believed to be multifactorial, including biological, genetic, environmental, and psychosocial factors. Clinical depression was earlier considered to be mainly due to abnormalities in the monoamine neurotransmitters, especially serotonin, norepinephrine, and dopamine. This has been evidenced by the use of different antidepressants such as selective serotonin receptor inhibitors, serotonin-norepinephrine receptor inhibitors, dopamine-norepinephrine receptor inhibitors in the treatment of depression.

GABA, an inhibitory neurotransmitter, and glutamate and glycine, both of which are major excitatory neurotransmitters are found to play a role in the etiology of depression as well. Depressed patients have been found to have lower plasma, CSF, and brain GABA levels. GABA is considered to exert its antidepressant effect by inhibiting the ascending monoamine pathways, including mesolimbic pathway (MLP). Drugs that antagonize NMDA receptors have been researched to have antidepressant properties. Thyroid and growth hormonal abnormalities have also been implicated in the etiology of mood disorders. Multiple adverse childhood experiences (ACEs) and trauma are associated with the development of depression later in life. (Bains N, Abdijadid S. 2023.).

Early severe stress, (tied to ACEs) can result in significant changes in neuroendocrine and behavioral responses, which can cause structural changes in the brain cerebral cortex. These changes have been associated with severe depression later in life. Structural and functional brain imaging of depressed individuals has shown increased hyperintensities in the subcortical regions, and reduced anterior brain metabolism on the left side, respectively (Bains N, Abdijadid S. 2023).

Family, adoption, and twin studies have indicated the role of genes in the susceptibility of depression. Genetic studies show a very high concordance rate for twins to have MDD, particularly monozygotic twins. Life events and personality traits have shown to play an important role, as well. The *learned helplessness theory* has associated the occurrence of depression with the experience of uncontrollable events. Per cognitive theory, depression occurs as a result of cognitive distortions in persons who are susceptible to depression.

**Treatment and Management of Clinical Depression**

The monoamine deficiency theory posits that the underlying pathophysiological basis of depression is a depletion of the neurotransmitters serotonin, norepinephrine or dopamine in the central nervous system. Serotonin is the most extensively studied neurotransmitter in depression.

Current neurobiological theories with the most valid empirical foundation and the highest clinical relevance are reviewed with respect to their strengths and weaknesses. The selected theories are based on studies investigating psychosocial stress and stress hormones, neurotransmitters such as serotonin, norepinephrine, dopamine, glutamate and gamma-aminobutyric acid (GABA), neurocircuitry, neurotrophic factors, and circadian rhythms. Because all theories of depression apply to only some types of depressed patients but not others, and because depressive pathophysiology may vary considerably across the course of illness, the current extant knowledge argues against a unified hypothesis of depression. As a consequence, antidepressant treatments, including psychological and biological approaches, should be tailored for individual patients and disease states. (Hasler G. 2010).

The serotonin hypothesis of depression, which suggests that depression is caused by abnormalities in serotonin levels in the brain, has been influential for decades. However, a 2022 review of previous research by scientists found no clear evidence that serotonin levels or activity are responsible for depression. Other experts have also cautioned that there is no scientifically established "balance" of serotonin

In recent years, while selective modification of serotonin neurotransmission has continued to be a therapeutic option in the treatment of mood and anxiety disorders, and the efficacy of the selective serotonin reuptake inhibitors (SSRIs) for a significant number of people (though not all) has been demonstrated (Cipriani A, et al. 2018 and Hieronymus F. 2020). the notion that a complex heterogeneous conditions such as clinical depression could be caused by deficient functioning of a single neurotransmitter has been regarded as implausible (Cowen PJ and Browning M. 2015.). Serotonergic agents continue to be widely employed in the treatment of a range of mental health conditions, particularly anxiety and depression. Indeed, one of the more dramatic demonstrations of the role of serotonin in mood and self-conscious experience comes from the study of psychedelic drugs, now being repurposed for the treatment of resistant depression.

As described, there are some reliable abnormalities in serotonin mechanisms in depressed patients but their potential role in the causation of illness remains to be determined. A likely aid in resolving this question will be the continued intense interest in pre-clinical studies of the role of serotonin in processes relevant to depression such as reward and punishment learning, decision-making, emotional regulation, and social cognition (Roberts C. 2020). Along with this, in clinical studies, there will be improvements in methods of assessing brain serotonin activity, as shown by recent investigations measuring serotonin release in the living human brain. Clearly, the role of serotonin in depression will need to be integrated into more complex neurobiological models than those originally envisaged. Nevertheless, the link between impaired serotonin activity and depression is likely to outlive its recent obituaries (Jauhar S, Cowen PJ, Browning M. 2023).

**Antidepressant Medications**
Major depressive disorder can be managed with various treatment modalities, including pharmacological, psychotherapeutic, interventional, and lifestyle modification. The initial treatment of clinical depression includes medications or/and psychotherapy. Combination treatment, including both medications and psychotherapy, has been found to be more effective than either of these treatments alone (Cuijpers P, Dekker J, Hollon SD, 2009 and Cuijpers

P, van Straten A, (2009). Electroconvulsive therapy is found to be more efficacious than any other form of treatment for severe major depression (Pagnin D, de Queiroz . 2004.

The major classes of antidepressant drugs include the tricyclic and related antidepressants (TCAs), selective serotonin re-uptake inhibitors (SSRIs), the selective serotonin and norepinephrine re-uptake inhibitors (SNRIs) and the monoamine oxidase inhibitors (MAOIs). A small number of drugs don't easily fall into this classification and are listed under Atypical antidepressants.

SSRIs are better tolerated and are safer in overdose than other classes of antidepressants and should be considered first-line for treating depression. Notably, sertraline has been shown to be safe in patients who have had a recent myocardial infarction or who have unstable angina. TCAs have similar efficacy to SSRIs, but their more troublesome side-effects leads to patients being more likely to discontinue treatment. TCAs are also more toxic in overdose than SSRIs. MAOIs have dangerous interactions with some foods and drugs, and should be reserved for use by specialists. Anxiolytics or antipsychotic drugs should be used with caution in depression which often presents as anxiety, as they can mask the true diagnosis, but are useful adjuncts in agitated patients.

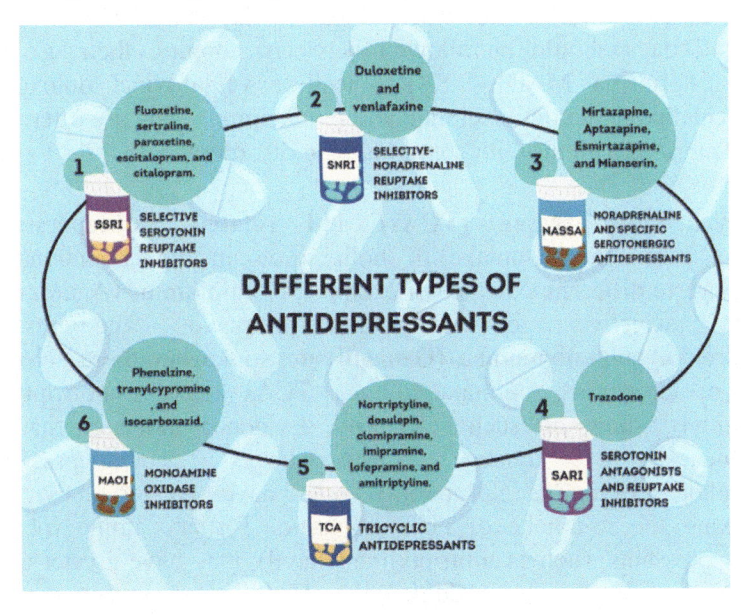

**DIFFERENT TYPES OF ANTIDEPRESSANTS**

1. SSRI — SELECTIVE SEROTONIN REUPTAKE INHIBITORS: Fluoxetine, sertraline, paroxetine, escitalopram, and citalopram.

2. SNRI — SELECTIVE-NORADRENALINE REUPTAKE INHIBITORS: Duloxetine and venlafaxine.

3. NASSA — NORADRENALINE AND SPECIFIC SEROTONERGIC ANTIDEPRESSANTS: Mirtazapine, Aptazapine, Esmirtazapine, and Mianserin.

4. SARI — SEROTONIN ANTAGONISTS AND REUPTAKE INHIBITORS: Trazodone.

5. TCA — TRICYCLIC ANTIDEPRESSANTS: Nortriptyline, dosulepin, clomipramine, imipramine, lofepramine, and amitriptyline.

6. MAOI — MONOAMINE OXIDASE INHIBITORS: Phenelzine, tranylcypromine, and isocarboxazid.

FDA-approved antidepressant medications for the treatment of clinical depression are equally effective but differ in side-effect profiles. However, combination treatment, including both medications and psychotherapy, has been found to be more effective than either of these treatments alone.

**Selective serotonin reuptake inhibitors (SSRIs).** SSRIs are the most commonly prescribed class of antidepressants. They are highly effective and generally well tolerated compared to other types of antidepressants. Side effects of SSRIs may include nausea, vomiting, diarrhea, sexual dysfunction, headache, weight gain, anxiety, dizziness, dry mouth, and insomnia. Caution should be used when prescribing SSRIs alongside other drugs that increase the risk of bleeding. SSRIs should not be used in patients with poorly controlled epilepsy or in patients entering manic phase. Common shared side-effects (often dose-related) include abdominal pain, constipation, diarrhea, dyspepsia, nausea and vomiting. An uncommon, but potentially serious side-effect is serotonin syndrome. SSRIs include fluoxetine, sertraline, citalopram, escitalopram, paroxetine, and fluvoxamine. They are usually the first line of treatment and the most widely prescribed antidepressants.

**Serotonin-norepinephrine reuptake inhibitors (SNRIs).** None of these drugs should be prescribed within 14 days of an MAOI and at least 7 days should be allowed between stopping their use and administering a MAOI. SNRIs include venlafaxine, duloxetine, desvenlafaxine, levomilnacipran, and milnacipran. They are often used for depressed patients with comorbid pain disorders.

**Tricyclic antidepressants (TCAs) and related antidepressants.** TCAs block the re-uptake of both serotonin and noradrenaline, although to different extents. For example, clomipramine (Anafranil) is more selective for serotonin re-uptake, and reboxetine (Endronax) and lofepramine (Gamanil) are somewhat more selective for noradrenaline re-uptake. Other TCAs such as nortriptyline (Aventyl), show no such selectivity. Evidence indicates that the secondary amine tricyclic antidepressants, including desipramine (Norpramin), may have greater activity in blocking the re-uptake of norepinephrine. Tertiary amine tricyclic antidepressants, such as amitriptyline (Elavil), may have greater effect on serotonin re-uptake. Additionally, TCAs block muscarinic $M_1$, histamine $H_1$, and alpha-adrenoceptors.

Tricyclic and related antidepressant drugs can be roughly divided into those with additional sedative properties and those that are less sedating. Agitated and anxious patients tend to respond best to the sedative compounds, whereas withdrawn and apathetic patients will often obtain most benefit from the less sedating ones.

TCAs are approved for treating several types of depression, obsessive compulsive disorder, and bedwetting (nocturnal enuresis). Also used for several off-label conditions such as panic disorder, bulimia, chronic pain (for example, migraine, tension headaches, diabetic neuropathy, and post herpetic neuralgia), phantom limb pain, chronic itching, and premenstrual symptoms. **NOTE:** Although effective, TCAs have largely been replaced by newer antidepressants that generally cause fewer side-effects.

**Monoamine oxidase inhibitor antidepressants (MAOIs).** MAOIs block the activity of monoamine oxidase, an enzyme that breaks down norepinephrine, serotonin, and dopamine in the brain and other parts of the body. The four most commonly prescribed MAOIs are **selegiline (Emsam), isocarboxazid (Marplan), phenelzine Nardil), and tranylcypromine Parnate).** MAOIs are used much less frequently than tricyclic and related antidepressants, or SSRIs and related antidepressants because of the dangers of dietary and drug interactions.

MAOIs exhibit some benefit for phobic patients and depressed patients with atypical, hypochondriacal, or hysterical features, but should only be prescribed by specialists. In general, MAOIs have been replaced by newer antidepressants that are safer and cause fewer side-effects. Common side-effects include postural hypotension, weight gain, and sexual side effects.

**Atypical antidepressants.** Each drug in this category has a unique molecular mechanism of action, or a chemical structure that excludes them from the classification above. However, like other antidepressants, atypical antidepressants affect the levels or effects of dopamine, serotonin, and norepinephrine in the brain.

- **Bupropion (Wellbutrin)**- used to aid smoking cessation in combination with motivational support in nicotine-dependent patients. This drug should not be used in patients with seizure disorders, eating disorders, and within 2 weeks of using MAOI. It generally does not cause weight gain or sexual problems.

- **Esketamine (Spravato)** - Esketamine is an NMDA glutamate receptor antagonist. Unlike other antidepressants, esketamine impacts glutamate levels and does not affect serotonin, dopamine, or norepinephrine. Glutamate is the most abundant neurotransmitter in the brain and affects mood, learning, memory, and communication between neurons. This medication is administered as a nasal spray.
- **Mirtazapine (Remeron)**- a presynaptic $\alpha_2$-adrenoceptor and serotonin 5-$HT_2$ receptor antagonist which increases central noradrenergic and serotonergic neurotransmission. Used to manage major depression.
- **Nefazodone** - a serotonin 5-$HT_2$ receptor antagonist also inhibiting serotonin and norepinephrine re-uptake. Used to manage depression, including major depressive disorder. Nefazodone should not be prescribed to patients with active liver disease.
- **Trazodone (Desyrel)**- principally a serotonin 5-$HT_2$ receptor antagonist, used to manage depressive illness, particularly where sedation is required.
- **Vilazodone (Viibryd)**- a potent serotonin 5-$HT_{1A}$ receptor partial agonist, with combined inhibitory action against serotonin re-uptake. Used to manage major depressive disorder. Vilazodone is not associated with significant weight gain or sexual dysfunction.
- **Vortioxetine (Trintellix)** - a partial agonist of 5-$HT_{1A}$ and 5-$HT_{1B}$ receptors and antagonist of the 5-$HT_7$ receptor used to manage major depressive disorder. May also inhibit re-uptake of serotonin.

## Side Effects of Antidepressant Medications

Side-effect profiles are as unique as their mechanisms of action. Some common side effects include dry mouth, constipation, dizziness, and light headedness. Mirtazapine and trazodone cause drowsiness and are usually taken at bedtime

The most common side effects reported by patients in the study by Hu et al of 401 outpatients taking SSRIs were drowsiness (38%), dry mouth (34%), and sexual dysfunction (34%)
- Fatigue or drowsiness
- Sexual dysfunction
- Nausea and stomach upset
- Constipation

- weight gain
- insomnia
- Fine and rapid tremors of the extremities
- apathy and indifference

Abrupt discontinuation of SSRIs, nefazodone, venlafaxine, and mirtazapine may precipitate a discontinuation syndrome that can occur hours to days following the termination of medication. The syndrome often includes flulike symptoms such as malaise, myalgias, nausea, dizziness, and headache, and may even include neurologic symptoms such as unsteady gait, dysesthesias such as unusual shock-like sensations, tremulousness, or vertigo

**Structured psychotherapies**
(Adapted from Karrouri R, Hammani Z, Benjelloun R, Otheman Y 2021).

**Cognitive and behavioral therapies:** Based on robust evidence, CBT is one of the most well-documented and validated psychotherapeutic methods available. Interventional strategies are based on modifying dysfunctional behaviors and cognitions]. CBT targets depressed patients' irrational beliefs and distorted cognitions that perpetuate depressive symptoms by challenging and reversing them. However, the effectiveness of CBT depends on patient's capacity to observe and change their own beliefs and behaviors.

**Interpersonal Therapy (IPT):** The goal of IPT is to identify the triggers of depressive symptoms or episodes. These triggers may include losses, social isolation, or difficulties in social interactions. IPT, like CBT, is a first-line treatment for mild to moderate major depressive episodes in adults; it is also a well-established intervention for adolescents with depression.

**Problem-solving therapy:** The problem-solving therapy (PST) approach combines cognitive and interpersonal elements, focusing on negative assessments of situations and problem-solving strategies. PST has been used in different clinical situations, like preventing depression among the elderly and treating patients with mild depressive symptoms, especially in primary care. Despite its small effect sizes, PST is comparable to other psychotherapeutic methods used to treat depression.

**Marital and family therapy:** Marital and family therapy (MFT) is effective in treating some aspects of depression. Family therapy has also been used to treat severe forms of depression associated with medications and hospitalization. Marital and family problems can make people more vulnerable to depression, and MFT addresses these issues. Marital therapy includes both members of the couple, as depression is considered in an interpersonal context in such cases. Some of the goals of this therapy are to facilitate communication and resolve different types of marital conflict. Family therapy uses similar principles as other forms of therapy while involving all family members and considering depression within the context of pathological family dynamics.

**Supportive Therapy (ST):** Although ST is not as well-structured or well-evaluated as CBT or IPT, it is still commonly used to support depressed patients. In addition to sympathetic listening and expressing concern for the patient's problems, ST requires emotionally attuned listening, empathic paraphrasing, explaining the nature of the patient's suffering, and reassuring and encouraging them. These practices allow the patient to ventilate and accept their feelings, increase their self-esteem, and enhance their adaptive coping skills.

**Psychodynamic therapy:** Psychodynamic therapy encompasses a range of brief to long-term psychological interventions derived from psychoanalytic theories. This type of therapy focuses on intrapsychic conflicts related to shame, repressed impulses, problems in early childhood with one's emotional caretakers that lead to low self-esteem and poor emotional self-regulation. Psychodynamic therapy's efficacy in the acute phase of MDD is well-established compared to other forms of psychotherapy.

**Group therapy (GT):** The application of group therapy (GT) to clinically depressed patients remains limited.

**Mindfulness-based Cognitive Therapy** (MBCT): MBCT is a relatively recent technique that combines elements of CBT with mindfulness-based stress reduction. Studies have shown that eight weeks of MBCT treatment during remission reduces relapse. Thus, it is a potential alternative to reduce, or even stop, antidepressant treatment without increasing the risk of depressive recurrence, especially for patients at a high risk of relapse (*i.e.*, patients with more than two previous episodes and patients who have experienced childhood abuse or trauma).

**Psycho-education:** This type of intervention educates depressed patients and (with their permission) family members involved in the patient's life about depression symptoms and management. This education should be provided in a language that the patient understands. Issues such as misperceptions about medication, treatment duration, the risk of relapse, and prodromes of depression should be addressed. Moreover, patients should be encouraged to maintain healthy lifestyles and enhance their social skills to prevent depression and boost their overall mental health. Many studies have highlighted the role of psycho-education in improving the clinical course, treatment adherence, and psychosocial functioning in patients with depression.

**Physical exercise:** Most guidelines for treating depression, including the National Institute for Health and Care Excellence, the American Psychiatric Association, and the Royal Australian and New Zealand College of Psychiatrists, recommend that depressed patients perform regular physical activity to alleviate symptoms and prevent relapses.. Exercise also promotes improvements in one's quality of life in general.. However, exercise is considered an adjunct to other anti-depressive treatments.

**Somatic Treatments**
In many situations, depression can also be managed *via* somatic treatments. ECT is the most well-known treatment for resistant depression, and solid evidence supports its effectiveness and safety. In recent decades, various innovative techniques have been proposed, such as repetitive transcranial magnetic stimulation (rTMS), transcranial direct current stimulation (tDCS), vagus nerve stimulation (VNS), deep brain stimulation (DBS), and magnetic seizure therapy, with varying efficiency levels.

**Electroconvulsive Treatment (ECT)**
ECT is perhaps the most effective treatment modality for clinical depression, and its superiority over pharmacotherapy for major unipolar depression is widely supported. ECT reduces the number of hospital readmissions and lightens the burden of depression, leading to a better quality of life. Moreover, ECT is considered safe. Advances in anesthesia and ECT techniques have decreased complications related to ECT while also improving cognitive outcomes and patient satisfaction. ECT is typically recommended for patients with severe

and psychotic depression, a high risk of suicide, or Parkinson's disease, as well as pregnant patients.

**rTMS**

This method, which is a type of biological stimulation that affects brain metabolism and neuronal electrical activity, has been widely used in research on depression. Recent literature shows a significant difference between rTMS and fictitious stimulation regarding its improvements in depressive symptoms. Treatments combining rTMS and antidepressants are significantly more effective than placebo conditions, with mild side effects and good acceptability. Although these results are encouraging, they remain inconsistent due to differences in rTMS treatment frequencies, parameters, and stimulation sites. Therefore, clinical trials with large sample sizes are needed to specify which factors promote favorable therapeutic responses

**Vagus Nerve Stimulation (VNS)**

VNS is a therapeutic method that has been used for the last sixteen years to treat resistant unilateral or bipolar depression. However, despite several clinical studies attesting to its favorable benefit-risk ratio and its approval by the Food Drug Administration in 2005, it is not used very often. VNS involves the implantation of a pacemaker under the collarbone that is connected to an electrode surrounding the left vagus nerve. Since the turn of the century, numerous studies have demonstrated the efficacy of VNS in resistant depression.

**Deep Brain Stimulation (DBS)**

According to the literature, DBS of the subgenual cingulate white matter (Brodmann area = BA 25) elicited a clinical response in 60% of resistant depression patients after six months and clinical remission in 35% of patients, with benefits maintained for over 12 mo. The stimulation of other targets, in particular the nucleus accumbens, to treat resistant depression has gained interest recently. Behavioral effects indicate the quick and favorable impact of stimulation on anhedonia, with significant effects on mood appearing as early as week one after treatment begins.

**Magnetic seizure therapy**

Magnetic seizure therapy involves inducing a therapeutic seizure by applying magnetic stimulation to the brain while the patient is under anesthesia. This technique is still being investigated as a viable alternative to ECT to treat many psychiatric disorders. Evidence supporting its effectiveness on depressive symptoms continues to grow, and it appears to induce fewer neurocognitive effects than ECT.

**Luxtherapy (phototherapy)**
The first description of reduced depression symptoms due to intense light exposure was presented in 1984. Optimal improvements were obtained with bright light exposure of 2500 Lux for two hours *per* day, with morning exposure shown to be superior to evening exposure. A review and meta-analysis showed that more intense (but shorter) exposures (10000 Lux for half an hour *per* day or 6000 Lux for 1.5 h *per* day) have the same efficacy. Importantly, this treatment method is effective both for those with seasonal and non-seasonal depression. Benefits of phototherapy related to sleep deprivation and drug treatments have also been reported..

**Prognosis for Clinical Depression**
Untreated depressive episodes in major depressive disorder can last from 6 to 12 months. About two-thirds of the individuals with MDD contemplate suicide, and about 10 to 15 percent commit suicide. Clinical depression is a chronic, recurrent illness; the recurrence rate is about 50% after the first episode, 70% after the second episode, and 90% after the third episode. About 5 to 10 percent of the patients with clinical depression eventually develop bipolar disorder. The prognosis of clinical depressive disorders is good in patients with mild episodes, the absence of psychotic symptoms, better treatment compliance, a strong support system, and good premorbid functioning. The prognosis is poor in the presence of a comorbid psychiatric disorder, personality disorder, multiple hospitalizations, and advanced age of onset.

## SUGGESTED READINGS ON THIS TOPIC

Bains N and Abdijadid S. Major Depressive Disorder. In: StatPearls. StatPearls Publishing; 2024. Available from: https://www.ncbi.nlm.nih.gov/books/NBK559078/

Bancroft PR and Ardley LB. Major Depression in Women. Nova Science Pub. 2008.
**ISBN-10 :** 1604562129

Chand SP, Arif H. Depression. In: StatPearls. StatPearls Publishing; 2024. Available from: https://www.ncbi.nlm.nih.gov/books/NBK430847/

Cuijpers P, Dekker J, Hollon SD, Andersson G. Adding psychotherapy to pharmacotherapy in the treatment of depressive disorders in adults: a meta-analysis. J Clin Psychiatry. 2009 Sep;70(9):1219-29. [PubMed]

Cuijpers P, van Straten A, Warmerdam L, Andersson G. Psychotherapy versus the combination of psychotherapy and pharmacotherapy in the treatment of depression: a meta-analysis. Depress Anxiety. 2009;26(3):279-88. [PubMed]

Dobson, KS. Clinical Depression. An Individualized, Biopsychosocial Approach to Assessment and Treatment. American Psychological Association. 2024. **ISBN:** 978-1-4338-3670-1

Gold PW. Breaking Through Depression: A Guide to the Next Generation of Promising Research and Revolutionary New Treatments. Twelve. 2023. **ISBN-10 :** 1538724618

Karrouri R, Hammani Z, Benjelloun R, Otheman Y. Major depressive disorder: Validated treatments and future challenges. World J Clin Cases. 2021 Nov 6;9(31):9350-9367.

Layton D. Depression: Clinical and Research Perspectives. American Medical Publishers. 2022. **ISBN:** 1639274383

McClintock SM and Choi J. Neuropsychology of Depression. Guilford Press. 2022.
**ISBN:** 9781462549276

Moncrieff, J., Cooper, R.E., Stockmann, T. *et al.* The serotonin theory of depression: a systematic umbrella review of the evidence. *Mol Psychiatry* **28**, 3243–3256. 2023.

Palazidou E.. The neurobiology of depression. *British Medical Bulletin*, Volume 101, Issue 1, March 2012, Pages 127–145.

Pagnin D, de Queiroz V, Pini S, Cassano GB. Efficacy of ECT in depression: a meta-analytic review. J ECT. 2004 Mar;20(1):13-20. [PubMed]

Strakowski S and Nelson E. Major Depressive Disorder. Oxford University Press. 2015.
**ISBN-10 :** 9780190206185

# CHAPTER 18
# ANXIETY DISORDERS
# SYMPTOMS, CAUSES AND TREATMENTS

## Key Concepts

| | |
|---|---|
| **Anticipatory Fears/Anxiety** | A fear of what lies ahead. It almost always involves a fear of failure, rejection, or uncertainty (i.e. bad things may or will happen). |
| **Cognitive Behavioral Therapy (CBT)** | Cognitive Behavioral Therapy focuses on the relationship between Thoughts, Behaviors, and Emotions (i.e. what we think affects how we act and feel, what we do affects what we think and feel, what we feel affects what we think and do). This form of therapy encourages people to examine and challenge distortive/irrational thoughts and change problematic behaviors. |
| **Cognitive Dissonance** | The distress one experiences when thinking of or engaging in some form of behavior that contradicts personal beliefs, values, ideals. Many people struggle with intrusive thoughts that create tremendous dissonance. These people are dealing not only with the exhaustion from having these thoughts repeatedly jumping into the mind (think of a time when a catchy jingle or song gets stuck in your head), they also are dealing with thoughts that go against their personal values or preferences. |
| **Cognitive Distortions** | Distorted or irrational thoughts that contribute to negative emotions or behaviors (avoidance). Common |

cognitive distortions of those who struggle with anxiety include: overvaluing thoughts, over-predicting the likelihood of negative outcomes, catastrophizing.

**Dialectical Behavioral Therapy (DBT)**

A form of Cognitive Behavioral Therapy. DBT in part focuses on skill development to help people achieve personal goals that will allow them to live a life they find meaning in. These DBT skills include: Mindfulness, Emotional Regulation, Distress Tolerance, and Interpersonal Effectiveness.

**Emetophobia**

Irrational and overriding fear of throwing up - particularly in front of others.

**Exposure Response**

A form of Cognitive Behavioral Therapy. Purposefully. confronting a fear, while not engaging in avoidant behaviors. The more one does this the more distress tolerance one develops/acquires. (Example: Think of getting in a cold pool. There are three different types of exposure: Imaginal (cognitive), Virtual (electronic presentation of visual and/or auditory stimuli), and In-vivo (in real life) situations.

**Executive Function**

Cognitive functions relating to a person's ability to plan ahead; make good judgments; learn from experience; adopt appropriate socio-emotional, internally guided behavior.

**Fear appraisal**

A person's ability to accurately and objectively evaluate the world around oneself for potential threats. People suffering from significant anxiety, struggle to make objective evaluations. While they are typically better at distinguishing the difference between overtly hostile or friendly interaction, they struggle in recognizing and interpreting neutral situations (i.e. anything that is not overtly positive or negative). The net result of a person with poor fear appraisal skills is that they frequently assign a strong likelihood for a negative outcome to a neutral event, or assign high probability of a negative outcome to a low probability event. (Example: "When I told a co-worker about a funny experience I had, she did not smile or nod her head, therefore she must think that I'm stupid, she probably does not like me, and I have made a fool of myself.")

**Generalized anxiety disorder** GAD usually involves a persistent feeling of anxiety or dread, which can interfere with daily life. It is not the same as occasionally worrying about things or experiencing anxiety due to stressful life events. People living with GAD experience frequent anxiety for months, if not years.

**Intrusive Thoughts** Unwelcome involuntary thought, image, or unpleasant idea that may become an obsession, is upsetting or distressing, and can feel difficult to manage or eliminate. Intrusive thoughts can become extremely disturbing and may induce panic as the thought becomes "stuck" and the individual is unable to let the thought go.. Individuals with Intrusive Thought Disorder often suffer in silence. They experience considerable

| | |
|---|---|
| | shame for experiencing the thought and are afraid to share the problem with others out of fear of being judged. |
| **Panic disorder** | People with panic disorder have frequent and unexpected panic attacks. Panic attacks are sudden periods of intense fear, discomfort, or sense of losing control even when there is no clear danger or trigger. Not everyone who experiences a panic attack will develop panic disorder. |
| **Perfectionism** | Striving for flawlessness; unrealistic expectations regarding performance. Individuals struggling with perfectionism will avoid handing in assignments even when completed, or are unable to finish assignments due to the amount of time spent trying to make it perfect. Often at the core of these issues is an inability to tolerate the uncertainty of how others will perceive their work |
| **Phobia-related disorders** | A phobia is an intense fear of—or aversion to—specific objects or situations. Although it can be realistic to be anxious in some circumstances, the fear people with phobias feel is out of proportion to the actual danger caused by the situation or object. There are several types of phobias and phobia-related disorders: Social anxiety disorder (previously called social phobia); Agoraphobia.; Separation anxiety disorder; Selective mutism |

# CHAPTER 18.

# Anxiety Disorders: Symptoms, Causes and Treatment

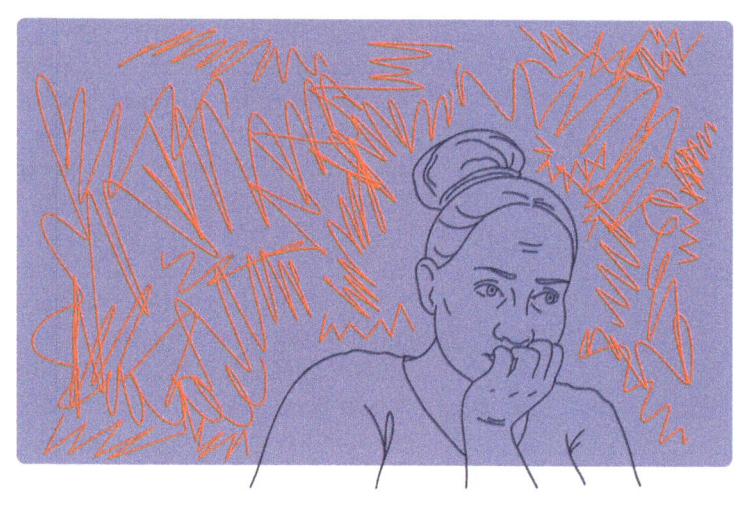

**ANXIETY DISORDERS**

*anxiety*

> *n.* an emotion characterized by apprehension and somatic (body) symptoms of tension in which an individual anticipates impending danger, catastrophe, or misfortune. The body often mobilizes itself to meet the perceived threat: Muscles become tense, breathing is faster, and the heart beats more rapidly. Anxiety may be distinguished from fear both conceptually and physiologically, although the two terms are often used interchangeably. Anxiety is considered a future-oriented, long-acting response broadly focused on a diffuse threat, whereas fear is an appropriate, present-oriented, and short-lasting.
> (American Psychological Association. 2023).

Ooccasional anxiety, according to the National Institute for Mental Health (NIMH) and the Substance Abuse and Mental Health Services Administration (SAMHSA), is an expected part of life. A person might feel anxious when faced with a problem at work, before taking an exam, or before making an important decision. But anxiety disorders involve more than temporary worry or fear. For a person with an anxiety disorder, the anxiety does not go away and often gets worse over time. The symptoms can interfere with daily activities such as job performance, schoolwork, and relationships. There are several types of anxiety disorders: generalized anxiety disorder, panic disorder with or without agoraphobia, specific phobias, agoraphobia, social anxiety disorder, separation anxiety disorder and selective mutism

**NOTE:** Obsessive-compulsive disorder (OCD) used to be classified as an anxiety disorder. But that changed with the fifth edition of the *Diagnostic and Statistical Manual of Mental Disorders*, published in 2013. It's now in a category called "Obsessive-Compulsive and Related Disorders." However, most people with OCD also have an anxiety disorder.

Unlike fear, which is a response to a realistic immediate danger, anxiety is a fearful response occurring in the absence of a specific danger, or it can be anticipatory anxiety. According to the National Institute of Health, anxiety disorders are the most common form of mental disorder in the population with a one-year prevalence of 9.7%. Patients experiencing anxiety may present with complaints of excessive fear or worry, or repetitive, intrusive thoughts including worrying about the future, health or relationships.

These people find it hard to relax, concentrate and sleep with physical symptoms such as heart palpitations, tension and muscle pain, sweating, hyperventilation, dizziness, faintness, headaches, nausea, indigestion and loss of sexual interest. In these disorders the symptoms associated with anxiety are accompanied by changes in thoughts, emotions and behavior that substantially interfere with the person's usual ability to live and work.

Anxiety usually begins in early adulthood and can be triggered by a series of life events. Anxiety disorders can be complicated by self-medication with alcohol and other substances. Similarly substance abuse may be complicated by the development of anxiety symptoms. Anxiety is common in withdrawal from alcohol, benzodiazepines, and opioids and is also common during intoxication with stimulants, marijuana and hallucinogens and, at times, can be very difficult to distinguish primary symptoms of anxiety from those caused by substance abuse. The failure to recognize and treat anxiety can lead to worsening of substance use and associated problems vice versa.

**Facts and Statistics about Anxiety Disorders**

- Generalized Anxiety Disorder (GAD) affects 6.8 million adults or 3.1% of the U.S. population, yet only 43.2% are receiving treatment. Women are twice as likely to be affected as men. GAD often co-occurs with major depression.

- Panic Disorder (PD) affects 6 million adults or 2.7% of the U.S. population. Women are twice as likely to be affected as men.

- Social Anxiety Disorder (SAD) affects 15 million adults or 7.1% of the U.S. population. SAD is equally common among men and women and typically begins around age 13. 36% of people with social anxiety disorder report - experiencing symptoms for 10 or more years before seeking help.

- Specific phobias affect 19.3 million adults or 9.1% of the U.S. population. Women are twice as likely to be affected than men. Symptoms typically begin in childhood; the average age of onset is 7 years old.

- 
  Obsessive-compulsive disorder (OCD) and posttraumatic stress disorder (PTSD) are closely related to anxiety disorders, which some may experience at the same time, along with depression.

- Stress. Everyone experiences stress and anxiety at one time or another. The difference between them is that stress is a response to a threat in a situation. Anxiety is a reaction to stress.

- Obsessive-Compulsive Disorder (OCD) affects 2.5 million adults or 1.2% of the U.S. population. Women are 3x more likely to be affected than men. The average age of onset is 19, with 25% of cases occurring by age 14. One-third of affected adults first experienced symptoms in childhood. OCD is clinically not an anxiety disorder but patients with OCD experience anxiety.

- Post-Traumatic Stress Disorder (PTSD) affects 7.7 million adults or 3.6% of the U.S. population. Women are 5x more likely to be affected than men. Rape is the most likely trigger of PTSD: 65% of men and 45.9% of women who are raped will develop the disorder. Childhood sexual abuse is a strong predictor of the lifetime likelihood of developing PTSD. PTSD is clinically not an anxiety disorder but patients with OCD experience anxiety. Obsessive-compulsive disorder (OCD) and posttraumatic stress disorder (PTSD) are closely related to anxiety disorders, which some may experience at the same time, along with depression.

There are several types of anxiety disorders, including generalized anxiety disorder, panic disorder, social anxiety disorder, and various phobia-related disorders (National Institute of Mental Health. 2022).

**Generalized anxiety disorder**
Generalized anxiety disorder (GAD) usually involves a persistent feeling of anxiety or dread, which can interfere with daily life. It is not the same as occasionally worrying about things or experiencing anxiety due to stressful life events. People living with GAD experience frequent anxiety for months, if not years.

**Symptoms of GAD include:**
- Feeling restless, wound-up, or on-edge
- Being easily fatigued
- Having difficulty concentrating
- Being irritable
- Having headaches, muscle aches, stomachaches, or unexplained pains
- Difficulty controlling feelings of worry
- Having sleep problems, such as difficulty falling or staying asleep

**Panic disorder**
People with panic disorder have frequent and unexpected panic attacks. Panic attacks are sudden periods of intense fear, discomfort, or sense of losing control even when there is no clear danger or trigger. Not everyone who experiences a panic attack will develop panic disorder. During a panic attack, a person may experience:
- Pounding or racing heart
- Sweating
- Trembling or tingling

- Chest pain
- Feelings of impending doom
- Feelings of being out of control

People with panic disorder often worry about when the next attack will happen and actively try to prevent future attacks by avoiding places, situations, or behaviors they associate with panic attacks. Panic attacks can occur as frequently as several times a day or as rarely as a few times a year.

**Social anxiety disorder**
Social anxiety disorder is an intense, persistent fear of being watched and judged by others. For people with social anxiety disorder, the fear of social situations may feel so intense that it seems beyond their control. For some people, this fear may get in the way of going to work, attending school, or doing everyday things.

People with social anxiety disorder may experience:
- Blushing, sweating, or trembling
- Pounding or racing heart
- Stomachaches
- Rigid body posture or speaking with an overly soft voice
- Difficulty making eye contact or being around people they don't know
- Feelings of self-consciousness or fear that people will judge them negatively

**Phobia-related disorders**
A *phobia* is an intense fear of—or aversion to—specific objects or situations. Although it can be realistic to be anxious in some circumstances, the fear people with phobias feel is out of proportion to the actual danger caused by the situation or object.
People with a phobia:
- May have an irrational or excessive worry about encountering the feared object or situation
- Take active steps to avoid the feared object or situation
- Experience immediate intense anxiety upon encountering the feared object or situation
- Endure unavoidable objects and situations with intense anxiety

There are several types of phobias and phobia-related disorders.

**Specific Phobias (sometimes called simple phobias)**: As the name suggests, people who have a specific phobia have an intense fear of, or feel intense anxiety about, specific types of objects or situations. Some examples of specific phobias include the fear of:
- Flying
- Heights
- Specific animals, such as spiders, dogs, or snakes
- Receiving injections
- Blood

**Agoraphobia:** People with agoraphobia have an intense fear of two or more of the following situations:
- Using public transportation
- Being in open spaces
- Being in enclosed spaces
- Standing in line or being in a crowd
- Being outside of the home alone

People with agoraphobia often avoid these situations, in part, because they think being able to leave might be difficult or impossible in the event they have panic-like reactions or other embarrassing symptoms. In the most severe form of agoraphobia, an individual can become housebound.

**Separation anxiety disorder:** Separation anxiety is often thought of as something that only children deal with. However, adults can also be diagnosed with separation anxiety disorder. People with separation anxiety disorder fear being away from the people they are close to. They often worry that something bad might happen to their loved ones while they are not together. This fear makes them avoid being alone or away from their loved ones. They may have bad dreams about being separated or feel unwell when separation is about to happen.

## TREATMENT AND MANAGEMENT OF ANXIETY DISORDERS

Anxiety disorders are generally treated with psychotherapy, medication, or both. There are many ways to treat anxiety, and in combination with the patient's input and treatment goals, the health care provider cooperatively develops the best treatment course.

## Psychotherapy
Psychotherapy or "talk therapy" can help people with anxiety disorders. To be effective, psychotherapy must be directed at the specific anxieties and tailored to the patient's needs.

## Cognitive behavioral therapy
Cognitive behavioral therapy (CBT) is an example of one type of psychotherapy that can help people with anxiety disorders. It teaches people different ways of thinking, behaving, and reacting to situations to help you feel less anxious and fearful. CBT has been well studied and is a *gold standard* for psychotherapy.

**Exposure therapy** is a CBT method that is used to treat anxiety disorders. Exposure therapy focuses on confronting the fears underlying an anxiety disorder to help people engage in activities they have been avoiding. Exposure therapy is sometimes used along with relaxation exercises.

## Acceptance and commitment therapy
Another treatment option for some anxiety disorders is acceptance and commitment therapy (ACT). ACT takes a different approach than CBT to negative thoughts. It uses strategies such as mindfulness and goal setting to reduce discomfort and anxiety. Compared to CBT, ACT is a newer form of psychotherapy treatment, so less data are available on its effectiveness.

## Antianxiety Medications
Medication does not cure anxiety disorders but can help relieve symptoms. Health care providers, such as a psychiatrist or primary care provider, can prescribe medication for anxiety. Some states also allow psychologists who have received specialized training to prescribe psychiatric medications. The most common classes of medications used to combat anxiety disorders are antidepressants, anti-anxiety medications (such as benzodiazepines), and beta-blockers.

## Antidepressants
Antidepressants are used to treat depression, but they can also be helpful for treating anxiety disorders. They may help improve the way the brain uses certain neurotransmitters that control mood or stress. Antidepressants can take several weeks to take effect so it's important to give the medication a chance before reaching any conclusion about effectiveness. In some cases, children, teenagers, and adults younger than 25 may experience increased suicidal thoughts or behavior when

taking antidepressant medications, especially in the first few weeks after starting or when the dose is changed. Because of this, people of all ages taking antidepressants should be watched closely, especially during the first few weeks of treatment.

**Anti-anxiety medications** (aka, anxiolytics the "reduction of anxiousness")
Anti-anxiety medications can help reduce the symptoms of anxiety, panic attacks, or extreme fear and worry. The most common anti-anxiety medications are called *benzodiazepines*. Although benzodiazepines are sometimes used as first-line treatments for generalized anxiety disorder, they have both benefits and drawbacks.

**Benzodiazepine**s are effective in relieving anxiety and take effect more quickly than antidepressant medications. However, some people build up a tolerance to these medications and need higher and higher doses to get the same effect. Some people even become dependent on them. To avoid these problems, health care providers usually prescribe benzodiazepines for short periods of time. If people suddenly stop taking benzodiazepines, they may have withdrawal symptoms, or their anxiety may return. Therefore, benzodiazepines should be tapered off slowly. The prescriber will determine the rate of a slow taper off of benzodiazepines.

**Beta-blockers**
Although beta-blockers are most often used to treat high blood pressure, they can help relieve the physical symptoms of anxiety, such as rapid heartbeat, shaking, trembling, and blushing. These medications can help people keep physical symptoms under control when taken for short periods. They can also be used "as needed" to reduce acute anxiety, including to prevent some predictable forms of performance anxieties. Atenolol (Tenormin), Metoprolol tartrate (Lopressor), Metoprolol succinate (Toprol XL), along with propranolol are the beta blockers used in anxiety disorders**.** Propranolol is also prescribed off-label for panic disorder, performance anxiety, and prevention of PTSD.

**Antianxiety Medications (BY GENERIC/TRADE NAME)**
(All of these antianxiety medications, except buspirone, are benzodiazepines)
* alprazolam/Xanax
* buspirone/BuSpar
* chlordiazepoxide/Librax, Libritabs, Librium

* clonazepam/Klonopin
* clorazepate/Tranxene
* diazepam/Valium
* halazepam/Paxipam
* lorazepam/Ativan
* oxazepam/Serax
* prazepam/Centrax

**Behavioral Treatments**
Anxiety disorders are generally treated with psychotherapy, medication, or both. There are many ways to treat anxiety. Psychotherapy can help people with anxiety disorders. To be effective, psychotherapy must be directed at the specific anxieties and tailored to each client's needs.

**Cognitive behavioral therapy.** Cognitive Behavioral Therapy (CBT) is an example of one type of psychotherapy that can help people with anxiety disorders. It teaches people different ways of thinking, behaving, and reacting to situations to help them feel less anxious and fearful. CBT has been well studied and is the gold standard for psychotherapy.

**Exposure therapy** is a CBT method that is also used to treat anxiety disorders. Exposure therapy focuses on confronting the fears underlying an anxiety disorder to help people engage in activities they have been avoiding. Exposure therapy is sometimes used along with relaxation exercises including mindfulness breathing.

**Support groups**
Some people with anxiety disorders might benefit from joining a self-help or support group and sharing their problems and achievements with others. Support groups are available both in person and online. However, any advice received from a support group member should be used cautiously and does not replace treatment recommendations from a health care provider.

**Stress management techniques**
Stress management techniques, such as exercise, mindfulness, and meditation, also can reduce anxiety symptoms and enhance the effects of psychotherapy.

# AN IMPORTANT NOTE ABOUT CO-OCCURRING DISORDERS

# What is a Co-Occurring Disorder?

When someone has one or more mental health issues along with one or more substance use or addiction issues.

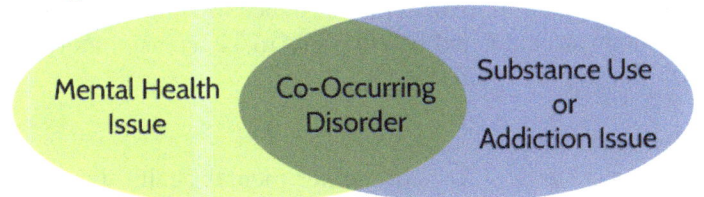

Mental Health Issue | Co-Occurring Disorder | Substance Use or Addiction Issue

Substance use disorder (SUD) is a treatable mental disorder that affects a person's brain and behavior, leading to their inability to control their use of substances like legal or illegal drugs, alcohol, or medications. Symptoms can be moderate to severe, with addiction being the most severe form of SUD.

People with a SUD may also have other mental health disorders, and people with mental health disorders may also struggle with substance use. These other mental health disorders can include anxiety, depression, schizophrenia, and bipolar disorder, among others. (National Institute on Drug Abuse. 2022).

Though people might have both a SUD and a mental disorder, that does not mean that one caused the other. Research suggests three possibilities that could explain why SUDs and other mental disorders may occur together:

- **Common risk factors can contribute to both SUDs and other mental disorders.** Both SUDs and other mental disorders can run in families, meaning certain genes may be a risk factor. Environmental factors, such as stress or trauma, can cause genetic changes that are passed down through generations and may contribute to the development of a mental disorder or a substance use disorder.
- **Mental disorders can contribute to substance use and SUDs.** Studies found that people with a mental disorder, such as anxiety, depression, or post-traumatic stress disorder (PTSD), may use drugs or alcohol as a form of self-medication. However, although some drugs may temporarily help with some symptoms of mental disorders, they may make

the symptoms worse over time. Additionally, brain changes in people with mental disorders may enhance the rewarding effects of substances, making it more likely they will continue to use the substance.
- **Substance use and SUDs can contribute to the development of other mental disorders.** Substance use may trigger changes in brain structure and function that make a person more likely to develop a mental disorder.

**Diagnosis and treatment**
When someone has a SUD and another mental health disorder, it is usually better to treat them at the same time rather than separately. People who need help for a SUD and other mental disorders should see a health care provider for each disorder. It can be challenging to make an accurate diagnosis because some symptoms are the same for both disorders, so the provider should use comprehensive assessment tools to reduce the chance of a missed diagnosis and provide the right treatment.

It also is essential that the provider tailor treatment, which may include behavioral therapies and medications, to an individual's specific combination of disorders and symptoms. It should also take into account the person's age, the misused substance, and the specific mental disorder(s). Talk to your health care provider to determine what treatment may be best for you and give the treatment time to work.

**Behavioral therapies**
Research has found several behavioral therapies that have promise for treating individuals with co-occurring substance use and mental disorders. Health care providers may recommend behavioral therapies alone or in combination with medications.

Some examples of effective behavioral therapies for adults with SUDs and different co-occurring mental disorders include:

- **Cognitive behavioral therapy (CBT)** is aimed at helping people learn how to cope with difficult situations by challenging irrational thoughts and changing behaviors.
- **Dialectical behavior therapy (DBT)** uses concepts of mindfulness and acceptance or being aware of and attentive to the current situation and emotional state. DBT also teaches skills that can help control intense emotions, reduce self-

destructive behaviors (such as suicide attempts, thoughts, or urges; self-harm; and drug use), and improve relationships.
- **Assertive community treatment (ACT)** is a form of community-based mental health care that emphasizes outreach to the community and an individualized treatment approach.
- **Therapeutic Communities** are a common form of long-term residential treatment that focuses on helping people develop new and healthier values, attitudes, and behaviors.
- **Contingency management (CM)** principles encourage healthy behaviors by offering vouchers or rewards for desired behaviors.

Source: The National Institute Mental Health. 2023.

## Integrated Treatment for Co-Occurring Disorders

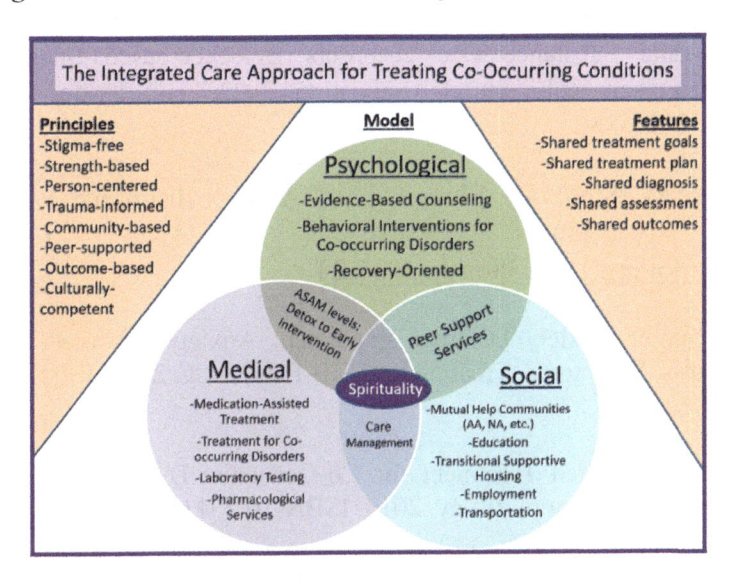

**The Integrated Care Approach for Treating Co-Occurring Conditions**

**Principles**
- Stigma-free
- Strength-based
- Person-centered
- Trauma-informed
- Community-based
- Peer-supported
- Outcome-based
- Culturally-competent

**Model**

*Psychological*
- Evidence-Based Counseling
- Behavioral Interventions for Co-occurring Disorders
- Recovery-Oriented

*Medical*
- Medication-Assisted Treatment
- Treatment for Co-occurring Disorders
- Laboratory Testing
- Pharmacological Services

*Social*
- Mutual Help Communities (AA, NA, etc.)
- Education
- Transitional Supportive Housing
- Employment
- Transportation

ASAM levels: Detox to Early Intervention
Peer Support Services
Spirituality
Care Management

**Features**
- Shared treatment goals
- Shared treatment plan
- Shared diagnosis
- Shared assessment
- Shared outcomes

In Integrated Treatment programs, the same treatment team provides both mental health and substance use interventions in an integrated fashion. Patients receive one consistent, integrated message about treatment and recovery. Services are integrated to meet the needs of people with co-occurring disorders. Co-occurring disorders can make it difficult for patients to cope with everyday life. Additionally, more than one mental health condition or substance use disorder may be involved, further complicating a person's life. Integrated treatment can address each issue to help patients cope and promote recovery.

# SUGGESTED READINGS ON THIS TOPIC

Anxiety & Depression Association of America (ADAA). Anxiety Disorders – Facts and Statistics. 2022.
Available at: https://adaa.org/understanding-anxiety/facts-statistics

APA Dictionary of Psychology. .Definition of anxiety. American Psychological Association (APA). Available at: https://dictionary.apa.org/anxiety

Andrews, G. The Treatment of Anxiety Disorders: Clinician Guides and Patient Manuals. Cambridge University Press. ISBN-10 : 0521788773.

Chandler TL, Dombrowski F and, Matthews TG. Co-occurring Mental Illness and Substance Use Disorders Evidence-based Integrative Treatment and Multicultural Application. 2022. Routledge. **ISBN** 9781032116518

Craske, M., Stein, M., Eley, T. *et al.* Anxiety disorders. *Nat Rev Dis Primers* **3**, 17024 (2017). https://doi.org/10.1038/nrdp.2017.24

Earlstein, F. Anxiety Disorder Explained: Anxiety Disorder Types, Diagnosis, Symptoms, Treatment. NRB Publishing. 2017. ISBN-10 : 1946286133.

Klott, J. Integrated Treatment for Co-Occurring Disorders: Treating People, Not Behaviors. Wiley. 2013. ISBN-10 : 1118205669

National Institute on Drug abuse (NIDA). Common Comorbidities with Substance Use Disorders Research Report 2022. Part 1: The Connection Between Substance Use Disorders and Mental Illness. Retrieved from https://nida.nih.gov/publications/research-reports/common-comorbidities-substance-use-disorders/part-1-connection-between-substance-use-disorders-mental-illness

National Institute for Mental Health (NIMH).
Available at: https://www.nimh.nih.gov/health/topics/anxiety-disorders

Penninx BW, Pine DS, Holmes EA, Reif A. Anxiety disorders. Lancet. 2021. 6;397(10277):914-927.

Robichaud, M. Cognitive Behavioral Treatment for Generalized Anxiety Disorder: From Science to Practice. Routledge. 2019. ISBN-10 : 1138888079.

Seif, MN. What Every Therapist Needs to Know About Anxiety Disorders: Key Concepts, Insights, and Interventions. Routledge. 2014. ISBN-10 : 0415828996

Substance Abuse and Mental Health Services Administration. Anxiety Disorders. 2023. Available at: https://www.samhsa.gov/mental-health/anxiety-disorders

TIP 42: Substance Use Treatment for Persons With Co-Occurring Disorders, by the Substance Abuse Mental Health Services Administration (SAMHSA). 2020. Publication ID PEP20-02-01-004. Available at: https://store.samhsa.gov/product/tip-42-substance-use-treatment-persons-co-occurring-disorders/pep20-02-01-004

# Appendix

## National Institute on Drug Abuse (NIDA) Principles of Drug Addiction Treatment: A Research-Based Guide (2018)

A message from Nora Volkow, MD. Director of NIDA

Drug addiction is a complex illness. It is characterized by intense and, at times, uncontrollable drug craving, along with compulsive drug seeking and use that persist even in the face of devastating consequences. This update of the National Institute on Drug Abuse's Principles of Drug Addiction Treatment is intended to address addiction to a wide variety of drugs, including nicotine, alcohol, and illicit and prescription drugs. It is designed to serve as a resource for healthcare providers, family members, and other stakeholders trying to address the myriad problems faced by patients in need of treatment for drug abuse or addiction.

Addiction affects multiple brain circuits, including those involved in reward and motivation, learning and memory, and inhibitory control over behavior. That is why addiction is a brain disease. Some individuals are more vulnerable than others to becoming addicted, depending on the interplay between genetic makeup, age of exposure to drugs, and other environmental influences. While a person initially chooses to take drugs, over time the effects of prolonged exposure on brain functioning compromise that ability to choose, and seeking and consuming the drug become compulsive, often eluding a person's self-control or willpower.

But addiction is more than just compulsive drug taking—it can also produce far-reaching health and social consequences. For example, drug abuse and addiction increase a person's risk for a variety of other mental and physical illnesses related to a drug-abusing lifestyle or the toxic effects of the drugs themselves. Additionally, the dysfunctional behaviors that result from drug abuse can interfere with a person's normal functioning in the family, the workplace, and the broader community.

Because drug abuse and addiction have so many dimensions and 4 disrupt so many aspects of an individual's life, treatment is not simple.

Effective treatment programs typically incorporate many components, each directed to a particular aspect of the illness and its consequences. Addiction treatment must help the individual stop using drugs, maintain a drug-free lifestyle, and achieve productive functioning in the family, at work, and in society.

Because addiction is a disease, most people cannot simply stop using drugs for a few days and be cured. Patients typically require long-term or repeated episodes of care to achieve the ultimate goal of sustained abstinence and recovery of their lives. Indeed, scientific research and clinical practice demonstrate the value of continuing care in treating addiction, with a variety of approaches having been tested and integrated in residential and community settings.

As we look toward the future, we will harness new research results on the influence of genetics and environment on gene function and expression (i.e., epigenetics), which are heralding the development of personalized treatment interventions. These findings will be integrated with current evidence supporting the most effective drug abuse and addiction treatments and their implementation, which are reflected in this guide.

Nora D. Volkow, M.D. Director
National Institute on Drug Abuse

## Principles of Effective Treatment

1. Addiction is a complex but treatable disease that affects brain function and behavior. Drugs of abuse alter the brain's structure and function, resulting in changes that persist long after drug use has ceased. This may explain why drug abusers are at risk for relapse even after long periods of abstinence and despite the potentially devastating consequences.

2. No single treatment is appropriate for everyone. Treatment varies depending on the type of drug and the characteristics of the patients. Matching treatment settings, interventions, and services to an individual's particular problems and needs is critical to his or her ultimate success in returning to productive functioning in the family, workplace, and society.

3. Treatment needs to be readily available. Because drug addicted individuals may be uncertain about entering treatment, taking advantage of available services the moment people are ready for treatment is critical. Potential patients can be lost if treatment is not immediately available or readily accessible. As with other chronic diseases, the earlier treatment is offered in the disease process, the greater the likelihood of positive outcomes.

4. Effective treatment attends to multiple needs of the individual, not just his or her drug abuse. To be effective, treatment must address the individual's drug abuse and any associated medical, psychological, social, vocational, and legal problems. It is also important that treatment be appropriate to the individual's age, gender, ethnicity, and culture.

5. Remaining in treatment for an adequate period of time is critical. The appropriate duration for an individual depends on the type and degree of the patient's problems and needs. Research indicates that most addicted individuals need at least 3 months in treatment to significantly reduce or stop their drug use and that the best outcomes occur with longer durations of treatment. Recovery from drug addiction is a long-term process and frequently requires multiple episodes of treatment. As with other chronic illnesses, relapses to drug abuse can occur and should signal a need for treatment to be reinstated or adjusted. Because individuals often leave treatment prematurely, programs should include strategies to engage and keep patients in treatment.

6. Behavioral therapies—including individual, family, or group counseling—are the most commonly used forms of drug abuse treatment. Behavioral therapies vary in their focus and may involve addressing a patient's motivation to change, providing incentives for abstinence, building skills to resist drug use, replacing drug-using activities with constructive and rewarding activities, improving problem-solving skills, and facilitating better interpersonal relationships. Also, participation in group therapy and other peer support programs during and following treatment can help maintain abstinence.

7. Medications are an important element of treatment for many patients, especially when combined with counseling and other behavioral therapies. For example, methadone, buprenorphine, and naltrexone (including a new long-acting formulation) are effective in

helping individuals addicted to heroin or other opioids stabilize their lives and reduce their illicit drug use. Acamprosate, disulfiram, and naltrexone are medications approved for treating alcohol dependence. For persons addicted to nicotine, a nicotine replacement product (available as patches, gum, lozenges, or nasal spray) or an oral medication (such as bupropion or varenicline) can be an effective component of treatment when part of a comprehensive behavioral treatment program.

8. An individual's treatment and services plan must be assessed continually and modified as necessary to ensure that it meets his or her changing needs. A patient may require varying combinations of services and treatment components during the course of treatment and recovery. In addition to counseling or psychotherapy, a patient may require medication, medical services, family therapy, parenting instruction, vocational rehabilitation, and/or social and legal services. For many patients, a continuing care approach provides the best results, with the treatment intensity varying according to a person's changing needs.

9. Many drug-addicted individuals also have other mental disorders. Because drug abuse and addiction—both of which are mental disorders—often co-occur with other mental illnesses, patients presenting with one condition should be assessed for the other(s). And when these problems co-occur, treatment should address both (or all), including the use of medications as appropriate.

10. Medically assisted detoxification is only the first stage of addiction treatment and by itself does little to change long-term drug abuse. Although medically assisted detoxification can safely manage the acute physical symptoms of withdrawal and can, for some, pave the way for effective long term addiction treatment, detoxification alone is rarely sufficient to help addicted individuals achieve long-term abstinence. Thus, patients should be encouraged to continue drug treatment following detoxification. Motivational enhancement and incentive strategies, begun at initial patient intake, can improve treatment engagement.

11. Treatment does not need to be voluntary to be effective. Sanctions or enticements from family, employment settings, and/or the criminal justice system can significantly increase treatment entry, retention rates, and the ultimate success of drug treatment interventions.

12. Drug use during treatment must be monitored continuously, as lapses during treatment do occur. Knowing their drug use is being monitored can be a powerful incentive for patients and can help them withstand urges to use drugs. Monitoring also provides an early indication of a return to drug use, signaling a possible need to adjust an individual's treatment plan to better meet his or her needs.

13. Treatment programs should test patients for the presence of HIV/AIDS, hepatitis B and C, tuberculosis, and other infectious diseases as well as provide targeted risk reduction counseling, linking patients to treatment if necessary. Typically, drug abuse treatment addresses some of the drug-related behaviors that put people at risk of infectious diseases. Targeted counseling focused on reducing infectious disease risk can help patients further reduce or avoid substance related and other high-risk behaviors.

Counseling can also help those who are already infected to manage their illness. Moreover, engaging in substance abuse treatment can facilitate adherence to other medical treatments. Substance abuse treatment facilities should provide onsite, rapid HIV testing rather than referrals to offsite testing—research shows that doing so increases the likelihood that patients will be tested and receive their test results. Treatment providers should also inform patients that highly active antiretroviral therapy (HAART) has proven effective in combating HIV, including among drug-abusing populations, and help link them to HIV treatment if they test positive.

Made in the USA
Las Vegas, NV
12 February 2025

18023354R10195